Long-Term Conditions

'We can envision in chronic illness and its therapy a symbolic bridge that connects the body, self and society. This network interconnects physiological processes, meanings and relationships so that our social word is linked recursively to our inner experience. Here we are privileged to discover powers within and between us that can either amplify suffering or disability or dampen symptoms and therefore contribute to care.'

Arthur Kleinman (1988:xiii)
The Illness Narratives – Suffering, Healing and the Human Condition
Basic Books, New York

Long-Term Conditions
Nursing Care and Management

Edited by

Liz Meerabeau

Dean of School of Health and Social Care
University of Greenwich, UK

Kerri Wright

Senior Lecturer
University of Greenwich, UK

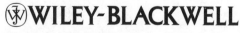

WILEY-BLACKWELL

A John Wiley & Sons, Ltd., Publication

This edition first published 2011 © 2011 by Blackwell Publishing Ltd

Blackwell Publishing was acquired by John Wiley & Sons in February 2007. Blackwell's publishing program has been merged with Wiley's global Scientific, Technical and Medical business to form Wiley-Blackwell.

Registered office: John Wiley & Sons, Ltd, The Atrium, Southern Gate, Chichester, West Sussex, PO19 8SQ, UK

Editorial offices: 9600 Garsington Road, Oxford, OX4 2DQ, UK
      The Atrium, Southern Gate, Chichester, West Sussex, PO19 8SQ, UK
      2121 State Avenue, Ames, Iowa 50014-8300, USA

For details of our global editorial offices, for customer services and for information about how to apply for permission to reuse the copyright material in this book please see our website at www.wiley.com/wiley-blackwell.

Library of Congress Cataloging-in-Publication Data
Long-term conditions : nursing care and management/edited by Liz Meerabeau and Kerri Wright.
    p. ; cm.
  Includes bibliographical references and index.
  ISBN 978-1-4051-8338-3 (pbk. : alk. paper)
  1. Chronic diseases–Nursing. 2. Long-term care of the sick. I. Wright, Kerri. II. Meerabeau, Liz.
  [DNLM: 1. Chronic Disease–economics. 2. Chronic Disease–therapy. 3. Health Care Costs.
4. Health Policy. 5. Patient Education as Topic. 6. Self Care. WT 500]
  RT120.C45L66 2011
  616′.044–dc22

                          2010049567

A catalogue record for this book is available from the British Library.

This book is published in the following electronic formats: ePDF 9781444341003; Wiley Online Library 9781444341034; ePub 9781444341010

Set in 10/12.5 pt Times by Aptara Inc., New Delhi, India
Printed and bound in Malaysia by Vivar Printing Sdn Bhd

1 2011

Contents

Foreword   vii
Notes on contributors   viii
Acknowledgements   x

Introduction   1

1 **Long-term conditions in perspective**   3
   Liz Meerabeau

2 **Case management**   23
   Kerri Wright

3 **Changing approaches to the management of long-term conditions**   36
   Kerri Wright

4 **Sociological insights**   45
   Liz Meerabeau

5 **Psychological effects of long-term conditions**   64
   Ben Bruneau

6 **Counselling skills**   87
   Val Sanders

7 **Living with long-term conditions: Tommy's story**   110
   Tommy Magee

8 **Self-management and current health care policies**   119
   Kerri Wright

9 **Managing common symptoms of long-term conditions**   135
   *Kerri Wright, Pia Sweet, Natasha Ascott, Harry Chummun and
   Jenny Taylor*

10   Medicines management   **173**
Shivaun Gammie

11   Management of heart failure   **194**
Susan Simpson

12   Management of respiratory disease   **225**
Liz Nicholls

13   Management of diabetes   **247**
Lynne Jerreat

Index   285

Foreword

This is a very important book. Although there have always been people with long-term conditions (LTCs) on nurses' caseloads, it is only in recent years that we have recognised the breadth and depth of these individuals' needs, and understood how much further we could go to meet them. For too many years, health professionals saw their interactions with people with LTCs as episodic, repetitive and unrewarding.

A better understanding of the nature and impact of these conditions on individuals has changed both attitudes and practice. We are more focused on prevention, both primary and secondary, for diseases once accepted as unavoidable. We are more proactive in finding people with LTCs, and instituting management to reduce their impact. And, most importantly, we now recognise that people with these conditions know a great deal about them, and are usually able and willing to take much more control than we had ever guessed. The advent of portable assistive technology, which can be used at home with minimal training, has helped enormously to shift the knowledge and power in disease management from the professional to the patient.

The timing of these changes is important. The number of people with LTCs in the United Kingdom and worldwide is set to grow exponentially. Lifestyle factors, including obesity and inappropriate diet, environmental challenges as well as some unknown causes, are all leading to sharp rises in conditions such as diabetes, asthma and heart disease. In a world with rising health care demand but caps on health care spending, managing LTCs well is a professional imperative for the sake of the individual patient and the wider health system.

This book is a very welcome tool, which will enable health professionals to understand the complexity, challenge and rewards of proactively managing LTCs. Putting this knowledge into skilled practice, in partnership with patients, will transform the lives of many individuals and their families, and thus fulfil the fundamental purpose of nursing.

Professor Rosemary Cook CBE, Honoris Causa, MSc, PGDip, RGN
Director, the Queen's Nursing Institute and Visiting Professor of Enterprise
University of Northumbria, Newcastle, UK

Notes on contributors

Natasha Ascott is a Clinical Nurse Specialist in pain management at Basildon and Thurrock University Hospital.

Ben Bruneau is a Senior Lecturer at the University of Greenwich. Ben has a broad interest in the field of personality research, and is a chartered psychologist.

Harry Chummun is a Senior Lecturer at the University of Greenwich. Harry has an interest in stress management and the genetics of health and well- being, and publishes in this area.

Shivaun Gammie is a registered pharmacist and currently works as a Clinical Lecturer at the Medway School of Pharmacy. Shivaun has worked as a senior medicines management pharmacist and has a strong interest in promoting evidence-based therapeutics.

Lynne Jerreat is the Lead Diabetic Specialist Nurse at Queen Elizabeth Hospital, South London. Lynne is also the author of the popular text 'Diabetes for Nurses' which is currently in its second edition. Lynne regularly teaches pre- and post-registration nurses at the University of Greenwich.

Tommy Magee lives in South-East London with his collie dog, Holly. Tommy set up the AA meeting currently still running in Hertfordshire, and is active on a number of committees, using his experiences to advise professionals on health issues. Tommy is an expert patient trainer on the Expert Patient Programme in South London, and regularly shares his story and insights with pre- and post-registration nurses at the University of Greenwich.

Liz Meerabeau is Dean of the School of Health and Social Care at the University of Greenwich. Liz has a clinical background as a health visitor and a research interest in the sociology of health and illness.

Liz Nicholls is an independent nurse practitioner, working in general practice for nearly 20 years. She has a very broad experience of helping clients to manage and control their long-term conditions (LTCs). Her main interests are nurse education and respiratory care.

Val Sanders is a senior accredited BACP counsellor and supervisor in private practice, in addition to her work as a senior lecturer in Therapeutic Counselling at the University of Greenwich. For the past 2 years she has delivered training sessions in counselling skills to post-registration nurses on an LTC course. She has a specialist interest in bereavement, death and dying, and has experience of working with people living with cancer.

Susan Simpson, Nurse Consultant in Cardiac Care at South London Healthcare Trust, is the nursing lead for the management of patients with heart failure for this Trust and has a large clinical caseload.

Pia Sweet is a Consultant Anaesthetist and Pain Specialist working at South London Health NHS Trust. Pia regularly teaches pain management on post-registration courses at the University of Greenwich.

Jenny Taylor is a Senior Physiotherapist and Head of the Allied Health Professions team at St Christopher's Hospice in South London.

Kerri Wright is a Senior Lecturer at the University of Greenwich. Kerri has a clinical background as a district nurse, and has an interest in the therapeutic relationship between nurses and patients and how this can enhance well-being.

Acknowledgements

Thanks to Rona Dury, Theresa Massey, Alice Neave for their helpful comments on drafts and to Garry Bodenham for recording the interview with Tommy. Also to Monique Petit, Louise Ramage and Emma Pattison for help in editing.

Introduction

It is a curious experience to have written a book during a time when the government was expected to change after many years, knowing that if that change came, many of the policy aspects of the book were likely to change as well, and the documents we refer to may fairly soon become unavailable. Organisations we refer to may also disappear. In addition, clinical guidance is also continually being updated and although we have used the most up-to-date guidance in this book, we are aware that this may soon be superseded and we would direct you to check for any updates.

As we write this Introduction, we do now know the new government's plans for the NHS, as the white paper, *Equity and Excellence: Liberating the NHS* appeared in July 2010. The most commented-upon intention is the devolution of health care commissioning in England to consortia of GPs and the abolition of primary care trusts and strategic health authorities – a high-risk strategy which may exacerbate health inequalities, since the quality of general practice is worst in many areas where the social disadvantage is greatest. There is, however, a stated aim in the white paper to put patients and the public first, in particular by making shared decision-making the norm: *no decision about me without me*. This fits well with the ethos of this book and supporting people with long-term conditions (LTCs).

There has also been much discussion about the election pledge 'the Big Society', in which communities will be encouraged to take action on problems rather than relying on the state; how this will work when many third sector organisations will be getting less funding remains to be seen. Local authority budgets will also be greatly reduced, putting the interface between health and social care at risk. In addition, public health measures such as minimum pricing for alcohol and improvements in food quality have been rejected, so we may return to an individualistic approach to public health, rather than the societal approach referred to in the discussion on health inequalities in our book.

Despite the future changes and the number of 'unknowns', the heart of the book, which is the experiences of people with LTCs, and the need for us to provide the best care we can, will not change. The demographic pressures of an older population, and more people developing LTCs, will remain, as will the complexity of care and support which many people need. In order to do justice to our subject, we have concentrated on the care of

Long-Term Conditions: Nursing Care and Management, First Edition. Edited by Liz Meerabeau and Kerri Wright.
© 2011 Blackwell Publishing Ltd. Published 2011 by Blackwell Publishing Ltd.

adults and on physical illnesses, although we recognise the importance of mental illness and the difficult interrelationship between social disadvantage, physical illness and mental illness, particularly depression.

The discussion in this book moves from a global and national perspective on some of the issues around LTCs, in chapters 1–3 ('Long-term conditions in perspective', 'Case management' and 'Changing approaches to the management of long-term conditions'), to a more personal and individualistic approach to supporting people living with an LTC with chapters 4 and 5 ('Sociological insights' and 'Psychological effects of long-term conditions') focusing on the effects that living with an LTC can have on individuals and their families. We also move from a generic approach to the care and management of people with LTCs in chapters 6–10, with many issues pertinent to all LTCs, to a more specific and clinical focus on three main LTCs in the final three chapters.

Due to the scope of this book, we have used a range of terminology according to the chapter focus and terms that are more commonly used. To this end, we have used such terms as illness, long-term conditions and chronic illness throughout the book, and referred to patients rather than people when more appropriate to do so.

The aim of this book is for nurses to gain a wider perspective on the issues and experiences of people who are living their life with LTCs. We are keen for the focus to be on the person with an LTC and the management and care of their condition to be aimed at enabling the person to live their life as they choose. With this aim there becomes not one truth for the best way to manage specific LTCs, but many truths which are individual to each person. These truths need to be understood and respected, and used *with* clinical knowledge to plan and manage care. To this end, the focus must be for nurses to develop a true partnership with people living with LTCs based on acceptance, empathy and respect. This involves nurses listening to people's stories and valuing their personal and unique understanding of their condition and how they manage their life with this.

Liz Meerabeau
Kerri Wright

Chapter 1

Long-term conditions in perspective

Liz Meerabeau

School of Health and Social Care, University of Greenwich, Eltham, London, UK

Introduction

All developed countries, whatever their political system and overall approach to health policy, face challenges in meeting the rising costs of health care. This increase in health care costs generally exceeds the rate of economic growth; contributing factors include increasing proportions of older people in the population, the development of expensive medical technologies and drugs, and increasingly well-informed people who demand access to these developments in health care. *High Quality Care for All* (Department of Health, 2008a), also known as the Darzi Report after the junior health minister who led the NHS Next Stage Review, identifies six challenges common to all advanced health care systems: rising expectations, demand driven by demographics, the continuing development of the 'information society', advances in treatments, the changing nature of disease and changing expectations of the health workplace (i.e. staff expect a better work-life balance).

An important element of the changing patterns of disease is the increase in prevalence of long-term conditions (LTCs); LTCs are one of the eight priorities for the NHS. Dowrick *et al.* (2005) consider that the management of what they term chronic illness is beginning to develop its own identity as an important component of health care, and that despite clinical differences, there are many similarities in the problems people with different LTCs face and the strategies needed in providing care. These include the proactive identification of relevant populations, supporting the relationships between people with LTCs and health and social care, the development of evidence-based guidelines intended to prevent exacerbations, and the promotion of empowerment, for example through self-management.

This chapter discusses changes in the need for health care due to demographic change and persistent inequalities in health, before going on to outline some of the changes both in service delivery generally and in the provision of health care for LTCs more specifically, such as the use of targets by governments, and the growth of patient-focused care. Generally, like the rest of this book, the chapter has an English focus, in which policy initiatives and service developments include user participation (Department of Health,

Long-Term Conditions: Nursing Care and Management, First Edition. Edited by Liz Meerabeau and Kerri Wright.
© 2011 Blackwell Publishing Ltd. Published 2011 by Blackwell Publishing Ltd.

2003) and National Service Frameworks (NSFs) with specific standards, for example for coronary heart disease (Department of Health, 2000a) and for LTCs (Department of Health, 2005a). Comparisons with the other three UK countries are also made briefly, and the global context is also discussed.

The global challenge: demographic change

Within the overall trend towards older populations, the most rapidly growing segment is that of people over 80: the Organisation for Economic Co-operation and Development (OECD)(1988) estimated that whereas in 1980 the cohort of older people was made up of 34% aged between 65 and 69, 48% between 70 and 79 and 18% 80 or over, by 2050 these percentages would be 26%, 43% and 31%, respectively.

More recently, *An Ageing World: 2008* (US Census Bureau, 2009) highlights a huge shift to an older population, with great consequences. In the next 30 years, the number of people over 65 in the world will almost double to 1.3 billion, and in 10 years time, older people will outnumber children for the first time. This will affect family structure, patterns of work and retirement. Europe has 23 of the 25 'oldest' countries in the world (including all of the countries of western Europe, with the exception of Ireland and Denmark). In the United Kingdom, the nineteenth 'oldest' country, by 2040 there will be 46 people aged 65 and over for every 100 people of working age (defined as aged 20 to 64); in Germany, the figure will be 58, and in Japan, 68. (This ratio is called the older dependency ratio.) This compares with 16 in South Africa and 23 in India. Japan, Singapore, France, Sweden and Italy all now have life expectancies at birth of more than 80 years. However, although the proportion of older people in the populations of developing countries is much lower, because of the size of these populations, overall most of the increase in the number of older people in the world is actually in these poorer countries. China is one of the fastest ageing countries in the world, since its fertility rate has been below the replacement rate since 1991, due to its long-standing one-child policy. In Japan, 22.5% of the 127 million people are over 65, whereas only 13% are under 15.

It should not be assumed that greater longevity automatically increases the burden of ill health; many people are likely to live relatively healthy lives until their last few years, although it is likely that they will be managing one or more LTCs. The Academy of Medical Sciences (2009) report *Rejuvenating Ageing Research* states that in the United Kingdom healthy life expectancy is increasing at least as quickly as overall life expectancy. Far fewer older people are disabled than was the case in the 1970s, and drug treatments for hypertension and cardiac problems have reduced the mortality from heart disease by 40% since the 1990s. Older people in many countries also contribute towards society in that they pay considerable tax and are major providers of care, both to children and to other older people. Nevertheless, the ageing of the population does result in higher health care costs. In most countries, people over 65 account for at least twice the health care expenditure that their proportion in the population would predict; in the United States, people over 65 constituted one-eighth of the population in 2000, but consumed nearly half of the health care expenditure (the UK figures were one-sixth and 43%, respectively). The OECD (1988) projection was that these figures for expenditure would rise to 63% for the United States and 54% for the United Kingdom, by 2040. Appleby (in Pilkington,

2009) estimates that the NHS needs about 1.5% extra funding every year just to cope with increased need due to demographic change.

The demand for health care

A second important factor in driving up health care costs is the growth of expensive medical interventions. Many medical innovations have not been fully assessed in terms of costs and benefits, although health technology assessment for potential new interventions is well established in Australia, Sweden, the Netherlands, the United Kingdom and the United States (in individual states such as Oregon, which was a pioneer in health technology assessment). In England, such assessment takes place through the National Institute for Health and Clinical Excellence (NICE). The costs of health technologies are assessed against the benefit, which is calculated primarily by means of quality-adjusted life years (QALYs). This measure has proved controversial; treatments for the terminal stages of diseases such as kidney cancer are likely to fall short of the threshold for NHS funding, since life expectancy is short, and in some instances QALYs have been recalculated to allow for this. Although NICE was set up to try to depoliticise decisions about expensive medical interventions, there has been intense lobbying in response to its decisions, and there is concern that services for other less vocal people, such as mentally ill or older people, may get displaced as a result. Arguments about the entitlement to treatment are likely to be tested in the courts, for example in 2006 in relation to Herceptin, a drug for certain types of breast cancer.

It has been recognised that a small percentage of people consume a large percentage of health care resources; therefore, managing LTCs has become an important element in health policy, both for humanitarian reasons and in an attempt to control costs. In England, one-third of the adult population has an LTC; in some areas this rises to half (Department of Health, 2008b). Even in younger age groups, 15% of children under 5 and 20% of children and young people aged 5–15 have an LTC (Wilson *et al.*, 2005). The British Household Panel Survey (2001) found that people with LTCs accounted for 80% of GP consultations; they also account for 72% of inpatient days in England and 65% of outpatient appointments (Haddad *et al.*, 2009). By 2030, the incidence of LTCs in people over 65 is estimated to more than double (Department of Health, 2005b). People with long-term physical conditions also have a 20% risk of depression, a rate which is two to three times higher than that for people in good physical health (Egede, 2007).

Globally, the most common LTCs are cardiovascular diseases such as hypertension, coronary artery disease, stroke and heart failure, various forms of arthritis, respiratory problems, diabetes and epilepsy; such illnesses contribute to nearly half of the prevalence of disability worldwide. HIV/AIDS has also become an LTC in countries where there is adequate treatment. Mental health problems such as depression are also increasingly viewed as LTCs. LTCs are collectively the largest cause of death globally (World Health Organisation, 2005), despite the prevalence of infectious diseases in poorer countries; by 2025, an almost 300% increase in deaths from ischaemic heart disease and stroke is predicted in Latin America, the Middle East and sub-Saharan Africa (Yach *et al.*, 2004). Chronic obstructive pulmonary disease is predicted to be the third main cause of death globally by 2020 (Murray and Lopez, 1997). About 2.8% of the global population has diabetes; this is likely to increase to 6.5% by 2030 (Murray and Lopez, 1996), and is linked to the increased incidence of obesity.

If current trends continue, 60% of men, 50% of women and 25% of children in the United Kingdom will be obese by 2050 (Foresight, 2007); excess weight is increasingly seen as the norm. It is beginning to be recognised in the United Kingdom that the environment is obesogenic, for example due to the availability of cheap, high-fat food, and that government intervention has not so far been effective; the chair of the International Obesity Task Force, Professor Philip James, gives the current English campaign, Change4Life, only a 10% chance of success (Dent, 2009). Change4Life is an example of a recent approach to addressing health-damaging behaviours which has been adopted from the United States, social marketing. A national centre for social marketing, a collaboration between the Department of Health and the National Consumer Council, was launched in 2006. The aim is not only to raise awareness but also to equip people with ways of changing their behaviour, using solutions which meet their needs, and where necessary, to change policies and structures which reduce people's capacity to live healthily.

As the example of obesity illustrates, reducing mortality and morbidity from LTCs requires individual engagement with lifestyle factors; Wanless (2002) has termed this the 'fully engaged' scenario, in which individuals take responsibility for their own health, and public health goals such as smoking cessation are achieved. If this scenario is not achieved, the costs of health care will become unaffordable. Public bodies also have a key public health role. *High Quality Care for All* (Department of Health, 2008a) refers to the legal duty for the NHS and local authorities to work together to address public health issues, and to cooperate in improving outcomes for their populations, on the basis of a formal assessment of people's needs (Joint Strategic Needs Assessment). These plans involve other agencies, such as the police, and focus not only on health priorities such as smoking but also on broader factors such as poor housing, education, local transport and recreational facilities.

Health inequalities

It has long been recognised that the risks of long-term health problems and premature death are not equally distributed in society throughout the developed world. Since the launch of the *Black Report* in England (Townsend *et al.*, 1992), there has been considerable debate and research to understand the relationship between social inequalities and health. There are two broad categories of explanation for the causes of health inequalities. Cultural/behavioural explanations stress differences in lifestyles and may imply that such differences are matters of choice; such explanations can lead to 'victim blaming' for illnesses which are obviously lifestyle related. However, comparisons between people with similar habits such as smoking show that there are still differences in the effects of these habits between the social classes (Department of Health, 1998a), indicating that structural factors also apply. Structural explanations stress the role of social circumstances; for example, mothers in poorer families tend to feed their families cheaper, higher fat foods, and are also reluctant to cook unfamiliar food which might be refused and therefore wasted. Housing conditions are also a major determinant of health; people in poor-quality housing suffer more from depression and respiratory disease. During the years of Conservative government in the 1980s and 1990s, the structural causes of health inequalities were not acknowledged in policy, and in the mid-1990s, the term used by the Department of Health was 'variations in health' rather than health inequalities. The establishment of the Acheson Inquiry (Department of Health, 1998b) by the incoming Labour government was recognised as a significant break with previous policy. However, recognising the structural causes of ill health has not led to a reduction in health inequalities, as most recently demonstrated in the strategic review of health inequalities led by Sir Michael Marmot (Marmot Review, 2010).

The 2009 House of Commons Health Committee report on health inequalities comments that a girl born in 2006 in the wealthy London boroughs of Kensington and Chelsea has a life expectancy of 87.8 years, compared with 77.1 years in Glasgow. Poor people have more years of poor health and also less access to health services, although it is socio-economic conditions, rather than poorer quality health care, which are thought to be the main factor in the greater prevalence of LTCs among disadvantaged people. There are also differences between ethnic groups. The 2001 census found that Pakistani and Bangladeshi men and women in England and Wales reported the highest rates of both poor health and limiting long-term illness, and Chinese men and women reported the lowest rates. South Asian people have high rates of heart disease and hypertension; Black Caribbean people have high rates of the latter, and also high rates of admission for severe mental illness, particularly for young men. All ethnic minority groups are reported to have high rates of diabetes. The Men's Health Forum in its evidence to the House of Commons Health Committee argued that men's life expectancy is more severely affected by deprivation than that of women; 67% of men are overweight or obese compared with 58% of women. People who are severely mentally ill, perhaps because they suffer from poverty and social exclusion, are also much more likely to have physical health problems. People with schizophrenia are 90% more likely to get bowel cancer and 42% more likely to get breast cancer. They also have higher rates of diabetes, coronary heart disease, stroke and respiratory disease, and on average die 10 years earlier (House of Commons Health Committee, 2009).

There has been debate for many years on the extent to which health-damaging behaviours such as smoking, poor diet and lack of exercise, which also show a socio-economic gradient, are amenable to change. In 1973, about 42% of the most affluent smoked; the figure in 2004 was about 15%. The figures for the poorest were 71% in 1973 and 61% in 2004, showing that whilst both figures have improved, the gap is now much wider (House of Commons Health Committee, 2009). The report comments that the reasons why poorer people are less likely to adopt beneficial health behaviours may be because they lack the information and material resources, other people in their environment may also have the same habits, making it harder to change, and changing health behaviours may not be a priority when there are more pressing problems such as poverty and local crime.

The poorer health of many black and minority ethnic communities was referred to in the House of Commons Health Committee report, and there is convincing evidence that this is mainly due to social and economic inequalities rather than ethnicity *per se* (Nazroo and Williams, 2005). Differences between dominant and minority cultures tend to be overemphasised in health policy, as if a person's ethnicity determined their whole identity (Ahmad and Bradby, 2007), whereas Atkin and Chattoo (2007) argue that policy makers and service providers should work with an individual's own definition of themselves. The interaction between religion and ethnicity has only recently been researched, partly because there were no large-scale data until the 2001 census (Beckford *et al.*, 2006), and there is also increasing recognition of the impact of racism on the health of minority groups (Nazroo *et al.*, 2007).

Many writers argue that relative poverty is an important cause of ill health (Wilkinson, 1996, 2005). Wilkinson and Pickett (2009) argue that in more unequal societies, the effects of inequality affect people throughout that society, not only the poorest people. The most equal of the developed countries are Japan, Sweden, Norway and Finland; the most unequal are the United States, Portugal, the United Kingdom, Australia and New Zealand. In less egalitarian countries, social relations and levels of trust deteriorate, and rates of obesity, mental illness and drug use are higher. Wilkinson and Pickett (2009) argue that relationships based on social exclusion inflict social pain. This is echoed by Mulgan and Buenfino (2006: 1), who state that 'in a society with relatively less risk of absolute malnourishment, psychic needs come to the fore: loneliness, depression, anxiety, and the misery caused by dangerous and unpleasant environments'. Income inequalities, measured by the Gini coefficient, have become much more pronounced in the United Kingdom since the election of a Conservative government in 1979 and were not remedied by the change of government in 1997; health policy in England has also moved away from the consensus of the post-war years, to a more market-oriented model, influenced by the United States.

Health care systems

As Blank and Burau (2004) discuss, variations in health care policy from one country to another can be explained by historical and cultural features; no two health care systems are identical, and within the United Kingdom, there are now divergences between Wales, Scotland, Northern Ireland and England, the latter having persisted with a much more market-oriented approach in which targets and strong performance management dominate (Greer, 2005). A recent report from the Nuffield Trust (Connolly *et al.*, 2010) has shown the English system to be more cost effective.

The location of political power in a country can be classified along a continuum (see Figure 1.1).

Where power is concentrated, rapid reform is possible; where it is fragmented, as in the United States, even small-scale change becomes almost impossible to implement and deeply contested, as the recent battles by President Obama to reform the US health care system demonstrate. The tendency to stalemate is exacerbated in systems such as the

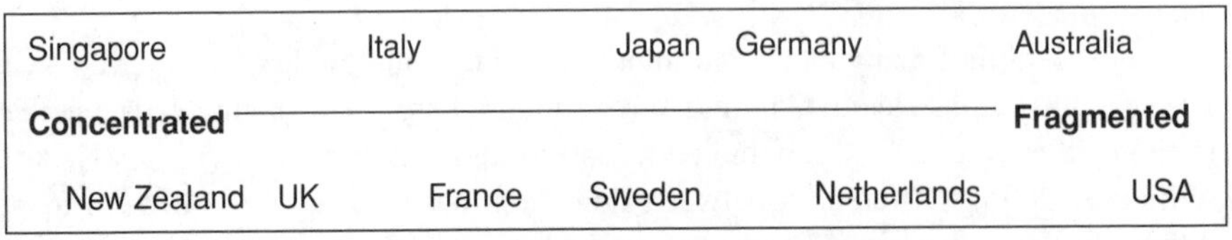

Singapore		Italy		Japan	Germany		Australia
Concentrated							**Fragmented**
New Zealand	UK		France	Sweden		Netherlands	USA

Figure 1.1   Location of political power (Blank and Burau, 2004).

United States where there is divided government with several branches or levels which different parties control. Conversely, in a highly centralised system such as the United Kingdom (or England) rapid change can destabilise the system. This was the case in New Zealand in the 1970s, where reform was nearly continuous (Martin and Salmond, 2001). Health care systems are always the focus of political struggle, since they are fundamental to society, and consume considerable resources.

Health care systems are obviously shaped by the wealth of the country, generally measured in Gross Domestic Product (GDP) per capita. In 2002, the average GDP per capita of all countries was $7,081, ranging from $498 in Sierra Leone to $22,801 in the United Kingdom and $35,831 in the United States. The majority of the fairly wealthy countries discussed by Blank and Burau (2004) spent between 7% and 9% of their GDP on health care, the United States being the exception at 12.9%. The percentage coming from public sources ranged from 67.3% in Italy to 83.8% in Sweden, the exceptions being the United States (44.8%) and Singapore (26%). However, the source of the public funding differs; whereas the United Kingdom, New Zealand and Sweden have national health systems funded from general taxation, countries such as Germany and the Netherlands fund their health care systems from compulsory social insurance (the so-called Bismarck system). Countries with the latter type of funding tend to have more private hospitals. Systems may also have a patchwork of funding; New Zealand funds hospital care through taxation, but primary care through direct payment. The United States is particularly notable for its high levels of expenditure on health care but very uneven provision. Millions of Americans have private health care plans, but 47 million have no insurance, and the systems designed to cover old people and the very poor are complex. Unmet health care bills are a major reason for bankruptcy in the United States (Harris, 2009).

Most, if not all, health care systems are now under additional pressure due to the global economic downturn. The United Kingdom has a relatively high use of hospital-based care (£1,009 per capita, compared to £766 in France; Gainsbury, 2009), and there are plans in England, as yet not clearly articulated, to transfer more care to 'polysystems', although the research evidence shows that it cannot be assumed that care in the community is cheaper (Roland *et al.*, 2007). The consultancy firm McKinsey has also modelled a reduction of 137,000 posts in the NHS, of which 1,600 would be district nurses (Gainsbury, 2009), based on assumptions about the 'productivity' of district nurses, i.e. the number of visits they undertake. It is not clear from the report whether these data took account of the relative complexity or acuity of the patients, and the district nursing service has had insufficient attention in formulating health care policy (Edwards and Dyson, 2003), as has home care in general.

Home care

Blank and Burau (2004: 149) argue that provision for LTCs has been marginal in the development of health policy:

'Health systems are concerned first and foremost with the provision of medical care and focus on acute illness. Doctors are the key professionals shaping the delivery of health care and hospitals are the primary location. The emphasis is on *curing* as opposed to long-term *caring*.'

In addition, much of the care for LTCs takes place in the home, where it, and deficits in care, are less visible than in acute settings which are by their nature much more public. Like other aspects of health care policy, home care policy varies from country to country, but it can be argued that it is more variable, and more influenced by cultural assumptions, than acute care. Blank and Burau (2004: 151) state:

'Home care policies are pushed by demography and costs, but are shaped by country-specific factors. Key factors include how the funding and provision of health care is organised, where health systems draw the boundary between health and social care; and cultural assumptions about appropriate divisions of labour between the state and the family.'

International statistics on home care are almost non-existent and it is difficult to know what is happening underneath the political rhetoric. The majority of countries spend very little on long-term care, generally around 1% of GDP, and home nursing is even more marginalised. Of the countries discussed by Blank and Burau (2004) only Britain and Sweden have public home nursing services. In other countries, the provision is more mixed; a legacy of informal care (Germany, Japan, Singapore), or liberalism (the United States and Australia). Sweden has a well-established home nursing system, but it is very localised and therefore variable. As in other countries, eligibility for home care has also become more restricted:

'Public funding is often not secure and hardly sufficient, and it has to be supplemented by out-of-pocket payments. Publicly funded services are also increasingly targeted ... and the entitlement to publicly funded services is being hollowed out. Furthermore, often the level of service provision is basic and involves a whole range of providers. As a result, the emphasis on welfare mix competes with the policy goal to integrate services across different providers and the boundary between health and social care.'

(Blank and Burau 2004: 167)

The percentage of people over 65 receiving formal help at home varies widely from 3% in Italy to 12% in the Netherlands, with the United States as an outlier at 16% (Jacobzone *et al.*, 1999). The latter is not a consequence of state generosity, but of the vigorous marketing of private insurance plans.

In England, a number of concerns have been raised about the provision of domiciliary services, although the picture is mixed. Overall, the evidence suggests some gains for people with complex needs, but fewer improvements for people with lower levels of dependency, and particular inadequacies in services for people from ethnic minorities (Patel, 1999). The number of home help hours purchased or provided by local authorities in England increased from 2.2 million in 1994 to 3.4 million in 2004 (Babb *et al.*, 2006), but whereas in 1994 81% of these were directly provided by the local authority, by 2004 this had fallen to 31%. The provision was also increasingly focused on the people with greatest need, which on the face of it is logical, but as with other targeted provision, can lead to the loss of preventative care.

A recent development is to pay cash benefits directly to dependent people, for them to purchase their own care. Personal budgets were first developed in social care under powers available to local authorities in England since 1996; uptake was slow until a pilot in 2006–2007 showed positive results. The possibility of extending the system to health care was ruled out in the white paper *Our Health, Our Care, Our Say* (Department of Health, 2006) on the grounds that it would erode the principle of the NHS as being free at the point of delivery, but this view was reversed in the NHS Next Stage Review and provision was made in the 2009 Health Bill, together with the announcement of a pilot scheme in 20 primary care trusts (PCTs). There are three ways in which a personal health budget could operate: a notional budget in which no money changes hands but the person talks to their clinician or care manager about the sum earmarked for them and how it should be spent, a real budget held by a third party, or direct payment. However, recent research (NHS Confederation, 2009) showed that health leaders were concerned that the scheme is not high priority nor likely to be welcomed by the NHS, may be complex to implement, and may compromise both patient safety and the quality assurance of services. These concerns were echoed in the experience of social care leaders, who concluded that achieving the cultural change needed was a far bigger challenge than the mechanics of implementing the scheme, that voluntary organisations were crucial as providers, trainers and advocates, and that a coordinated approach across health and social care was also needed.

A particular focus for policy analysts for many years has been the coordination, or lack of it, between health and social services in England, whereas in Northern Ireland structures have been integrated since 1973 (House of Commons Health Committee, 1998). This lack of focus was considered to result in duplication, fragmentation and delays in providing services, issues which may often impact upon people with LTCs. Intermittent attempts have been made to achieve more 'joined-up' government (Bogdanor, 2005) and to address policy 'silos' both nationally and locally. Legislation has permitted the pooling of budgets for several years, and the most recent attempt to coordinate local public sector budgets is the Total Place pilots, one of which, in Dorset, addresses services for older people (Smulian, 2009). It remains to be seen whether this is successful, whether it can be rolled out, and indeed whether it survives a change in government; however (premature) projections from the 13 pilots have already been made to argue that public service costs could be cut by 15% (Curtis, 2010).

Informal care and social care

Duff (2001) states that the costs of home care are largely borne by the community (so-called informal care). Whilst the role of the state is generally residual in the provision of home care, this is particularly marked in countries which have a strong cultural heritage, such as Germany where the role of women in providing care is still heavily influenced by Catholicism, and Japan, where the cultural honouring of older people results in a legal requirement for near relatives to provide financial support. Politicians and policy makers assume that families should want to take on the care of dependent members. Land (1991: 18) refers to this expectation, which falls particularly on women, as 'compulsory altruism' in that it is difficult to decline. The balance between individual and state responsibility in welfare, established after the Second World War, shifted in the 1980s back to a greater emphasis on the individual. This was explicitly expressed in the National Health Service and Community Care Act 1990, which greatly curtailed state expenditure on residential care.

The 2001 census identified 1.9 million unpaid carers in the United Kingdom, who each provided at least 20 hours of care a week. The highest levels of unpaid care were mainly in poorer areas such as South Wales, Merseyside, and in the London boroughs of Newham and Tower Hamlets. Estimates suggest that in the United Kingdom carers save the government £34 billion a year (Pickard *et al.*, 2003). Therefore, supporting carers has become an important policy goal, and in 1995 the Conservative government passed The Carer (Recognition and Services) Act. *Caring about Carers: A National Strategy for Carers* (Department of Health, 1999) recognised the need for primary care teams to improve communication with carers, provide support, and with the consent of the cared-for person, work collaboratively with them. Explicit standards and guidelines for supporting carers were also part of the NSFs, such as the NSF for Coronary Heart Disease (Department of Health, 2000a) and for Older People (Department of Health, 2001a). For example, para 3.28 of the latter states that 'The care plan should demonstrate user and carer involvement in decision making and each user and carers should hold their own copies of the care plan.'

Financial benefits for carers in the United Kingdom did not exist until the 1970s, when the invalid care allowance was introduced; it was a means-tested benefit for people under retirement age who gave up paid employment to care for a dependent, although married women were unable to claim until 1986, when the European Court ruled that their exclusion was sex discrimination. The introduction of the carer's allowance in the 1990s has improved the levels of support since the 1980s, when they were severely criticised (Glendinning, 1983), but they are not generous and there are concerns that higher levels might encourage carers with inappropriate motivations. Carers also suffer loss of income, since they are less likely to be in employment, and when employed, tend to be in lower paid jobs (Carmichael and Charles, 2003).

Although care homes fulfil a key role in providing social care, Henwood (2002) considers that we are ambivalent about them, through guilt at 'putting away' older people or people needing care. The sector has been placed under considerable pressure, squeezed between the need to invest and improve the physical fabric, the inadequate fee paid by local authorities, and a mobile workforce. In Henwood's view, the Royal Commission on Long-term Care, established under Sir Stewart Sutherland in 1997, could have addressed fundamental questions about the provision of care, but its terms of reference were limited to examining funding. Its recommendation, that the costs of care arising from frailty or disability should be met by the state, was accepted in Scotland but not in England (and is currently under review in the former due to financial pressures). More recently, the Wanless review of social care (Wanless, 2006) proposed a new funding model, but the issues remain the subject of considerable debate, since many people have not made sufficient provision for old age or illness, and the state is limited in its capacity unless more money is raised by taxation. A National Care Service was proposed in a 2009 green paper, which proposed that on retirement, people who could afford it should pay a lump sum of about £20,000 to pay for future care; this was superseded by an unaffordable promise of free care for 'critical' needs. In early 2010, a personal care at home bill was proposed, but with no published regulations on how it would work; a political row then ensued when it was suggested that £20,000 should be deducted from estates after death to help pay for the system.

Policy and practice developments in managing LTCs

The reforms of the NHS enacted by the Labour government elected in 1997 were set out in the white paper, *The New NHS* (Department of Health, 1997), followed by *The NHS Plan* (Department of Health, 2000b); key elements were greater partnership, and the elimination of unacceptable variations in care. Developments included new national standards, greater performance management, improved clinical governance and the creation of organizations such as NICE, the National Institute for Clinical Excellence which later subsumed the Health Development Agency, and the Modernisation Agency (which later merged with other elements to become the NHS Institute for Innovation and Improvement). A more recent example is NHS Evidence (www.evidence.nhs.uk). These are examples of the development of knowledge transfer, aided by the growth of information technology; knowledge transfer has also been promulgated through the creation of clinical networks and collaboratives, of which the first was the cancer network, set up after the Calman–Hine report (1995). The Coronary Heart Disease Collaborative, part of the Modernisation Agency, started in 2000 with 10 programmes, and expanded to 30, one in each cardiac network. Edwards (2002) considered that networks could make the best use of scarce clinical expertise, standardise care, improve access, and enable a faster spread of innovation.

NSFs have also been an important means of standardising care and promoting innovation. The Diabetes NSF was published in December 2001, followed by a delivery strategy, providing a 10-year programme of change. The progress of the Diabetes NSF was reviewed after 2 years (Department of Health, 2005c), as was the Coronary Heart Disease NSF (Department of Health, 2005d) exemplifying the process of service audit which has become central both to performance management in the NHS, and as a source of data for lobbying by clinical interest groups. A further example of the former is *Getting to the Heart of It* (Commission for Healthcare Audit and Inspection, 2005), a review of progress on the Coronary Heart Disease NSF. Examples of the latter are the third national COPD audit, funded by The Health Foundation (Royal College of Physicians *et al.*, 2008), the national audit of services for people with multiple sclerosis (Royal College of Physicians and Multiple Sclerosis Trust, 2008) and the pilot audit of intermediate care services carried out by the British Geriatric Society (Greenwood, 2009).

Since the NHS Plan, a whole suite of policy documents, such as *Commissioning a Patient-Led NHS* (Department of Health, 2005e) have developed patient choice and patient information as a means to driving up quality. Patient and public engagement are supposed to be integral to the work of the NHS, and from April 2010 a new system, run by the Care Quality Commission, will legally require all health and social care providers to gather the views of their service users. Currently, the evidence from the Picker Institute Europe (2009) is that the standard of engagement is variable.

As discussed in other chapters, the concept of the expert patient (Department of Health, 2001b) has been an important feature of the new approach to managing LTCs. The original programme, developed at Stanford University in California, recognised that many issues were common across a range of illnesses, including cognitive symptom management, exercise, nutrition and communication with professionals. There are two main types of self-management programme, those which are professionally led and usually condition specific, focusing on adherence to treatment regimes, and those which are user led and take a wider view on how people can take more control over their lives. A randomised controlled trial of the Expert Patients Programme by the National Primary Care Research and Development Centre (Kennedy *et al.*, 2007) found that it increased self-efficacy and energy, although it did not change patterns of health service use.

By 2010 everyone with an LTC should be offered a personalised care plan, which enhances self-care and records the discussion between the patient and the health care professional, and decisions made. The five elements of self-care support are information, healthy lifestyle choices, support networks, skills and confidence training, and tools such as self-monitoring devices, also called assistive technology. *2020 Vision* (Queen's Nursing Institute, 2009) considers that the use of this technology is vital. A £30 million programme of assistive technology is being piloted in three sites in Kent, Cornwall and the London borough of Newham, involving more than 6,000 people with LTCs and focusing on COPD, heart failure and diabetes. The experience in Cornwall has been positive (Lyndon and Tyas, 2010); patients have reported being able to manage their condition better, and feeling more empowered and confident.

A range of initiatives has been developed nationally to improve clinicians' skills in working in partnership with patients, for example the Department of Health (2009a) publication, *Your Health, Your Way*, and partnership is also at the heart of recent NICE (2009) guidance on medicines adherence, which highlights a 'no-blame' approach. The Health Foundation has invested over £6 million in a 3-year-demonstration programme of partnership based on eight sites, called Co-creating Health.

Another key element in the Labour government reforms of public services has been the use of targets. A national Public Service Agreement (PSA) target was set by the government to reduce emergency bed days by 5% by 2008 through improved care in primary and community settings, coupled with a PSA target to increase the number of people over 65 supported to live at home, by 1% per year in 2007 and 2008. *Supporting People with Long-Term Conditions: An NHS and Social Care Model to Support Local Innovation and Integration* (Department of Health, 2005f) builds on the intention stated in the *NHS Improvement Plan* (Department of Health, 2004) to move away from reactive care based in acute systems, to a systematic, patient-centred approach. It argues that improved support for people with LTCs requires wholesale change in the way that both health and social care services deliver care. They are required to identify all people with LTCs in their community and identify the level of care they need, using a model of care based on that used by the US health care provider, Kaiser Permanente. The case management of people in level 3 is discussed in Chapter 2.

Level 3: Case management for the most vulnerable people and those with highly complex needs, to anticipate and coordinate care.

Level 2: Disease-specific care management, which involves providing people who have a complex single need or multiple conditions with responsive, specialist services using multi-disciplinary teams and disease-specific protocols and pathways.

Level 1: Supported self-care, developing knowledge, skills and confidence.

As discussed in Chapter 2, in addition to the Kaiser Permanente model, another American model which has been used in England is Evercare, which is reported to have reduced hospitalisation and improved care in the United States, although the evaluation of both models in England has been inconclusive (Hutt *et al.*, 2004). This may be because the comparator arm of the clinical trials, i.e. existing primary and community care services, are already more comprehensive in England than in the United States and so elements of case management are already in place.

As concerns about the affordability of health care have deepened with the huge growth in the national debt, it is increasingly being argued that much care takes place in inappropriate, and expensive settings. For example, currently the ability of GPs to provide care for people with type 2 diabetes varies widely, and as a result outpatient clinics, which should be concerned mainly with people with type 1 diabetes and complex diabetes, are seeing patients who should be managed in primary care. The Darzi Report (Department of Health, 2008a) introduced the concept of polyclinics as a way of providing some hospital services and also aggregating primary care services, although there are no evaluations of their cost-effectiveness (Imison *et al.*, 2008) and the concept has proved vulnerable, since it was closely linked to a Labour junior minister. More recently, the concept has been modified to the polysystem, where services may be networked rather than co-located. Again, the Department of Health has not marketed its vision with any degree of clarity or energy, and as a result the debate is captured by the campaigners against hospital closures.

Pharmacy services are being developed, under a contract which has three categories; essential, advanced and enhanced. The white paper *Pharmacy in England; Building on Strengths – Delivering the Future* (Department of Health, 2008c) encouraged a move from dispensing to clinical services, such as 'compliance support'. However, there has been little development to date as pharmacists have generally required financial help to minimise the risk of the shift (Clews, 2009).

Ambulance services are also being reconfigured in some parts of England, moving from being the medical part of emergency services to being the emergency part of medical services, that is, part of a system which can triage 999, NHS Direct and GP out-of-hours calls (Kendall, 2009). Three quarters of the increase in 999 calls in the last decade has been due to four problems; falls, breathing problems, chest pain and unconsciousness (often alcohol related). The second and third of these have particular relevance to the management of LTCs; the government is determined that more health care should be managed effectively in primary care (Department of Health, 2009b), for example through the development of paramedic practitioners who can assess, treat and maintain the person in their own home.

It is widely considered that community services, which cost about £10 billion a year, or 10 per cent of the NHS budget, are key to reducing health care costs, although the evidence base is slim and the workforce implications are often not fully spelt out. Six *Transforming Community Services* guides were launched by the Department of Health (2009c) in June 2009, of which one concerns the care of people with LTCs:

- Use a proven tool to stratify risk.
- Support and enable people to manage their own health needs.
- Use case managers to proactively manage very high intensity users and those with complex needs. Develop shared care planning.
- Invest in telehealth and telecare to empower patients to take, maintain and maximise their health potential.
- Develop personalised care planning using joint or integrated assessments.
- Engage service users by offering choice and personalisation through expert patient programmes or encouragement to hold individualised budgets.

Nursing provision

Currently, it can be argued that practice nurses (and primary care in general) have a clearer policy focus than their colleagues in district nursing (and community care). A recent study (Griffiths *et al.*, 2010) found that after controlling for a number of practice and population characteristics, higher levels of nursing staffing in general practice were associated with better outcomes in relation to the clinical indicators used in the Quality and Outcomes Framework for reimbursing GP practices, of COPD, CHD, diabetes and hypertension. There is little research evidence on the impact of the increasing use of health care assistants.

Community matrons have also been proposed by the government as a key element in managing people with LTCs. *Supporting People with Long-term Conditions: Liberating the Talents of Nurses Who Care for People with Long-Term Conditions* (Department of Health, 2005g) set out the principles of case management and the skills required of a community matron, such as managing risk, medicines management, and managing cognitive impairment. PCTs were required to have 3,000 community matrons in post by March 2007 and to implement the Expert Patients Programme. More generally, in the report of the Prime Minister's Commission on the Future of Nursing and Midwifery (2010) LTCs are one of the six dimensions identified.

Overall, then, there is currently considerable turmoil in the NHS, but amidst this change there are perhaps more opportunities for nursing. Corner (2010) proposes that nurses should move fast to acquire skills such as prescribing, assessment and motivational interviewing, and that (using a phrase from Christensen *et al.*, 2009) we should become a 'disruptive technology' which has a widespread impact on the services in which we work. However, as the examples above demonstrate, there has, perhaps, been a policy overload. *Commissioning a Patient-Led NHS* (Department of Health, 2005e), which required PCTs to divest themselves of their community staff, was heavily criticised by the Commons Health Select Committee (HSC, 2006) in its report *Changes to Primary Care Trusts*. In particular, it was criticised for lack of consultation and poor timing, since it was issued in late July. Overall, the committee felt that the proposals anticipated the outcome of consultations to shape out-of-hospital care, and that this 'made a mockery of the consultation process' and created an impression of 'policy-making on the hoof'. Its effect in destabilising a valuable workforce was also recognised. In the intervening time, the timescale for implementing the change has been extended, and at the time of writing a variety of models, such as social enterprises and becoming part of another NHS Trust (such as an acute Trust or a mental health Trust) have been created, in some cases causing considerable union disquiet. In recognition of this, the *Operating Framework for the NHS in England 2010/11* (Department of Health, 2009b) stated that direct provision would remain an option, and also that 'commissioners and providers must maximise security of employment across their health economies' (para 3.47). Recently there have also been mixed messages from the Department of Health as to whether the NHS is the 'preferred provider' for services, or whether other organisations, such as those within the third sector, can also bid with a reasonable hope of success.

The role of the third sector

The term 'third sector' covers both voluntary and not-for-profit organisations, and also social enterprises, defined as businesses with primarily social objectives, whose surpluses are reinvested in the business or in the community. This sector is diverse, and ranges from very large organisations such as Macmillan to small charities with few or no paid staff, but common principles include operating on trust, management by values rather than by rules or profit margins, and user involvement. A growing role for voluntary organisations has been in developing expertise and lobbying, for example in relation to AIDS (Epstein, 1996).

In the nineteenth and early twentieth centuries, voluntary organisations played a central role in meeting welfare needs such as unemployment benefits, health insurance, and beds in the voluntary hospitals, by both mutual aid and charitable giving. Both district nursing and health visiting had their origins in such philanthropic provision and, as with other voluntary provision, both were absorbed into state provision. With the founding of the welfare state in 1948 the voluntary sector became marginalised, but the late 1960s saw a renaissance as campaign groups such as Shelter were established, influenced by the civil rights movement in the United States. As noted in Chapter 4, campaign groups have been important in addressing issues such as stigma, and disability groups have campaigned successfully for the reform of services through the provision of personal budgets.

The most recent phase has been the participation of the voluntary/third sector in the mixed economy of care. In the 1990s, the Conservative government used both incentives and pressures to 'roll back the state', arguing that it did not provide care which was tailored to people's needs. A market was created, and local authorities were required to shift much of their commissioning to the independent sector, defined as any provider not owned, managed or controlled by the local authority. The public, however, did not support a wholesale shift in provision, preferring that voluntary provision should complement, not replace, the statutory provision (Jowell *et al.*, 1995). The Labour government which came to power in 1997 also embraced the voluntary sector, not only on economic grounds but also as a way of addressing the decline in active citizenship (Fyfe and Milligan, 2003).

In relation to health care, it went further than its Conservative predecessor in creating markets and encouraging a range of provision. This has not only advantages but also risks in that the voluntary sector is often underfunded and too reliant on short-term contracts. This is illustrated in end-of-life care. The first modern hospice in the United Kingdom was founded in 1967, and funded mainly from public subscription. Dean (2005), reflecting on the death of its founder, Dame Cicely Saunders, argued that the hospices have never been properly funded by the NHS. They raise about £300 million of their own funding a year, with the equivalent of another £100 million in volunteer time; however, they have been hit by rising costs and the financial crash (Stratton, 2009). It is, therefore, essential that core services continue to be provided by the state, in order to provide stability.

Conclusion

This chapter has considered the context in which the care and management of people with LTCs takes place, by briefly reviewing the global context such as demographic and epidemiological change, and the social and health inequalities which result in increased morbidity and mortality for disadvantaged people. Health policy in all the developed countries is grappling with these issues, although the main focus tends to be on acute services. Home-based health care is generally more hidden from view and is more vulnerable to cuts as there are greater – though culturally variable – expectations of the role the family should play in providing care.

In the United Kingdom, and England in particular, the health service has been through a period of great instability with even greater to follow. However, there are also optimistic developments, such as a growing emphasis on patient involvement, and the legacy of the great investment in the NHS in the early years of the twenty-first century will hopefully be an infrastructure which includes better sources of data and assistive technology to enable this involvement to grow.

References

Academy of Medical Sciences (2009) *Rejuvenating Ageing Research*. Available at: www.academicmedicine.ac.uk.

Ahmad, W. I. U. & Bradby, H. (2007) Locating ethnicity and health: exploring concepts and contexts, *Sociology of Health and Illness*, 29(6), pp. 793–811.

Atkin, K. & Chattoo, S. (2007) The dilemmas of providing welfare in an ethnically diverse state: seeking reconciliation in the role of a 'reflexive practitioner', *Policy and Politics*, 35(3), pp. 379–395.

Babb, P., Butcher, H., Church, J. & Zealey, L. (2006) *Social Trends*. Office for National Statistics, London. Available at: www.statistics.gov.uk.

Beckford, J. A., Gale, R., Owen, D., Peach, C. & Weller, P. (2006) *Review of the Evidence Base on Faith Communities*. Office of the Deputy Prime Minister, London. Available at: http://www.communities.gov.uk/documents/corporate/pdf/143816.pdf.

Blank, R. H. & Burau, V. (2004) *Comparative Health Policy*. Palgrave Macmillan, Basingstoke.

Bogdanor, V. (2005) *Joined Up Government.* Oxford University Press, London.

British Household Panel Survey (2001). Available at: www.iser.essex.ac.uk/survey/bhps.

Calman, K. & Hine, D. (1995) *A Policy Framework for Commissioning Cancer Services.* NHS Executive, Leeds. Available at: http://www.dh.gov.uk/prod_consum_dh/groups/dh_digitalassets/@dh/@en/documents/digitalasset/dh_4014366.pdf.

Carmichael, F. & Charles, S. (2003) The opportunity costs of informal care: does gender matter? *Journal of Health Economics,* 22, pp. 781–803.

Christensen, C. M., Grossman, J. H. & Hwang, J. (2009) *The Innovator's Prescription – A Disruptive Solution for Health Care.* McGraw-Hill, New York.

Clews, G. (2009) Powerful chemistry, *Health Service Journal,* 17 July, pp. 22–24.

Commission for Healthcare Audit and Inspection (2005) *Getting to the Heart of It.* Commission for Healthcare Audit and Inspection, London.

Connolly, S., Bevan, G. & Mays, N. (2010) *Funding and Performance of Healthcare Systems in the Four Countries of the UK before and after Devolution.* The Nuffield Trust, London.

Corner, J. (2010) This is the perfect time for nurses to spearhead change, *Nursing Times,* 106(6), p. 25.

Curtis, P. (2010) Public services could cut costs by up to 15%, *Guardian,* 25 January, p. 12.

Dean, M. (2005) It is time to consider the future for hospices and how they are financed, *Guardian,* 20 July, p. 5.

Dent, E. (2009) The fat of the land, *Health Service Journal,* 26 March, pp. 18–20.

Department of Health (1997) *The New NHS: Modern, Dependable.* Available at: www.dh.gov.uk/publications.

Department of Health (1998a) *Our Healthier Nation a Contract for Health.* Available at: www.dh.gov.uk/publications.

Department of Health (1998b) *Acheson INQUIRY: Independent Enquiry into Inequalities in Health.* Available at: www.dh.gov.uk/publications.

Department of Health (1999) *Caring about Carers: A National Strategy for Carers.* Available at: www.dh.gov.uk/publications.

Department of Health (2000a) *National Service Framework for Coronary Heart Disease.* Available at: www.dh.gov.uk/publications.

Department of Health (2000b) *The NHS Plan: A Plan for Investment, a Plan for Reform.* The Stationery Office, London.

Department of Health (2001a) *National Service Framework for Older People.* Available at: www.dh.gov.uk/publications.

Department of Health (2001b) *The Expert Patient: a New Approach to Chronic Disease Management for the 21st Century.* Department of Health, London.

Department of Health (2003) *Making Partnership Work for Patients, Carers and Services Users.* Available at: www.dh.gov.uk/publications.

Department of Health (2004) *NHS Improvement Plan: Putting People at the Heart of Public Services.* Available at: www.dh.gov.uk/publications.

Department of Health (2005a) *The National Service Framework Long Term Conditions.* Available at: www.dh.gov.uk/publications.

Department of Health (2005b) *Independence Wellbeing and Choice: Our Vision for the Future of Social Care for Adults in England.* Department of Health, London.

Department of Health (2005c) *Improving Diabetes Services – The NSF Two Years On.* Available at: www.dh.gov.uk/publications.

Department of Health (2005d) *The Coronary Heart Disease National Service Framework.* Available at: www.dh.gov.uk/publications.

Department of Health (2005e) *Commissioning a Patient-Led NHS*. Available at: www.dh.gov. uk/publications.

Department of Health (2005f) *Supporting People with Long Term Conditions: An NHS and Social Care Model to Support Local Innovation and Integration*. Available at: www.dh.gov.uk/cno.

Department of Health (2005g) *Supporting People with Long Term Conditions: Liberating the Talents of Nurses Who Care for People with Long Term Conditions*. Available at: www.dh.gov.uk/cno.

Department of Health (2006) *Our Health, Our Care, Our Say*. Department of Health, London.

Department of Health (2008a) *High Quality Care for All: NHS Next Stage Review Final Report*. The Stationery Office, London.

Department of Health (2008b) *Raising the Profile of Long Term Conditions Care, A Compendium of Information*. Department of Health, London. Available at: Tinyurl.com/compendium-ltc.

Department of Health (2008c) *Pharmacy in England: Building Strengths – Delivering the Future, White Paper*. Available at: www.dh.gov.uk/publications.

Department of Health (2009a) *Your Health, Your Way – a Guide to Long Term Conditions and Self Care*. Available at: www.dh.gov.uk/publications.

Department of Health (2009b) *The NHS Operating Framework for England 2010/11*. Available at: www.dh.gov.uk/publications.

Department of Health (2009c) *Transforming Community Services*. Available at: www.dh.gov. uk/publications.

Dowrick, C., Dixon-Woods, M., Holman, H. & Weinman, J. (2005) What is chronic illness? *Chronic Illness*, 1, pp. 1–6.

Duff, J. (2001) Financing to foster community health care: a comparative analysis of Singapore, Europe, North America, and Australia, *Current Sociology*, 49(3), pp. 135–54.

Edwards, N. (2002) Clinical networks, *British Medical Journal*, 324, p. 63.

Edwards, M. & Dyson, L. (2003) Is the district nursing service in a position to deliver intermediate care? A national survey of district nursing provision, *Primary Health Care Research and Development*, 4, pp. 353–364.

Egede, L. E. (2007) Major depression in individuals with chronic medical disorders: prevalence, correlates and association with health resource utilization, lost productivity and functional disability, *General Hospital Psychiatry*, 29, pp. 409–416.

Epstein, S. (1996) *Impure Science: AIDS, Activism and the Politics of Knowledge*. University of California Press, Berkeley, CA.

Foresight (2007) *Tackling Obesities: Future Choices – Project Report*. Foresight, London. Available at: tinyurl.com/foresight-project.

Fyfe, N. R. & Milligan, C. (2003) Space, citizenship, and voluntarism: critical reflections on the voluntary welfare sector in Glasgow, *Environment and Planning*, 35, pp. 2069–2086.

Gainsbury, S. (2009) McKinsey exposes hard choices to save £20bn, *Health Service Journal*, 10 September 2009, pp.12–13.

Glendinning, C. (1983) *Unshared Care: Parents and Their Disabled Children*. Routledge and Kegan Paul, London.

Greenwood, L. (2009) The national standard for intermediate care, *Health Service Journal*, 3 December 2009, pp. 24–25.

Greer, S. (2005) *Territorial Politics and Health Policy: UK Health Policy in Comparative Perspective*. Manchester University Press, Manchester.

Griffiths, P., Murrells, T., Maben, J., Jones, S. & Ashworth, M. (2010) Nurse staffing and quality of care in UK general practice: cross sectional study using routinely collected data, *British Journal of General Practice*, 60(570), pp. 36–48.

Haddad, M., Taylor, C. & Pilling, S. (2009) Depression in adults with long term conditions 1: how to identify and assess symptoms, *Nursing Times*, 7 December 2009, 105(48), pp. 14–17.

Harris, P. (2009) Whistleblower tells of America's hidden nightmare for its sick poor, *Observer*, 26 July 2009, p. 19.

Henwood, M. (2002) 'No grey areas', *Health Service Journal*, 12 December 2002, pp. 24–27.

House of Commons Health Committee (1998) *The Relationship between Health and Social Services*. The Stationery Office, London.

House of Commons Health Select Committee (HSC) (2006) *Changes to Primary Care Trusts*. The Stationery Office, London.

House of Commons Health Committee (2009) *Health Inequalities*. The Stationery Office, London.

Hutt, R., Rosen, R. & McCauley, J. (2004) *Case-Managing Long-Term Conditions: What Impact Does It Have on the Treatment of Older People?* King's Fund, London.

Imison, C., Naylor, C. & Maybin, J. (2008) *Under One Roof. Will Polyclinics Deliver Integrated Care?* King's Fund, London. Available at: www.kingsfund.org.uk.

Jacobzone, S., Cambois, E, Chaplain, E. & Robine, J. M. (1999) *The health of older persons in OECD countries: is it improving fast enough to compensate for population ageing?* OECD Labour Market and Social Policy Occasional Papers 37. OECD, Paris.

Jowell, R., Curtis, J., Park, A., Brook, L., Ahrendt, D. & Thomson, K. (eds) (1995) *British Social Attitudes: The 12th Report*. Dartmouth Publishing, Aldershot.

Kendall, L. (2009) Take the fast track to efficiency, *Health Service Journal*, 19 November, p. 17.

Kennedy, A. Reeves, D. Bower, P. *et al.* (2007) The effectiveness and cost effectiveness of a national lay led self care support programme for patients with long-term conditions: a pragmatic randomised controlled trial, *Journal of Epidemiology and Community Health*, 61, pp. 254–261.

Land, H. (1991) Time to care. In: *Women's Issues in Social Policy*. (eds M. Mclean & D. Groves). Routledge, London.

Lyndon, H. & Tyas, D. (2010) Telehealth enhances self care and independence in people with long term conditions, *Nursing Times*, 106(26), pp. 12–13.

Marmot Review (2010) *Fair Society, Healthy Lives: Strategic Review of Health Inequalities in England Post-2010*. London.

Martin, J. & Salmond, G. (2001) Policy making: the 'messy reality.' In: *Health and Public Policy in New Zealand* (eds P. Davis & T. Ashton). Oxford University Press, Auckland.

Mulgan, G. & Buenfino, A. (2006) Pressing needs, *Society Guardian*, 12 July, p. 1.

Murray, C. & Lopez, A. (1996) *The Global Burden of Disease*. Harvard School of Public Health, Boston, MA.

Murray, C. J. L. & Lopez, A. D. (1997) Alternative projections of mortality and disability by cause 1990–2020: global burden of disease study, *Lancet*, 349(9064), pp. 1498–1504.

National Institute for Health and Clinical Excellence (NICE) (2009) *Medicines Adherence: Involving Patients in Decisions about Prescribed Medicines and Supporting Adherence*. NICE Clinical Guideline 76. Available at: www.nice.org.uk.

Nazroo, J. Y., Jackson, J., Karlsen, S. & Torres, M. (2007) The black diaspora and health inequalities in the US and England: does where you go and how you get there make a difference? *Sociology of Health and Illness*, 29(6), pp. 811–830.

Nazroo, J. Y. & Williams, D. R. (2005) The social determination of ethnic/racial inequalities in health. In: *Social Determinants of Health* (eds M. Marmot & R. G. Wilkinson). Oxford University Press, Oxford.

NHS Confederation (2009) *Shaping Personal Health Budgets*. NHS Confederation, London.

OECD (1988) *Ageing Populations: Social Policy Implications*. OECD, Paris.

Patel, N. (1999) Black and minority ethnic elderly: perspectives on long-term care. *Royal Commission on Long Term Care – Research Volume 1*. Stationery Office, London.

Pickard, S. Jacobs, S. & Kirk, S. (2003) Challenging professional roles: lay carers' involvement in health care in the community, *Social Policy and Administration*, 37(1), pp. 82–96.

Picker Institute Europe (2009) *Patient and Public Engagement – the Early Impact of World Class Commissioning. A survey of Primary Care Trusts*. Available at: www.pickereurope.org.

Pilkington, E. (2009) World faces age of dependency as over 65s outnumber young, *Guardian*, 21 July 2009, pp. 16–17.

Prime Minister's Commission on the Future of Nursing and Midwifery in England (2010) *Front Line Care*. Central Office of Information, London.

Queen's Nursing Institute (2009) *2020 Vision*. QNI, London.

Roland, M., McDonald, R. & Sibbald, B. (2007) *Can Primary Care Reform Reduce Demand on Hospital Outpatient Departments?* NHS Service Delivery and Organisation R&D Programme. Available at: www.sdo.lshtm.ac.uk.

Royal College of Physicians and Multiple Sclerosis Trust (2008) *National Audit of Services for People with Multiple Sclerosis*. Royal College of Physicians, London.

Royal College of Physicians, *et al.* (2008) *National COPD Audit 2008*. Royal College of Physicians, London. Available at: tinyurl.com/copd-audit-2008.

Smulian, M. (2009) Pooling Power, *Health Service Journal*, 17 December, pp. 30–31.

Stratton, A. (2009) Millions for charities hit by recession, *Guardian*, 9 February 2009, p. 1.

Townsend, P., Whitehead, M. & Davidson, N. (eds) (1992) *Inequalities in Health: the Black Report and the Health Divide*. Penguin, Harmondsworth.

US Census Bureau (2009) *An Ageing World: 2008*. US Government Printing Office. Available at: www.census.gov/prod/2009pubs/p95-09-1.pdf.

Wanless, D. (2002) *Securing our Future Health: Taking a Long-Term View*. Final report. Her Majesty's Treasury, London. Available at: www.dh.gov.uk/assetRoot/04/07/61/34/04076134.pdf.

Wanless, D. (2006) *Securing Good Care for Older People*. King's Fund, London.

Wilkinson, R. G. (1996) *Unhealthy Societies: the Afflictions of Inequalities*. Routledge, London.

Wilkinson, R. G. (2005) *The Impact of Inequality: How to Make Sick Societies Healthier*. Routledge, London.

Wilkinson, R. & Pickett, K. (2009) *The Spirit Level: Why More Equal Societies Almost Always Do Better*. Allen Lane, London.

Wilson, R., Buck, D. & Ham, C. (2005) Rising to the challenge: Will the NHS support people with long term conditions? *British Medical Journal*, 330, pp. 657–661.

World Health Organisation (2005) *Preventing Chronic Diseases: A Vital Investment: WHO Global Report*. World Health Organisation, Geneva. Available at: tinyurl.com/disease-investment.

Yach, D., Hawkes, C., Gould, C. & Hofman, K. (2004) The global burden of chronic diseases: overcoming impediments to prevention and control, *Journal of the American Medical Association*, 291, pp. 2616–2622.

Chapter 2

Case management

Kerri Wright
School of Health and Social Care, University of Greenwich, Eltham, London, UK

Introduction

The increase in the numbers of people living with long-term conditions (LTCs) in the United Kingdom and the implications of this for present and future health care resources have led to a radical rethink of health care provision in the United Kingdom (Wanless, 2004, 2007). The previous focus on cure and the episodic treatment of people as and when they became unwell is untenable, especially with the expected increases in LTC prevalence within future populations. Health care provision for LTC care has required a new approach and a new system for caring for and managing the health needs of people living with LTCs. The new approach is discussed in Chapter 3 and details the necessity of moving away from cure-focused care to the management of LTCs within the context of the individual's life. The new approach also incorporates the increased focus on self-management and self-care; developing expert patients and increasing patient choice within health policies and the necessity for people to take increasingly more responsibility and action to promote health for themselves (Department of Health, 2005a, 2005b, 2009a). This is discussed in detail in Chapter 8. Finally, the management of LTCs requires a change to the health care system if it is to build the infrastructure to allow care to move away from a 'reactive, unplanned and episodic approach to care' (Department of Health, 2005a: 8) to one which is based on the continuous care of people with LTCs by teams that combine 'specialist expertise with generalist capabilities' (World Health Organisation, 2002). One approach to try to achieve this aim has been the introduction of case management for people with LTCs.

Case management overview

Case management is a process or method of delivering care that ensures that people are 'provided with whatever services they need in a co-ordinated, effective and efficient manner' (Intagliata, 1982: 657). The aim of case management is to provide supportive care continuously, so that services or care can be implemented in a timely way and

Table 2.1   Common LTC case management models.

United healthcare – Evercare Identified population of high risk elderly people who had two or more admissions in previous year or nominated by GP as meeting local criteria agreed. Population identified as high risk, case managed by advanced primary nurses (APN) along with the redesign of services and processes to enable effective management. Evercare teams developed a range of processes and tools to assist with case management, for example Early Alert poster for patients and families to use and medicine review sheets (Evercare 2004).	**Pfizer health solutions** This model has developed highly customised services in the United States to address at risk populations. In the United Kingdom, Pfizer can work with PCTs to identify areas of service need and develop bespoke services and solutions to address issues in relation to LTC. Pfizer's focus is on encouraging self care through developing ways of improving engagement between people with LTCs and the health care providers. For example, Pfizer has just developed a telephone-based care management service, Birmingham OwnHealth, in collaboration with Birmingham PCTs, which is specifically designed for people with diabetes, COPD, cardiovascular disease or heart failure. Pfizer Health Solutions website has more information about bespoke services that they have developed.
Kaiser Kaiser Permanente is a United States model that provides and manages care for populations according to disease. Kaiser integrates primary and secondary care enabling people to move easily between the two depending on their needs, and focuses on empowering people to take more responsibility for managing their conditions. Kaiser uses advanced technology to manage people at all stages of their conditions and ensures continuity and rapid response to changes. Aspects of the Kaiser Model have been implemented within the United Kingdom and are discussed on the National Primary and Care Trust Development Centre (NatPaCT) website.	**Castlefields** The Castlefields model predates the Evercare pilots and involves an integrated case management approach across health and social care. The model includes a district nurse and a social worker working together to coordinate and arrange appropriate support and care. The district nurse provides assessment, coordinates care and offers advice and education to the patient and their family (Lyon *et al.,* 2006).

prevent crises or acute episodes occurring that may result in hospitalisation. The method of delivering care could be a team approach or one person who is responsible for working with the person involved. There are a number of different case management models being used across a range of health and social care areas. The key models related to LTCs are outlined in Table 2.1. In addition, other services are continually being developed to provide continuous care for people with LTCs, such as telecare or telehealth systems (Department of Health, 2009b) (see Box 2.1) or to provide intensive care for people who are at 'high risk' of unplanned admissions on virtual wards (Robinson, 2008) (see Box 2.2). The key components of case management are finding the right people to case manage, with case finding being an important part of this, assessment, care planning, monitoring and review of the individual (Challis *et al.,* 1990). Some models also include a clinical component, where the case manager has a clinical role, for example advanced nurses in the Evercare Model.

Box 2.1   Telemedicine/Telecare/Telehealth (Department of Health 2009b).

The use of technology to support people in their own homes has expanded recently and there are now a host of different systems in use to provide this service. The Department of Health launched a Whole Systems Denominators programme in 2007 to evaluate the use of these systems in healthcare. Three pilot sites using telehealth and telecare were set up in 2007 in the London borough of Newham, Cornwall and Kent and will provide the largest evaluation of telecare in the world to date. The terms for this new technology are often used interchangeably and inconsistently in the literature. Brief definitions of these services are:

Telecare describes any service that uses information or communication technology to support someone to live at home, for example motion or falls monitors that trigger a warning to a response centre.

Telehealth uses equipment to monitor someone's health remotely, for example clinical details such as blood pressure or glucose levels can be recorded and monitored by a response centre, usually a nurse who can then act on these results.

Telemedicine allows clinical consultations remotely, often by video conference.

Box 2.2   Virtual community wards.

The concept of a 'virtual ward' was first developed by Croydon PCT and is an approach to provide support and care to people with LTCs who are most at risk of being admitted to a hospital as an unplanned admission. The virtual ward has the same systems and staff available as a hospital ward, but without the person being in that physical space. Virtual wards consist of approximately 100 beds. Once someone is admitted they receive an assessment from a community matron and access to a range of professionals in the virtual ward team, for example community nurses, social workers, GP, pharmacist and other allied professionals such as physiotherapists and occupational therapists and a ward administrator. Ongoing progress and care is discussed at regular meetings and is communicated to the person's GP and local hospital to ensure continuity of care between these services. When a bed becomes available predictive risk models, for example PARR tools, are used to identify the next person in the local area who is most at risk of an unplanned admission and they are admitted to the virtual ward.

An important element of the community ward is that it arose from data on patients' reasons for calling emergency services, for example the perception that a hospital ward was safer, and addressed these in the community (Ioannou, 2010).

Case management is not a new concept in health and social care. Case managers were introduced to work with older people in the 1990s following the *National Health Service and Community Care Act, 1990* and the integration of a number of client groups into the community. These case managers were usually trained in social work and worked with vulnerable elderly people to support them in living in the community; potentially the same group is now felt to require case management under the LTC agenda (Murphy, 2004). Within mental health, there is a long history of case management following the closure of large psychiatric hospitals and the move to integration within the community. Case management has been used in mental health teams since the 1970s and as a consequence this service has a wealth of experience and knowledge relating to this provision of care (Simpson *et al.*, 2003). In relation to LTC, case management has been used in the United States and Canada to support frail older people with chronic conditions since the early 1990s. In the United Kingdom, the government has embraced the concept of case management within LTCs to work in partnership with individuals who are most vulnerable and intensive users of the health care system (Department of Health, 2006). As part of this initiative, the government has created a new advanced nurse role of community matron to provide clinical-focused case management.

The case management model introduced in the United Kingdom is based on the Kaiser Permanente model (see Table 2.1) and categorises people living with LTCs according to their level of risk of using inappropriate episodic care to manage their condition (Department of Health, 2005a) (see Chapter 1 for more information on this model). People felt to be at high risk could already be high-intensity users of secondary care or at risk of this without case management. Case managers are tasked with proactively identifying those people with LTCs who are felt to be most vulnerable and then working in partnership with them and relevant health care professionals to coordinate and manage their care (Department of Health, 2006). Community matrons are tasked to provide complex case management to those identified as being at level 3 of this model in order to 'treat patients sooner, nearer to home and earlier in the course of their disease' (Department of Health, 2005a: 7). Thus, community matrons have an advanced clinical role which helps in the long-term management of conditions, early detection of problems and appropriate and timely treatment. Initially, community matrons were working with a Public Service Agreement (PSA) target of reducing the number of emergency bed days by 5% by 2008 (Department of Health, 2004, 2005a). Although this target has reportedly been achieved and emergency bed days have decreased by 10.1% between 2003–2004 and 2006–2007 (HM Treasury, 2007), it is difficult to equate this decrease with the case management initiative alone.

Evaluating case management

The evaluations of case management are often focused on the successful achievement of targets or aims set for the service. The role of the community matron in case management has been based in part on the successful Evercare model used in the United States (Table 2.1). This model was successful in reducing the number of emergency bed days and hospital admissions in the United States (Kane *et al.*, 2003; Hutt *et al.*, 2004). Several

Evercare pilot sites were set up across the United Kingdom, based on the US success, and used to form the current community matron initiative. Perhaps unfortunately, the introduction of case management by community matrons was implemented before formal evaluations of the Evercare pilots were completed. These evaluations demonstrated that the Evercare project and case management by an advanced clinical nurse was not successful in reducing bed days or emergency admissions for the population being case managed (National Primary Care Research and Development Centre, 2005; Gravelle *et al.,* 2006). Indeed, reviews of studies examining the effectiveness of case management approaches have also found that it is not an effective approach in reducing hospital usage in the United Kingdom (Hutt *et al.,* 2004; Marshall *et al.,* 1998).

With many case management approaches the desired outcome is the reduction of episodic and unplanned care, and this is often measured through the reduction of emergency bed days in hospitals (Department of Health, 2005a). A systematic Cochrane review of case management approaches within mental health services identified that case management was effective in increasing the number of people who had contact with the mental health service, but actually doubled the number of people admitted to hospital (Marshall *et al.,* 1998). There were no advantages noted with case management as compared to standard care approaches and no cost savings to the health service evidenced using this approach.

Evaluations of case management approaches to care are, however, difficult to tease out, due to an absence of definitions and details of the case management role in studies and a focus on targets where case management cannot have a direct causal effect (Sargent *et al.,* 2007). Evaluations often focus on measurable outcomes, for example evidence of improved clinical outcomes and decreased use of health care services and subsequent cost savings (Hutt *et al.,* 2004; Sargent *et al.,* 2008). Other concerns mainly focus on the narrow scope of studies included, for example reviews only including randomly controlled trials and not other research methods that may have included different outcome measures as part of their evaluations (Ziguras and Stuart, 2000).

Case management approaches

As discussed above, there is a wealth of experience and literature on case management of people with long-term mental illness which is useful to explore in relation to LTCs. However, it is important to note that with mental health services the issue of compulsory treatment for some people with severe mental illness can limit the transferability of some of the literature, although many of the principles of case management still remain the same. The development of case management in mental health services is similar to the current needs for the health service in relation to LTCs; to find an alternative approach to manage people's health continuously in the community to prevent untimely and inefficient uses of acute hospital resources. The approaches developed to achieve this aim within mental health services were diverse, but have been categorised into three basic core models (Mueser *et al.,* 1998). These are summarised in Table 2.2. These approaches have been studied extensively and evaluated in relation to many different outcomes, from service specific outcomes such as the use of health care services to user

Table 2.2 Models of case management in mental health and comparison with LTC initiatives.

Case management core model	Description	Similarities with LTC initiatives
Clinical case management	The case manager assesses and provides ongoing support and clinical care to individuals and facilitates the person's management and adaptation to their condition.	Community matron 'clinical interventions as well as care coordination' (Department of Health, 2005a: 16) to patients with 'very complex and intensive clinical needs' (Department of Health, 2006: 3).
Strengths model	This model grew in response to concerns that traditional approaches to case management and psychiatric treatment focused on the person's impairments and problems to the detriment of acknowledging the person's strengths and resources used to manage their life with their conditions. The aim is to focus and continue developing the individual's strengths, rather than their pathology, through collaborative working towards agreed short- and long-term goals. The ultimate aim is that the individual is able to engage and integrate within the local community and that this community support can replace the case manager.	Supported self-care 'With the right support people can be empowered and learn to be active participants in improving existing symptoms, avoiding flare-ups, slowing deterioration and preventing development of complications and other conditions. This can help them in achieving a better quality of life while living with and taking care of their conditions' (Department of Health, 2005b: 4).
Intensive and assertive community treatment (ACT)	Both these models involve intensive treatment to small numbers of people who are unable or unwilling to cooperate with standard mental health services. ACT involves a multidisciplinary approach and provides all required interventions as a team in the person's home, including practical support such as shopping. Intensive case management can be described as a more intensive version of clinical case management with smaller caseloads directed towards people who have increased 'needs' and require intensive support.	Intermediate care 'rapid assessment, diagnosis and treatment in response to a crisis or impending crisis and referral to most appropriate service' for example Hospital at home – 'intensive support at home for a short period, including community nursing, community therapy services and home care support' (Department of Health, 2001: 3).

perceptions of their health, and there has been debate regarding the effectiveness of a case management approach (NHS Centre for Reviews and Dissemination, 2001; Ziguras and Stuart, 2000).

The different case management models used in mental health are useful to explore since there are similarities between the CPA and the LTC case management agenda, for example the current case management role for LTCs highlights the requirements of the role and the training needs expected (Department of Health, 2006), but does not stipulate how this role is to be implemented (Sargent *et al.*, 2007). There are benefits of not being prescriptive regarding case management 'tasks' as it leaves heath services flexibility to provide a case management service that meets local needs, yet still retains the core principles of case management. This has resulted in the different LTC case management models and facets of these models being used across different primary care trusts (Hutt *et al.*, 2004) which are arguably providing care that is more appropriate to local needs. However, the lack of definition of exactly what case management models are being used and how these are implemented across individuals, teams and services mean that the evaluation and comparison of these case management approaches can be problematic (Sargent *et al.*, 2007). This can hinder the process of teasing out what exactly the 'active ingredients' are within the case management models that are beneficial and produce positive outcomes (Simpson *et al.*, 2003: 476).

Active ingredients of case management

The effectiveness of a case management approach can be due to a number of different variables. These variables are discussed below under the broad headings of individual case managers, case management structure and health and social care infrastructure.

Individual case managers

The requirements of the case management role are standardised, with core competencies identified so that all case managers have been assessed as having the necessary skills to carry out the role. However, as case managers are all individuals with differing personalities, experiences and clinical backgrounds, there will obviously be differences in the approaches and standards of care implemented by individuals (Cooper and Yarmo Roberts, 2006). These differences can impact on the effectiveness of the case management approach. The case manager is highlighted as someone who is 'accessible, approachable and emotionally engaged' (Simpson *et al.*, 2003: 477), which encourages the development of a therapeutic relationship. The quality of the relationship between the individual and the case manager has been suggested as vital to the success of case management approaches (Burns and Santos, 1995, Williams and Cooper, 2008, Cooper and Yarmo Roberts, 2006). Developing a relationship is also instrumental in providing psychosocial support which has been highlighted in reducing stress and increasing confidence in both people with LTC and their carers (Allen and Fabri, 2005; Sargent *et al.*, 2007):

'When I know she's coming to see her [patient] then it relaxes me as well ... that's where she's been very helpful, she's helped me to unbottle and get rid of the tension that I'm feeling.'

(Sargent *et al.*, 2007: 516)

Despite the importance of psychosocial support in LTC care, there is no core domain within the competency framework for the case manager's role related to this aspect of care. Therefore, this area of care will be implemented according to the case manager's previous experiences and will result in variability across individuals and case management models. The requirement of training in psychosocial interventions is highlighted in several studies on case management and is an arguably important omission in the present LTC case management model (Sargent *et al.*, 2007; Williams and Cooper, 2008).

Case management structure

The organisational structure of the case management model implemented can impact on the care of people with LTCs. The quality of relationship developed can be affected by the size of the caseload of the case manager and the continuity of care the case manager is able to give to people on their caseload. The case management policy for community matrons and other care managers indicates that their caseload is expected to be between 50 and 80 people (Department of Health, 2005a). Studies have demonstrated that the size of the caseload can impact on the quality of the care offered to each person, with larger caseloads reducing the quality of care, increasing hospital admissions and shifting the focus from proactive to reactive care (Sargent *et al.*, 2008). The exact effect that different caseload size has on the care implemented and how this impacts on the overall quality and effectiveness of case management offered to people is still unknown. Williams and Cooper (2008) point out that the optimum 'dosage' of case management is not known, and therefore, it is difficult to determine the impact that changes to the organisational structure have on the effectiveness of case management in individual cases. However, there is some indication that the care given during contact as well as the indirect care that is required outside contact time, for example making telephone calls and writing letters, also needs to be considered (Simpson *et al.*, 2003).

Health and social care infrastructure

The effectiveness of case management is also influenced by the local infrastructure of health and social care services. Effective case management in the past has been found to have close links with secondary care, allowing access to clinical assessments by specialists (Challis and Hughes, 2002), and is thought to depend on the active involvement of hospital specialists, social services and developing a vertically integrated system of care from primary to secondary care, with the same financial incentives (Murphy, 2004). At present, there are differing financial incentives for case managing people with LTCs between primary care trusts (PCTs) and acute hospitals. The Payment by Results (PbR) initiative, that was introduced to improve efficiency within acute hospitals, rewards hospitals according to the number of patients and types of conditions they treat (Department of Health, 2002). The financial incentives effectively encourage acute trusts to admit and treat people with LTCs and could be a disincentive for case managing people in the community. The challenge for PCTs is to establish incentives across the primary and secondary care divide (Murphy, 2004). In addition, care received by individuals with LTCs is dependent on local variables such as the GP and the threshold at which they will send people to accident and emergency departments as well as the doctor's threshold for admitting the individual into hospital. Billings *et al.* (2006a, 2006b) found a 20% variation in the decisions made by doctors caring for people with LTCs. This variable impacts on the evaluation of case management models, yet is unrelated to the case management interventions given.

Case finding

One of the challenges for case management is case finding; identifying those people assessed as being at high risk and in need of complex case management. The goal of case finding is to 'target and calibrate resources for interventions to those who will benefit most, allowing savings from reduced subsequent resource use' (Billings *et al.,* 2006a: 1). In order to be effective any method employed to identify this population must be sensitive enough so that it does not omit people who are at risk and would benefit from case management, yet not be so sensitive that resources are used up case managing people who would not be at risk. Within LTCs, the aim of case management is to reduce emergency bed days. Therefore, effective case finding for LTC case management involves identifying those people who are most likely to be admitted to hospital and are at the greatest risk of longer hospital stays. Case finding requires case managers and PCTs firstly to decide on the criteria for identifying high-risk populations in their area and then to develop systems to allow this population to be identified and provide appropriate care. These requirements have resulted in challenges for primary and secondary care and led to new systems and sharing of information to be developed and agreed. The initial criteria for the Evercare pilots identified the over 65 population who had required two or more emergency admissions that year. These criteria have since been shown to be oversensitive and identified too many people who may not actually be at risk (National Primary Care Research and Development Centre, 2005; Roland *et al.,* 2005).

Case finding tools are now available for local trusts to use in order to identify their 'at risk' population for case management. Case finding software has been developed which utilises a number of factors that could contribute towards someone being at risk of emergency hospital admission in the next 12 months, called the Patient at Risk of Re-Hospitalisation (PARR) tool (Billings *et al.,* 2006b). This software has since been commissioned by the Department of Health and NHS and is now available as an online tool for local health communities to use. The tool utilises a range of information about a person using a list of factors that could contribute towards their risk of being re-admitted to hospital (see Table 2.3) and then assigns a numerical figure out of 100, known as their PARR score. The PARR score is only a guide to the person's level of risk. Case managers need to use their own clinical judgement alongside this score to determine whether complex case management is required. The PARR tool is activated by a hospital

Table 2.3   Variables included in PARR case finding algorithm (Billings *et al.* 2006a: 3).

Alcohol-related diagnoses
Cerebrovascular disease
Chronic obstructive pulmonary disease
Connective tissue disease/rheumatoid arthritis
Developmental disability
Diabetes
Ischaemic heart disease
Peripheral vascular disease
Renal failure
Sickle cell disease
Previous admission for respiratory infection
Number of different treatment specialists seen
Age 65–74, age 75+
Sex
Ethnicity
Previous admission for a reference condition
Number of emergency admissions in previous 90, 180 and 365 days
Number of non-emergency admissions in previous 365 days
Total number of previous emergency admissions in previous three years
Average number of episodes per spell for emergency admissions
Observed: expected ratio for GP decision making (which takes into account the GP's usual practice)
Observed: expected ratio for rate of readmissions for hospital of current admission
Diagnostic cost groups/hierarchical condition category

admission and can only predict the risk of someone being readmitted to hospital in the next 12 months. The King's Fund has developed another tool, known as the Combined Predictive Model, which uses information from the community to highlight if someone is deteriorating and at risk of emergency hospital admission, thereby identifying them before the PARR tool would pick them up. This tool does not have an online interface, although full instructions are available for PCTs to commission this tool to be built by programmers. The Combined Predictive Model aims to help PCTs to target their care more effectively to those most at risk.

Risk

The focus on risk within case management can lead to conflicts between providing a person-centred or service-led approach to LTC management. The case management initiative is arguably service-led with an aim to reduce the inefficient and unplanned use of secondary care services by people with LTCs. Although there is a benefit to the individual, who gains continuous care through case management and perhaps prevention of exacerbations which cause distress, primarily the measure of case management effectiveness is unplanned hospital admissions with the focus of care then becoming service-led. Case finding tools identify people deemed to be at risk of emergency readmissions to hospital, based on data gathered about them, and place them into a 'high-risk population' requiring complex case management. This high-risk population is deemed to require case management to minimise the risks of inappropriate and costly health care interventions which are viewed as preventable and undesirable. This perception can result in people with LTCs who are identified as 'high risk' being perceived as 'problematic' by health care providers and can lead to a focus on the individual's impairments or limitations in attempts to eradicate risks (Clarke, 2009). This can trivialise the successes and adaptations that a person has made to their lives to manage their LTC and was one of the reasons that the strengths model was developed within mental health services, as shown in Table 2.2 (Simpson *et al.,* 2003).

If all risk is removed from an individual's life, this can also remove those components of life which are valued and provide meaning, thus compromising a person's quality of life (Clarke, 2009). However, if risks are left unmanaged then physical deterioration and crises can occur, resulting in more intensive care being required. This care is costly and affects the well being of the individual and their family. Risks from a health care perspective are determined by the adherence to medical and nursing care, based on current evidence based practice (EBP) and this information is used to advise on how to manage the LTCs. However, risk management for an individual in relation to their life is more than a rational weighing up of objective technical information from EBP, for example the effects of smoking on lung function, but involves the person embedding the information into their own knowledge and life context (Clarke, 2009). Therefore, case finding based on risk alone is a service-led strategy that identifies people who are deemed to be expensive users of the health care service, rather than people identifying themselves as requiring case management. However, studies evaluating the perceptions of case management from the service user's perspective have highlighted general satisfaction with the service given, which gives some indication that, however the patient is identified, case management may still be perceived as beneficial (NPCRDC, 2005). The challenge within case management, therefore, is to try to marry up risk from a service perspective, to ensure better clinical outcomes and prevention of hospital admissions, with risk from an individual's perspective from within the context of their life.

Conclusion

This chapter has discussed the challenges to providing and evaluating a case management approach to people with LTCs. Despite there being inconclusive evidence relating to the effectiveness of case management and lack of clarity about case management components, the principle of case management is sound. People with ongoing health needs, such as LTCs, require continuous support and care, not reactive and episodic treatment. However, the debate still remains as to what this care and support should be, how it should be delivered, and the organisational structure required to best support this approach. It is important throughout this debate, as pressures increase on resources and targets, that we do not lose sight of the person living with an LTC, but try to find a balance between meeting the needs of the service and providing person-centred care.

References

Allen, J. & Fabri, A. (2005) An evaluation of a community aged care nurse practitioner service, *Clinical Nursing*, 14, pp. 1202–1209.

Billings, J., Dixon, D., Mijanovich, T. & Wennberg, D. (2006a) Case finding for patients at risk of readmission to hospital: development of algorithm to identify high risk patients, *British Medical Journal*, 333(7563), pp. 327–330. Available at: http://dx.doi.org/1136/bmj.38870.657917.AE.

Billings, J., Mijanovich, T., Dixon, J., Curry, N., Wennberg, D., Darin, B. & Steinort, K. (2006b) Case finding algorithms for patients at risk of rehospitalisation PARR1 and PARR2 Kings Fund, Health Diag Analytic Solutions and New York University for Health and Public Service Research.

Burns, T. & Santos, A. (1995) Assertive Community Treatment: an update of randomised trials, *Psychiatric Services*, 46, pp. 669–675.

Challis, D., Chessum, R., Chesterman, J., Luckett, R. & Traske, K. (1990) *Case Management in Health and Social Care*. Personal Social Services Research Unit, The University of Kent, Canterbury.

Challis, D. & Hughes, J. (2002) Frail old people at the margins of care: some recent research findings, *British Journal Psychiatry*, 180, pp. 126–130.

Clarke, C. (2009) Risk and long-term conditions: the contradictions of self in society, *Health, Risk and Society*, 11(4), pp. 297–302.

Cooper, B. & Yarmo Roberts, D. (2006) National case management standards in Australia – purpose, process and potential impact, *Australian Health Review*, 30, pp. 12–16.

Department of Health (2001) *National Service Framework for Older People*. Department of Health, London.

Department of Health (2002) *Reforming NHS Financial Flows: Introducing Payment by Results*. Department of Health, London.

Department of Health (2004) *Spending Review 2004 Public Service Agreement*. Department of Health, London.

Department of Health (2005a) *Supporting People With Long-Term Conditions: An NHS and Social Care Model to Support Local Innovation and Integration*. Department of Health, London.

Department of Health (2005b) *Self care – A real choice: Self care support – A practical option*. Department of Health, London.

Department of Health (2006) *Caring for People with Long-term Conditions: An Education Framework for Community Matrons and Case Managers*. Department of Health, London.

Department of Health (2009a) *Improving the Health and Well being of People with Long-term Conditions*. Department of Health, London.

Department of Health (2009b) *Whole Systems Demonstrators An Overview of Telecare and Telehealth*. Department of Health, London.

Evercare (2004) *Implementing the Evercare Programme*, Interim Report. Available at: www.natpact.info/cms/186.php.

Gravelle, H., Dusheiko, M., Sheaff, R. *et al.* (2006) Impact of case management (Evercare) on frail elderly patients: controlled before and after analysis of quantitative outcome data, *British Medical Journal*, Available at: http://dx.doi.org/10.1136/bmj.39020.413310.55.

HM Treasury (2007) *PSA Delivery Agreement 19: Ensure Better Care for All*. HM Stationery Office, London.

Hutt, R., Rosen, R. & McCauley, J. (2004) *Case-Managing Long-term Conditions: What Impact does It have in the Treatment of Older People?* King's Fund, London.

Intagliata, J. (1982) Improving the quality of community care for the chronically mentally disabled: the role of case management, *Schizophrenia Bulletin*, 8, pp. 655–674.

Ioannou, M. (2010) Virtual Reality, *Health Service Journal*, 15 July, p. 23.

Kane, R., Keckhafer, G., Flood, S., Bershadsky, B. & Siadaty, M. (2003) The effect of Evercare on hospital use, *Journal of the American Geriatrics Society*, 51, pp. 1427–1434.

Lyon, D., Miller, J. & Pine, K. (2006) The castlefields integrated care model: the evidence summarised, *Integrated Care*, 14(1), pp. 7–12.

Marshall, M., Gray, A., Lockwood, A. & Green, R. (1998) Case management for people with severe mental disorders, *Cochrane Database of Systematic Reviews*, Issue 2, Available at: http://dx.doi.org/10.1002/14651858.CD000050.

Mueser, K., Bond, G., Drake, R. & Resnick, S. (1998) Models of community care for severe mental illness, a review of research on case management, *Schizophrenia Bulletin*, 24, pp. 37–74.

Murphy, E. (2004) Case management and community matrons for long-term conditions, *British Medical Journal*, 329, pp. 1251–1252.

National Primary Care Research and Development Centre (NPCRDC) (2005) *Evercare Evaluation Interim Report: Implications for Supporting People With Long-Term Conditions*. Available at: http://www.natpact.nhs.uk/uploads/2005_Feb/Evercare_evaluation_interim_report.pdf last accessed 30/5/10

NHS Centre for Reviews and Dissemination (2001) *CRD Report 21 – Scoping Review of the Effectiveness of Mental Health Services (Executive Summary)*, University of York, York.

Robinson, P. (2008) *Reducing Avoidable Emergency Admissions*. Croydon PCT. Available at: http://www.productivity.nhs.uk/caseStudies.aspx last accessed 26/6/10.

Roland, M., Dusheiko, M., Gravelle, H. & Parker, S. (2005) Follow up of people aged 65 and over with a history of emergency admissions: analysis of routine admission data, *British Medical Journal*, 330, pp. 289–292.

Sargent, P., Pickard, S., Sheaff, R. & Boaden, R. (2007) Patient and carer perceptions of case management for long-term conditions, *Health and Social Care in the Community*, 15(6), pp. 511–519.

Sargent, P., Boaden, R. & Roland, M. (2008) How many patients can community matrons successfully case manage? *Nursing management*, 16, pp. 38–46.

Simpson, A., Miller, C. & Bowers, L. (2003) Case management models and the care programme approach: how to make the CPA effective and credible, *Journal of Psychiatric and Mental Health Nursing*, 10, pp. 472–483.

Wanless, D. (2004) *Securing Good Health for the Whole Population*. Final Report. HM Treasury, The Stationery Office, London.

Wanless, D. (2007) *Our Future Health Secured?* Kings Fund, London.

Williams, A. & Cooper, B. (2008) Determining caseloads in the community care of frail older people with chronic illness, *Nursing and Healthcare of Chronic Illness in association with Journal of Clinical Nursing*, 17 (5a), pp. 60–66.

World Health Organisation (2002) *The World Health Report 2002: Reducing Risks, Promoting Healthy Life*. World Health Organisation, Geneva. Available at: www.who.int/whr/2002/en/.

Ziguras, S. & Stuart, G. (2000) A meta-analysis of the effectiveness of mental health case management over 20 years, *Psychiatric Services*, 51, pp. 1410–1421.

Chapter 3

Changing approaches to the management of long-term conditions

Kerri Wright

School of Health and Social Care, University of Greenwich, Eltham, London, UK

Introduction

The approach to managing people with long-term conditions (LTCs) is changing. The increasing population of older adults, advances in medicine which prolong life and the increase in conditions which are long term and incurable have led to a large population of people in the United Kingdom living with an LTC and predictions that this is likely to increase (Department of Health, 2009). These changes to the demographic and illness patterns of people living in the United Kingdom are discussed in more detail in Chapter 1. They highlight that the current approaches to managing people with LTCs are untenable in view of finite health care resources (Wanless, 2004) and point to the urgent need for a changing approach to people living with an LTC. This chapter briefly critiques the current medical approach to illness and how this approach alone is ineffective for people with LTCs.

A critique of the medical model

Within modern medicine, the focus on physical aspects of health is still paramount and minimises the emotional and spiritual components of health which were once given equal credence. The exclusive role of physical health has developed in part through both the mind–body divide and the growth of science in medicine. The idea of humans having a separate mind and body was first proposed by Descartes in 1641. This mind–body divide, or Cartesian dualism as it is also known, is important as it sparked the beginning of a focus on the physical body, which has become embedded in the practice of medicine and still pervades today. Descartes proposed that humans were divided into two parts: the mind or soul which he described as a 'thing that thinks' and the body (Rozemond, 2002). The body is distinguished by the fact that it occupies space and is, therefore, observable and measurable. For example, temperature can be measured to identify an infection. In contrast, although subjective experiences can be noted and behaviours observed, these cannot be easily measured. With traditional medicine, it is possible to carry out baseline observations, carry out treatment and then repeat the measurement in order to show that

Long-Term Conditions: Nursing Care and Management, First Edition. Edited by Liz Meerabeau and Kerri Wright.
© 2011 Blackwell Publishing Ltd. Published 2011 by Blackwell Publishing Ltd.

the treatment has made a change to the person and their health has improved. The effect of the treatment is tangible. However, when considering the effect of someone's mind or soul on health, this cannot be measured. Although behaviours can be observed, the mental processes and effect that these have on health cannot be proved. The absence of observable mental processes and emotions arguably has led to the importance of these being minimised within health, a view that has continued with the move towards a scientific culture in health care.

The scientific revolution of the nineteenth century resulted in more value being given to science and measurable interventions. The dominance of science led to the positivist approach to evaluation of treatments where scientific evidence, based on objective and measurable information, became increasingly important, although the scientific method became fully developed only in the mid-twentieth century. This scientific preeminence was further enhanced by government policy which stipulated that medicine and health care should be based on sound evidence to ensure that evidence-based medicine or care was always given to patients (Department of Health, 1997). The scientific approach to medicine and care fits well into the medical model of health. The medical approach is successful at managing many diseases and illnesses and can be credited with the reduction of mortality and morbidity in many areas, for example infectious diseases through antibiotics and vaccinations. However, a difficulty with this approach becomes apparent when medicine cannot identify a tangible cause to the ill health or the symptoms someone is experiencing, or when the cause is known but no medical treatment is available.

Society, one can argue, depends on medicine to sanction illness and legitimise exemptions from life's roles. An illness for which the medical profession can find no physical cause or no measurable physical symptoms to support the person's subjective experience can result in the doctor professing that the person does not have an illness. Without this medical sanction, an individual is unable to, for example, be legitimately sick from work or claim benefits. In addition, without medical sanction it is difficult for the individual to legitimately enter into the 'sick role' and be exempt from other personal roles such as parenting (Parsons, 1951). The 'sick role' is discussed more in Chapter 4. The difficulty in requiring medical sanction to legitimise subjective experiences of ill health is highlighted by conditions such as myalgic encephalopathy (ME) (also known as chronic fatigue syndrome (CFS)). Initially, this condition was not acknowledged by the medical profession and many people were left frustrated and struggling to manage their lives having been told that there was nothing wrong with them (Working Group on CFS/ME, 2007) (see Box 3.1). Although there are still doubts about this condition due to the absence of observable and measurable physical signs and identified causes, ME is generally now recognised as a condition by the medical profession (defined as a disease in 1988) and the person accepted as legitimately 'ill' by society.

Box 3.1 Experiences of Rose Perkins (pseudonym) (Savage 2007).

'I was diagnosed with ME when I was 14, after every other possible condition was ruled out. I had doctors telling me to go to school because I didn't have a temperature. They would look at me like I was faking the symptoms to get a day off school. But I was lucky enough to have one doctor who knew what she was doing. She got me an appointment with the local paediatric doctor because I had been back every two weeks during a six-month period. . . .

Someone with ME can be feeling like they have been hit by a truck and yet it doesn't show, because you look completely normal; you don't have a sign over your head saying: "Girl with ME". Maybe that's a curse not to have our illness defined in a certain physical way, such as cancer patients who undergo chemotherapy.'

The increasing dominance of medicine and the use of the medical model in western society was highlighted by Ivan Illich (1975) who wrote critically about the medicalisation of society and argued that medicine had taken over many of life's natural events such as birth, death, ill health and ageing. Illich felt that the involvement of medicine at these times reduced our ability to cope with and manage these natural events and created a dependence on the medical profession. For example, in the early twentieth century, people would commonly die at home, cared for by their family. This was viewed as a normal part of the life cycle and accepted. Today most people die in hospitals, under the care of the medical profession. Their families are removed from the responsibility of caring and look to the medical profession to direct and inform them about their loved one's progress and plans (Gomes and Higginson, 2008). Not all medicalisation has been negative, and it cannot be disputed that the advances in medicine have been beneficial in curing and treating more diseases and conditions, allowing people to die in comfort through advances in pharmacology and medical interventions, and reducing the child mortality rate significantly. However, what Illich highlights is important in raising awareness of the medical perspective in shaping our beliefs and the danger of becoming reliant on this to explain everyday life experiences.

This dependency can encourage people to seek medical help for everyday ailments which are a normal part of life; for example, an active child who dislikes sitting for long periods, who would in the past be managed independently without medical intervention, today may be labelled as having 'attention deficit hyperactivity disorder (ADHD)'. In addition, the overreliance on medicine, and demands for medicine to explain experiences of ill health, have arguably led to an increase in people being 'labelled' with conditions and illnesses which render them 'life-long patients' (Illich, 1975). This can also lead to exclusion and stigma for those people who have been given a medical label as being 'ill' and has led to many groups actively fighting against this medicalisation of their lives (see Chapter 4).

For some conditions where there is no medical 'cure', the dependence on medicine and the wait for a medical 'breakthrough' can be detrimental. This overreliance on medicine can create a culture where ill health is viewed as the domain of doctors, and therefore, better health can only be achieved by following medical treatment and advice. This leads to an overreliance on medical care to improve a person's health and can prevent the person actively taking on responsibility for managing their condition and improving their health. The medical approach seeks an organic cause for the experience of ill health and prescribes treatments that aim to remove or control this cause to provide better health for the individual. The attempts to address the physical causes of the ill health can sometimes occur to the detriment of the individual's quality of life. Many medicines have side effects which for some people can be experienced as more problematic than the illness itself, for example anti-depressants.

Illich (1975) first coined the phrase 'clinical iatrogenesis' to describe the illness created by medicine in its attempts to cure and manage conditions. A further example of this is the management of advanced cancer with chemotherapy and radiotherapy which causes prolonged episodes of ill health as a result of the body's reaction to the treatment rather than the cancer itself. Generally, people accept short-term illness and discomfort if they know that their long-term health or life chances will be improved. However, the focus on organic causes to explain ill health can lead to extreme attempts to achieve 'cure', in particular historically in mental health through practices such as ECT. Such focus on organic causes to explain and find treatments for ill health can result in health care losing sight of other potential and sometimes coexisting causes of conditions and more appropriate approaches to treatment.

The search for an organic cause to explain an illness can lead to reliance on medical treatment alone to alleviate it and potentially prevent people from learning to manage and adjust to life with the illness. The management of depression is an example of this difficulty. Depression is viewed by many medical doctors as resulting from a chemical imbalance in the brain, and the treatment prescribed is generally anti-depressants to alter the balance of chemicals. This can lead to the expectation that depression can be cured by taking the medicine alone and reliance on the medicine to alleviate the illness rather than the individual believing that their individual actions can also have an effect. Current evidence demonstrates that depression can be more effectively managed by the use of 'talking therapies' than anti-depressants and that individuals can contribute greatly to improving their depression through activities such as exercise (NICE, 2009). The approach to the management of depression now advocated by most medical doctors supports the subjective experiences and accounts of many people who have experienced depression, but were not previously acknowledged by medical doctors (NICE, 2009).

The medical management of illness based on objective and scientific principles can also deny the subjective experiences of people who have found alternative and more effective ways to improve their health. Evidence-based medicine is based on scientific experiments that prove with a degree of certainty the effectiveness of particular treatments to alleviate ill health or symptoms. The experiments do not show that every person who undertakes that treatment will improve. They only demonstrate that there is a high probability that the treatment will work. Therefore, it can be said that evidence-based medicine deals with populations, but clinicians need to deal with individuals (O'Donnell, 2000). In addition, most medications have side effects, and these may prevent some people from continuing this treatment, for example the use of the cholesterol-lowering drugs statins (Hope, 2009). The limitations of the medical management of some illnesses and conditions and the rejection of medical treatments have led to some individuals taking more responsibility for their condition and seeking alternative ways to manage and improve their health. These alternative treatments and management, although found to be effective by individuals, were originally met with scepticism by the medical profession as they were based on subjective experiences rather than sound scientific evidence. The use of complementary therapies such as acupuncture, reiki and reflexology to alleviate symptoms of ill health have been the subject of much derision from the medical profession over recent years and are evidence of the preference for scientific treatments.

The limitations of the medical profession in managing certain conditions and the increase in finding alternative treatments led to the development of self-help groups, which allow members to share experiences of their condition and strategies that worked for them, and offer support and encouragement to others who have similar conditions. They also offer a powerful collective voice and can advocate for better quality health services specific to the needs of the condition. An example of a self-help group is the Sickle Cell Society which supports people living with sickle cell disease, informs health care professionals, undertakes research and informs national policy on the management of sickle cell disease (Sickle Cell Society, 2008, 2009). In addition, self-help groups also provide opportunities for people to begin to adjust to and accept conditions that are lifelong and start to find ways to live their life with the condition. However, concerns have been expressed that the focus on self-management as a new concept ignores the experiences built up over many years; it is argued that self-management as a core feature of LTC management needs to build more on self-help groups (Kendall and Rogers, 2007).

Medicine does, however, have a vital role in managing ill health. Some illnesses are purely biological in origin, for example bacterial infections. The most effective way of treating illnesses with a clear biological origin is by treating the biological cause, in this example with antibiotics. Likewise, some conditions cause symptoms as a result of the alteration of biological processes in the body, and again, the most effective method of treating these can be medicine, for example asthma and the use of inhalers to alleviate the tightening of the airways and improve breathing. However, as already discussed, there can be difficulties if medicine is relied on to alleviate and explain every imperfection we experience in life, from sadness and loneliness to ageing and dying. Medicine cannot solve these problems (Smith, 2002). All that results is a medicalisation of life which leads to responsibility for our health being devolved to medicine, an increase in the population who are labelled as unwell and an increase in treatments aimed at 'cure' which can divert people away from finding better ways to adjust and manage their ill health (Illich, 1975; Kleinman, 1988). Therefore, the biological approach to health is effective in some cases, but needs to be balanced with an approach which embraces the whole individual and their subjective experience of health and be open to the possibility that medicine is not always the right approach.

The necessity of a new approach to health has been brought about by the increasing population of people with LTCs, which by nature of the definitions are conditions which are lifelong and cannot be cured. The medical approach to LTCs has been to prescribe medical treatments that 'cure' the presenting symptoms (Kleinman, 1988). This can be successful when conditions are more biological in nature such as diabetes or asthma and can lead to many people managing their lives successfully through minimal adjustment and use of medicine to control the condition, for example controlling blood glucose levels or keeping airways open. For other conditions where the symptoms are more difficult to manage, such as fatigue or deformity of joints, the medical approach is less successful. However, even in conditions where medical treatment is effective in managing the condition, the actual symptom still has not been 'cured'. An individual with well-controlled type 1 diabetes through twice-daily insulin injections and careful monitoring of dietary intake still has diabetes. The high blood glucose levels, the 'symptom' of diabetes, are controlled, but only as a result of the person making adjustments to their life and managing the condition as part of that. If the insulin were not taken, then the symptom of high blood glucose levels would come back. The person will always have diabetes and will always be a patient requiring health care. This has implications for health care resources and the finite nature of these. With more of the population being diagnosed with lifelong conditions and relying on medical care, the medical approach alone is unsustainable.

The biological approach also does not take into account the impact that an LTC has on an individual's whole life. The biological management of a symptom, such as insulin injections, cannot take place in isolation. The injections and dietary management pervade all aspects of the person's life, from the practicalities of achieving this to the psychological and social adjustments necessary to manage the condition, for example exclusion from social drinking or the cultural stigma of being 'ill'. People are also individuals and construct their own meaning and reality in which to live their lives (Kleinman, 1988).

The biopsychosocial model

The new approach to the management of LTCs needs to include the biological, psychological and sociological impact of the condition on individuals' lives; this is known as the biopsychosocial model (Engel, 1980). We also need to start with the person's experience of living with the condition and use this to determine, in collaboration with the person, what problems the person is facing and how best to manage these. For example, a person living with arthritis may say that their inability to reach the toilet in time and subsequent incontinence is the most difficult thing for them to accept and manage. An agreed gentle exercise regime to increase joint mobility, referral to the continence service for advice and a review of analgesics to reduce pain on mobility could be an agreed plan of action to resolve this issue. The management of the individual takes a biological, psychological and social approach to the condition of arthritis through appreciating the biological effect of the arthritis on the person's joints which causes pain and loss of mobility, the psychological effect of embarrassment and distress of incontinence, and the social impact this could have on social events and possible isolation. Although the action may have been planned by a doctor or nurse generally for someone with arthritis, the difference with this plan is that it stems from the individual and is based on alleviating a symptom of the condition that is meaningful for them in the context of their lives (Kleinman, 1988; Wasson *et al.*, 2008).

Therefore, the way a person views and ultimately manages to live with an LTC is dependent on how the condition relates to the meaning and purpose they derive from their life (Kralik *et al.*, 2004; Whittemore and Dixon, 2007). For example, an LTC that affects the fine motor control of an individual who is a pianist may have a greater impact than the same symptom for someone who is a counsellor. In the same way, the medical management offered for a symptom of an LTC may be declined due to the effect the treatment has on an aspect of the person's life. Management of LTCs is not just about the medical 'curing' of symptoms, but of appreciating and understanding the meaning of the LTC and any symptoms for the individual and their lives (Kralik *et al.*, 2004).

Therefore, applying the biopsychosocial model and ensuring that management is person centred requires a change to the way that health care professionals have been managing patients. Previously, management of ill health was directed by health care professionals, and patients were 'passive recipients' of this care. This approach still pervades health care as the medical model continues to dominate (Wilson *et al.*, 2006, 2007). However, there has been an increasing acknowledgement that the medical or biological approach, in particular to LTCs, is no longer always effective, and the realisation that other approaches to managing conditions could be more effective (Department of Health, 2008, 2010). This has led to support for people to have a more active role in the management of their care and for their expertise in managing their conditions to be recognised. Thus, the health care professional's role in LTCs has moved from being a director of care and manager of the person's medical condition to someone who supports and facilitates a person to manage their lives with this condition (Department of Health, 2006). This is discussed in more depth in Chapter 8.

However, there have been some initial difficulties with embracing a new approach to the management of LTCs. Firstly, some nurses feel threatened by the expertise of some patients and find it difficult to adapt to a new way of working (Wilson *et al.*, 2006) and a much more proactive patient (see Box 3.2). Secondly, the new approaches require new skills and knowledge to facilitate and support people with LTCs. Psychosocial aspects of this management are not always valued as highly as biological aspects and have led to the recommendation that nurses need to be trained in the importance and use of psychosocial skills (MacDonald *et al.*, 2008; Wilson *et al.*, 2006). Thirdly, a person-centred approach can lead to conflicts between evidence-based practice and individual management, for example accepting that a person does not want to take medication to reduce the risk of developing a future condition and would rather live with this risk (Wilson *et al.*, 2006). In addition, individual management requires health care professionals to be more flexible and to help the person to find a balance between the necessities of some treatments and the negative effect they could have on their life. The chapters on diabetes and heart failure in particular highlight how medicine regimes do not need to be rigid and can be adjusted to fit with individual requirements. Acknowledging and addressing these areas of concern will be a challenge for health care professionals and education providers.

Box 3.2   An account of a community nurse's visit to an 'expert patient' requiring wound care.

'George is a 64-year-old gentleman who presented with an open wound to the top of his foot. Referred to the district nursing service by podiatrist at local hospital. George is an insulin-controlled diabetic and has been totally self-caring for many years. George is totally concordant with diet and medication. . . . On further questioning regarding past medical history, it became apparent George had an enormous amount of knowledge of diabetes. When asked about his methods of blood glucose monitoring, George produced computer-generated tables, graphs and pie charts to show how they compare for set times of the months. He even had a charted result sheet whereby he averaged his blood glucose results on a monthly basis . . . . he gave me a folder to browse through.

Every month for the last 2 years all charts and figures as referred to previously, all filed in date order also included action taken each month, that is, changes to medication, insulin doses, why, when, visits, attendance at clinics. . . . I asked for permission to photograph George's foot the following day . . . I returned the next day camera in hand. I didn't need it. George provided me with a set of photographs of his foot taken from every conceivable angle, all reproduced on computer. . . . During the course of time that George was our patient, he educated himself about wound care and the healing process, and continued to photograph his wound at regular intervals to keep a photographic profile to be used by the hospital staff and us. In my opinion, George is the textbook expert patient. His knowledge of his illness and in particular diabetes is exceptional. He has actually now become an expert patient teacher, teaching fellow patients and passing on his own personal knowledge and skills' (Wright, 2005: 114).

Conclusion

As discussed in Chapter 1, there has been a shift in the way that ill health is managed in the western world. This shift is in part a result of the increase in the population living with LTCs and the finite health care resources available to meet this current and future need, and a growing realisation that the mind–body split and the focus on biological aspects of health are no longer totally effective. This has led to a changing approach to the way that health care is managed. These changes include the following: the acknowledgement of the effect LTCs can have on all aspects of a person's life and the necessity of a biopsychosocial approach to LTC management; the acknowledgement of the expertise that people living with an LTC have; and the focus on health care professionals to help facilitate people to self-manage their conditions. These changes hope to reduce the impact of LTCs on health care resources and allow people with LTCs to effectively manage their life with the condition.

References

Department of Health (1997) *The New NHS: Modern, Dependable*. Department of Health, London.
Department of Health (2006) *Our Health, Our Care, Our Say*. Department of Health, London.
Department of Health (2008) *Your Health, Your Way—A Guide to Long-Term Conditions and Self Care*. Department of Health, London.
Department of Health (2009) *Improving the Health and Well-being of People with Long-Term Conditions*. Department of Health, London.
Department of Health (2010) *Improving the Health and Well-being of People with Long-Term Conditions. World Class Services for People with Long-Term Conditions: Information Tool for Commissioners*. Department of Health, London.
Engel, G. (1980) The clinical application of the biopsychosocial model, *American Journal of Psychiatry*, 137, pp. 535–544.
Gomes, B. & Higginson, I. (2008) Where people die (1974–2030): past trends, future projections and implications for care, *Palliative Medicine*, 22, pp. 33–41.

Illich, I. (1975) *Medical Nemesis, the Expropriation of Health*. Calder and Boyars, London.

Hope, J. (2009) Side effects alert for all statin users as drug is linked to depression and memory loss. *Daily Mail*. Available at: http://www.dailymail.co.uk/health/article-1226238/Side-effects-alert-statin-users-drug-linked-depression-memory-loss.html (accessed on 24 March 2010).

Kendall, E. & Rogers, A. (2007) Extinguishing the social? State sponsored self-care policy and the chronic disease self-management programme, *Disability and Society*, 22(2), pp. 129–143.

Kleinman, A. (1988) *The Illness Narratives Suffering, Healing and the Human Condition*. Basic Books, New York.

Kralik, D., Koch, T., Price, K. & Howard, N. (2004) Chronic illness self management: taking action to create order, *Journal of Clinical Nursing*, 13, pp. 259–267.

MacDonald, W., Rogers, A., Blakeman, T. & Bower, P. (2008) Practice nurses and the facilitation of self management in primary care, *Journal of Advanced Nursing*, 62(2), pp. 191–199.

National Institute for Health and Clinical Excellence (NICE) (2009) *Depression in Adults (update). Depression: The Treatment and Management of Depression in Adults*. National Clinical Practice Guideline, 90, NICE.

Parsons, T. (1951) *The Social System*. Routledge and Kegan Paul, London.

O'Donnell, M. (2000) Evidence-based illiteracy: time to rescue "the literature", *Lancet*, 355, pp. 489–491.

Rozemond, M. (2002) *Descartes' Dualism*. Harvard University Press, Cambridge.

Savage, C. (2007) Surviving ME, *Guardian*. Available at: http://www.guardian.co.uk/lifeandstyle/2007/sep/18/health-and-wellbeing (accessed on 27 June 2010).

Sickle Cell Society (2008) *Standards for the Clinical Care of Adults with Sickle Cell Disease in the UK*. Sickle Cell Society, London.

Sickle Cell Society (2009) *History of the Sickle Cell Society*. Available at: http://www.sicklecellsociety.org/history.html (accessed on 25 March 2010).

Smith, R. (2002) Spend (slightly) less on health and more on the arts. Health would probably be improved. *British Medical Journal*, 325, pp. 1432–1433.

Wanless, D. (2004) *Securing Good Health for the Whole Population: Final Report*. Department of Health, London.

Wasson, J., Johnson, B. & Mackenzie, T. (2008) The impact of primary care patients' pain and emotional problems on their confidence with self management, *Journal of Ambulatory Care Management*, 31(2), pp. 120–127.

Whittemore, R. & Dixon, J. (2008) Chronic illness: the process of integration. *Journal of Nursing and Healthcare of Chronic Illness* in association with *Journal of Clinical Nursing*, 17(7b), pp.177–187.

Wilson, P., Kendall, S. & Brooks, F. (2006) Nurses' responses to expert patients: the rhetoric and reality of self-management in long-term conditions: a grounded theory study. *International Journal of Nursing Studies*, 43, pp. 803–818.

Wilson, P., Kendall, S. & Brooks, F. (2007) The expert patient programme: a paradox of patient empowerment and medical dominance, *Health and Social Care in the Community*, 15(5), pp. 426–438.

Working group on CFS/ME (2007) *A Report of the CFS/ME Working Group*. Department of Health, London.

Wright, K. (2005) Impact of a course on community nurses' practice: an evaluation, *British Journal of Community Nursing*. 10(3), pp. 110–117.

Chapter 4

Sociological insights

Liz Meerabeau

School of Health and Social Care, University of Greenwich, Eltham, London, UK

Introduction

The aim of this chapter is to provide sociological concepts which can help practitioners to gain wider insights into the experiences of their patients with long-term conditions (LTCs), and also personal accounts from the literature which augment those provided elsewhere in this book. This chapter discusses the sociological literature on the doctor–patient relationship, deviance and stigma, help seeking, illness as biographical disruption and consumerism in health care, relating these topics to the care of people with LTCs.

The doctor–patient relationship

The sick role

In the current policy climate, in which the concept of the expert patient is promoted, it is salutary to look back over 60 years to see how thinking on the doctor–patient relationship has evolved. This may also remind us that for many patients there is still a gulf of knowledge and understanding between them and health professionals, and that if a whole systems approach is to be implemented, many changes in the organisation of care are still required (Rogers *et al.,* 2005).

In his work *The Social System,* Parsons (1951) examined the complementary roles of doctor and patient, and between 1951 and 1958 developed the concept of the sick role. He was a functionalist and, therefore, interested in how systems in society generally work to prevent conflict and to maintain social order; the obligations of the sick role helped to prevent the social problem of people evading other obligations such as work. He was also writing at a time in the United States when there was a (short-lived) shift to a 'collectivity orientation', replacing the 'business ethic', and a rise in the importance of the professions. Gerhardt (1987) states that Parsons considered health to be the most important issue in a democratic social structure.

Long-Term Conditions: Nursing Care and Management, First Edition. Edited by Liz Meerabeau and Kerri Wright.
© 2011 Blackwell Publishing Ltd. Published 2011 by Blackwell Publishing Ltd.

'Certainly by almost any definition health is included in the functional needs of the individual member of the society so that from the point of view of the functioning of the social system, too low a general level of health, too high an incidence of illness, is dysfunctional.'

(Parsons, 1951: 430)

Parsons (1964) also recognised that patterns of illness were changing, from a predominance of infectious diseases to illnesses with a more psychosomatic element (he was, unusually for a sociologist, a trained psychoanalyst). Urbanism, industrialisation and the growth of technology were increasing the demands on individuals, which in Parsons' view accentuated the motivation to retreat into ill health. This would remove them from the workforce and be dysfunctional for society.

In Parsons' model, sick people have certain rights and obligations; failure to comply with the latter may result in the loss of the former. These rights and obligations were:

- Exemption from everyday responsibilities.
- Not being held responsible for their illness.
- An expectation that they will not find illness rewarding and will be motivated to get better.
- An expectation that they will seek medical help and will comply with advice and treatment.

Parsons also identified (although less clearly) a corresponding medical role, with privileges and obligations. Since doctors have intimate access both to the body and to private information, Parsons considered that the patient needed to be protected from exploitation. Safeguards included the doctor's formal education, professional detachment, professional standards and self-regulation, and the ethical obligation to act in the patient's best interests.

Parsons was criticised by other sociologists who, in Gerhardt's (1987) view, largely misinterpreted him. In particular, he was criticised for having failed to grasp the complexities of social interaction, the potential conflict of interest between doctor and patient, and the great variety both in medical practice and in illness behaviour (Strong and Davis, 1977). There was also considerable debate as to whether the sick role could be applied to the situation of chronic illness; Parsons (1978) conceded that its application might be limited, but using the example of his own diabetes, he argued that it was still applicable, since the diabetes did not exempt him from the demands of life and there was an obligation to prevent the diabetes worsening by adherence to medical treatment.

Conflict theorists

Whereas Parsons' work promulgated a consensus model of the doctor–patient relationship, during the 1960s and 1970s, sociologists began to be more critical of medicine, a reflection of the general questioning of authority in that time period. Bury (1997: 77) questions the very term doctor–patient relationship, suspecting that it probably arose within medicine, from doctors' claim that they had a special place within the health care system. 'Put this way, the term seems more ideological than descriptive, rendering clinical judgement and medical claims over the patient benign, and conveying a "medico-centric" image of trust and public acceptability.' There were several strands to this critique of medicine. McKeown (1976) used epidemiological evidence to argue that medicine had played only a small part in reducing mortality from infectious diseases, with a greater role played by improved living conditions and nutrition. Illich (1975) argued vociferously that medicine disempowered and deskilled people by taking over problems which they could manage themselves.

Freidson (1970), writing about the US system of care, argued that medicine was not only financially dominant but it also dominated other related occupations, such as nursing. Freidson's major point was that medicine not only controlled the treatment of illness but also its definition, and that doctors could, therefore, exercise social control. This critique was particularly powerful in relation to the definition of mental illness; Scheff (1966) argued that the doctor inadvertently applied a lifelong stigmatising label to the patient, spoiling his or her identity and life chances, although his argument was overstated (Gove, 1970). Stimson (1976) identified that doctors did not show 'affective neutrality', as Parsons' concept of the sick role had stated. Behind the scenes they were clear on which patients they disliked; women, particularly those with children, and patients presenting with emotional problems. Bloor and Horobin (1975) argued that doctors, particularly GPs, had contradictory, and therefore unfair, expectations of their patients, since they expected them to have sufficient knowledge to know when to consult, but then ignored patients' views within the consultation.

Marxists such as Waitzkin (1979) made links between the doctor–patient relationship and the wider structures of capitalist society, in particular examining the way in which the deleterious effects of poverty and occupational illnesses were ignored in the medical encounter, and patients were rendered 'mute' in challenging the oppressive conditions in which they lived. This line of argument did not become popular in the United Kingdom, although an analogous line of argument was used by feminist writers to examine the relationship between the medical encounter and the dominant assumptions of patriarchal society (e.g. Oakley, 1980).

The negotiation model

This model overlaps with the conflict model, since negotiation presupposes an existing potential degree of conflict. The model recognises that the relationship may shift over time and will be affected by the social characteristics of both doctor and patient (for example, it is possible that the 'feminisation' of medicine in the United Kingdom has altered the general tone of consultations). In the 1970s, there was also a growing body of research drawing on interactionism, which examined the exchanges between doctors and patients, including the covert ways in which patients may be critical of their doctors (e.g. Stimson and Webb, 1975). Stimson and Webb found that patients may rehearse what they intend to say, and think carefully how to present a problem, in order to try to achieve their desired outcome, although time pressures create constraints on the consultation. On many occasions, patients discussed the consultation afterwards in their own social network, and recounted 'atrocity stories' which belittled or made fun of the doctor. Patients might be satisfied with part of the consultation, but not the rest; there was no simple relationship with patient expectations, which were often reconstituted in the discussion after the event.

In a later study, Tuckett *et al.* (1985) found less negotiation; doctors explained issues, but showed little interest in patients' views.

Bury (1997) points out that much of the discussion of the doctor–patient relationship has not been set in its social context, which is changing, and that we can expect evolution to a contractual model in which the expectations of both parties are clearer. Dingwall *et al.* (1991) argue that in a formal contractual relationship, doctors are likely to be more careful, although poor and chronically ill patients are unlikely to be able to realise the benefits of a contract. The context for changes in medical care includes the following: the shift in illness patterns, requiring the long-term management of illness; the growing expertise of patients; the fact that many treatments now require active patient cooperation; and the growing importance of self-help groups. Bury (1997) also points out that patients may actively seek 'medicalisation', or the application of a medical label, partly because it may give access to benefits such as compensation (Arksey, 1994).

Role theory

The functionalist sociology exemplified by Parsons used the concept of social roles. This concept derives from the theatre, where there is generally a script, and it has been used extensively in anthropology to capture the 'multiplex relationships held to exist in primitive societies' (Strong and Davis, 1977: 796). In the 1960s, role theory occupied a central position in social theory, but it has now almost disappeared; in Strong and Davis's view, this was because it served as bridge between social interaction and social structure, but as views on both of these elements shifted, the 'bridge' collapsed. In these authors' view, the balance then shifted too far towards an emphasis on negotiation between doctor and patient, without recognising the context in which that occurred, and the constraints that context imposed. Strong and Davis proposed the concept of role format, derived from Goffman (1961, 1968a), which is less rigid than the concept of role, but provides a structure built from the expectations of both parties. Strong and Davis (1977) also use Goffman's term 'the ceremonial order', based on a working consensus between the partners on the nature of social reality, for present purposes. Norms are generated by a particular balance of resources; where this balance exists over a wide range of encounters, behaviour becomes routinised as role formats, so avoiding uncertainty and the need for negotiation. One such role format may be the portrayal of deference to the doctor, whatever the private feelings of the patient, as Stimson and Webb found in their research.

Strong (1979) used both the ceremonial order and role formats in his work on Scottish paediatric clinics. The dominant format in these clinics was what Strong termed the bureaucratic format, in which all parents were assumed to be well motivated, parents rarely voiced direct criticism, doctors were treated as virtually interchangeable and there was what Strong termed a 'general air of gentility' or politeness. There was little opportunity for parents to express their view or feelings, even though some were likely to be distressed by their child's disabilities. Silverman (1987) confirms Strong's findings in a wide variety of paediatric clinics and refers to the 'inescapable asymmetry' of the doctor–patient relationship; my study of infertility clinics in the mid 1980s (Meerabeau, 1998) identified similar constraints such as the inhibiting effect of long clinic waits, as does a much more recent study by Rogers *et al.* (2005) of attempts to introduce patient-centred care for patients with irritable bowel disease.

Seeking help

Many long-term illnesses begin with symptoms which are fairly non-specific, and the illness may not be diagnosed for some time. Most people experience quite frequently symptoms (such as a headache) which could be interpreted as being due to illness, yet only a small proportion seek medical help. Zola (1973) proposed that seeking medical help generally requires a prompt, or trigger. His study identified five types of triggers (although since it concerned patients who consulted, it could not account for those who did not seek medical help):

- An interpersonal crisis calling attention to the symptom.
- Perceived interference with social life.
- Sanctioning of the intention to consult by another person.
- Perceived interference with work or physical activity.
- Deciding that the problem had gone on for too long.

Freidson (1970) argues that whether a person decides to seek medical help depends firstly on whether he or she recognises symptoms of illness, and secondly on his or her culture and social network. If the person comes from a similar culture to that of the practitioner and has a truncated referral system, then he or she is likely to either self-treat or go directly to the doctor; if he or she comes from a similar culture and has an extended referral system, it is likely to encourage referral. If the professional service is not only foreign to the person's culture but also seen as stigmatising (for example psychiatric services), it may only be sought if the person is fairly independent from his or her network. The research evidence for this argument is mixed, and it is likely that the process varies depending on factors such as the particular problem.

Nettleton and Hanlon (2006) review Zola's work in the light of the development of e-health information (studied by Nettleton *et al.*) and also NHS Direct (studied by Hanlon *et al.*). They conclude that these technologies modify and enhance, rather than replace, the previous social processes of help seeking. Nevertheless, the cultural assumptions, norms and values of the sick role remain; callers to NHS Direct were keen to present themselves as rational and deserving of care. The new technologies have increased men's participation in health care, although not by a great extent, and as previously they often had to be cajoled into consulting by women family members. Furthermore, although some social commentators have portrayed internet access to information as a means to engage with doctors on more equal terms, in these studies, the Internet was used mainly to supplement and enhance consultations, for example by seeking further information afterwards. Lastly, people managed their information seeking, concentrating on information they needed rather than dwelling on future complications, and were also careful to seek out trustworthy forms of information.

The relatively slow shift of cultural norms is also demonstrated in Arksey and Sloper's (1999) study of disputed diagnoses, using the examples of repetitive strain injury and childhood cancer. They conclude: 'While the exercise of rigorous diagnostic standards is an important element of clinical practice, this should not be at the expense of denying patients' perceptions' (Arksey and Sloper, 1999: 495).

Deviance and stigma

Deviance was an important concept in sociology in the 1960s (Freidson, 1972); although it has since dropped from fashion in mainstream sociology, it is useful for exploring disability and chronic illness. In the 1960s, many sociologists saw themselves as part of the counter-culture; although this movement became generally discredited by a turn towards neo-conservatism in the 1980s, it can be argued that the refusal by many disadvantaged or disabled people to accept society's definition of their situation originated in the 1960s and is gradually gaining momentum. Becker (1963), one of the leading writers on the sociology of deviance, argued that deviance was not a quality of the act the person committed (or of the person), but rather a consequence of the application of rules and sanctions by others. There is a distinction between primary deviance, the initial act or aspect of difference, and its subsequent labelling as secondary deviance, as a consequence of which the person may become increasingly separated from the rest of society. An example from the earlier part of the twentieth century would be people who were admitted to psychiatric asylums for minor misdemeanours or pregnancy outside marriage, who then became institutionalised.

Therefore, deviant behaviour is not inherently deviant, but has been given that label by other people. Thus, it may sometimes be possible to reject these rules and labels. For example, in the first half of the twentieth century homosexuality was defined as a mental illness, but that label, and the stigma of homosexuality, are being gradually overthrown by movements such as Gay Pride (see Box 4.1).

Box 4.1   Rejecting the label of deviance.

Up until 1967 homosexuality was recognised as a mental health disorder and listed as a disease on the Diagnostic and Statistical Manual of Mental Disorders (DSM). People who were sexually attracted to the same sex could be diagnosed as mentally unwell and treated to 'cure' this disease. Despite the weight of evidence to support homosexuality not being a form of mental illness the belief is still held in some countries and religions. In addition, research within sexuality studies has focused on genetics and identifying a 'gay gene' to try to rationalise and find a biological explanation for homosexuality.

The 'deviance paradigm' in sociology was scrutinised and contested by disability activists and theorists such as Oliver (1996) and Shakespeare (1993), writing within the 'oppression paradigm'. Oliver (1996) uses a mix of social constructionism and Marxism to argue that disability does not originate from the body, but from the consequences of social oppression; in his view, capitalist societies exercise 'exclusionary practices' against bodies which are deemed to be unproductive. Bury had an ongoing debate with Oliver on these issues for several years, and considers: 'Such an approach can easily gloss over social realities and reduce the complexities of individual and social responses to a unidimensional view of disability' (Bury, 1997: 138). It should also be noted that the view of disability as a social construction promulgated by the disability theorists cited above is essentially one of a healthy adult who is young or middle aged, whereas the majority of disabled people are older and experience several illnesses for which they are generally on complex regimes of medication. Bury also argues that in embracing individual empowerment, the radical disability movement 'finds itself championing individual rights and autonomy, without examining closely the moral and ideological ambiguities involved' (Bury, 1997: 140). More recent disability theorists have moved away from Oliver's distinction between impairment (characteristics of the body) and disability (social restrictions placed upon them) to argue that the two are intertwined. Hughes and Paterson (1997: 335) state that 'Disability is experienced in, on and through the body, just as impairment is experienced in terms of the personal and cultural narratives that help to constitute its meaning' (see Box 4.2).

Box 4.2   Deaf culture.

There has been resistance and opposition to the medicalisation of hearing loss over recent years. The medical view assumes that being deaf or having a degree of hearing loss is unwanted and strives to find cures to alleviate the loss of hearing. This has become marked over the last 10 years with advances in medicine offering cochlear implants to babies with the possibility that they will develop listening and speaking skills as they get older. The Deaf community however hold a view that being Deaf doesn't make you unwell or ill and see being Deaf as something to be shared and celebrated. This has led to a strong Deaf Culture within Britain, in particular, with a shared identity, language and community. The development of cochlear implants and the reasonable success of these could threaten the Deaf community with erosion of their shared culture and language.

The person who is different may also be stigmatised. The concept of stigma was developed in sociology by Goffman (1968b) as part of a wider development of theory on the presentation of self (Goffman, 1969). It was derived from the mark placed on a Greek slave or criminal to single them out as inferior. Goffman distinguished three types of stigma: those of the body, of the character and of social collectivities such as ethnic groups. He argued that we tend to impute a wide range of imperfections on the basis of the original one, and may then perceive the person's defensive response to his situation as a direct expression of his defect. This may occur regardless of whether the deviance is voluntary or involuntary. The stigmatised person is also likely to be aware of society's norms and how he or she falls short of them, so is, in Goffman's view, likely to feel shame. Stigma may also spread to other closely connected people, which Goffman terms a 'courtesy stigma'.

Goffman (1968b) distinguishes between the discredited, whose stigma is obvious, and the discreditable, whose stigma is not obvious and who may 'pass' as normal. The primary problem for the first is impression management, and for the second, the management of information. The discredited person needs to be able to manage the tension generated during social interaction, as other people often find it difficult to know how to react; the ambiguity and unease can result in avoidance, rejection or withdrawal. The commonest reaction is 'careful disattention'.

As Davis (1964: 122, 123) states:

'[W]hether the handicap is overtly and tactlessly responded to as such or, as is more commonly the case, no explicit reference is made to it, the underlying condition of heightened, narrowed, awareness causes the interaction to be articulated too exclusively in terms of it. This is usually accompanied by one or more of the familiar signs of discomfort and stickiness: the guarded reference, the common everyday words suddenly taboo, the fixed stare elsewhere, the artificial levity, the compulsive loquaciousness, the awkward solemnity.'

This may be a particular problem where the person has a facial disfigurement, since conversational norms in many cultures involve looking at the face.

The discreditable person has the dilemma of whether to reveal his or her problem by revealing information or bodily signs. This may lead to a high level of anxiety about the possibility of revelation; 'What are unthinking routines for normals can become management problems for the discreditable' (Goffman, 1968b: 110). Another, potentially less stressful strategy, which may however require more interactional skill, is that of covering, by admitting the stigma but ensuring that it does not loom large in the interaction. 'The individual's object is to reduce tension that is, to make it easier for himself and the others to withdraw covert attention from the stigma, and to sustain spontaneous involvement in the official context of the interaction' (Goffman, 1968b: 125, 126). Such techniques are part of the work of organisations such as Changing Faces, the leading UK charity that supports and represents people who have disfigurements to the face, hand or body from any cause.

Goffman also addresses the effects of stigma on the person's own identity, such as the ambivalence the person may feel about identifying with other people who have the same problem. Most difficult is the double bind in which society may put the person, requiring 'good adjustment', including withdrawing from situations where acceptance would be difficult.

'This means that the unfairness and pain of having to carry a stigma will never have to be presented to them: it means that normals will not have to admit to themselves how limited their tactfulness and tolerance is . . . The stigmatised individual is asked to act so as to imply neither that his burden is heavy nor that bearing it has made him different from us . . .'

(Goffman 1968b: 146, 147)

Scambler (2009) argues that what is missing from Goffman's account of interaction is the social structure or 'social facts' which surround and constrain it, including an account of the power relations involved in labelling. He also draws a distinction between the onto-logical deficit (or deficit of being), which leads to stigma and shame, and the moral deficit which equates to deviance, and blame. Both are embedded in social structures, as Scam-bler (2006) demonstrates in his discussion of the British 'welfare-to-work' programmes for people with chronic illnesses or disabilities. Based on the premise that worklessness led to poverty and social exclusion, they offered a range of strategies such as education and work placements (Bambra *et al.*, 2005). However, the policy has to be understood in the context of the growth of neo-liberalism and the concern to control the welfare bill referred to below, in which the 'stigma' of the chronically ill person is partially transmuted into the 'deviance' of the person who could work but does not wish to.

Stigma in chronic illness

Fabrega and Manning (1972) state that there are four major dimensions to illness: (1) the duration, (2) the possibility of cure, (3) the degree of discomfort or disability and (4) the potential for stigmatisation. Drawing on their work, Field (1976) distinguishes between acute illness, long-term non-stigmatised illness, long-term stigmatised illness and mental illness, which is perhaps the most stigmatising, becoming a 'master status' which dominates the rest of the person's identity. Freidson (1972) claims that in the case of acute illness, normal people need to adjust to the sick person and the latter is exempt from his or her usual duties (as in Parsons' sick role), whereas the person with a stigmatised long-term illness is obliged to adjust to 'normal' people. Strauss (1975) uses Goffman's work to develop the concept of 'normalisation', the strategies which people with long-term illnesses use to minimise stigmatisation. Strauss also focuses on problems of daily living, such as the control of symptoms, managing therapeutic regimens, and the risk of social isolation.

In Scambler's (1984) UK study, adults with epilepsy were usually very upset to have the diagnosis confirmed, and felt that they might then be rejected by normal people; some attempted to negotiate a different diagnosis. Scambler distinguished between felt stigma, the shame associated with being epileptic, and enacted stigma, or actual discrimination. Many people used concealment, particularly in relation to employment. In an earlier study of people with epilepsy in the United States, Schneider and Conrad (1981) distinguished between what they called adjusted and unadjusted modes of adaptation. In adjusted adaptation, people were able to neutralise the impact of epilepsy, at least to some extent, and had a sense of control. Schneider and Conrad delineated three subtypes of adjusted adaptation: the pragmatic type, in which the existence of epilepsy was rarely denied or concealed, but its impact was minimised; the secret type, in which often elaborate procedures were used to conceal information and the quasi-liberated type, in which the person with epilepsy took on a role to educate others and to overturn stereotypes. In the unadjusted mode of adaptation, people seemed to be overwhelmed by their epilepsy, and did not develop any strategies for stigma management.

Williams (1987) concludes that the concept of stigma is fundamentally important for understanding the social dynamics of illness. He also discusses the potential marginalisa-tion of many people with long-term illness or disability, and the risk that professionals may be unaware of the difficulties that patients experience. In particular, since the biomedical model of disease cannot encompass the notion of stigma, doctors may ignore the fact that it exists and the social consequences which it has for patients.

Economic effects of long-term illness

Long-term illness is a major factor in causing poverty, even in countries where medical treatment is largely free. Grewal *et al.* (2006) examine the economic effects of disability. These include the effects of limited participation in the labour market. There are also increased costs, such as housing alterations, heating costs, dietary requirements and home help, and these are unlikely to be covered in full by state benefits. Indirect costs may include the need to rely on more expensive small local shops, or taxis for shopping. Other family members may also have to give up paid employment. In addition, people with LTCs are more likely to be in occupations lower in the hierarchy (Bajekal *et al.,* 2006) and therefore less likely to have accumulated savings. Although the current economic climate may not be conducive to its implementation, the 2008 report *Working for a Healthier Tomorrow* by the National Director for Health and Work, Dame Carol Black, may help to rehabilitate people in employment by recommending the use of an electronic 'fit note' concentrating on what the person can do. The policy context is that the national cost of sickness absence and worklessness associated with ill health is currently over £100 billion a year, which is greater than the entire budget of the National Health Service (NHS) (Topping, 2009). However, GPs may need further occupational health training, since not all are active in managing fitness for work (Mowlam and Lewis, 2005; Hiscock and Ritchie, 2005), and the effectiveness of such approaches has to be set in the context of wide national variations in income, levels of employment, and health inequalities (Shaw *et al.,* 1999). As alluded to above, there is concern that this policy can put pressure on disadvantaged people living in places where work is not readily available even for those who are well, and that it ignores the uncertainties about day-to-day wellness and capacity which long-term illness often entails.

Illness as biographical disruption

Modern cultures are based on a general expectation of health and a long life, and a future which can, to a large extent, be planned. Changes in our body can disrupt these taken-for-granted expectations about everyday life, and much of the sociology of health and illness is built around personal accounts of such experiences, which provide an important resource for practitioners to help their understanding. Bury (1982), who interviewed patients with rheumatoid arthritis, emphasises that illness is a biographical disruption, involving the disruption of everyday behaviours, the need to rethink one's self-concept and the need to mobilise resources to face an uncertain future; 'The onset of illness, especially that which is not evidently self-limiting, fractures this social and cultural fabric, exposing the individual to threats to self-identity and potentially damaging loss of control' (Bury, 1997: 124). Carel (2008: 61, 62), a lecturer in philosophy, provides a powerful account of her own diagnosis at the age of 35 and her experience of illness (see Box 4.3).

Box 4.3   The experience of illness (Carel 2008).

'In the morning I was still happily navigating the world as a healthy person although I got breathless easily. That afternoon I learned I had LAM [lymphangioleiomyomatosis]. The next day I was told that my prospects were poor, that there was no treatment for LAM and that I would probably die within the next ten years . . .When I learned that there was nothing I could do to prevent my lung function from declining and that at the end of my illness lay death from respiratory failure, the extent of my tragedy became clear. How could it be? How could there be no treatment?'

'The thought that was truly novel for me was this: I will never get better. All the usual rules that governed my life – that trying hard yields results, that looking after yourself pays off, that practice makes perfect – seemed inoperative here. . . . No matter what I did I would only get worse.'

(Carel, 2008: 63)

'I still remembered doing everything . . . without oxygen. The memory was alive not only in my mind, but in my body. My body rushed forwards, only to be halted by a force stronger than it, chained to its dying lungs.'

(Carel, 2008: 63)

'Life ceases to be a long, gently flowing river. The future no longer contains the vague promise of many more decades. Death is no longer an abstract, remote notion. The soft-focus lens is replaced by a sharp magnifying glass through which terminal stages of illness can be viewed in nauseating detail.'

(Carel, 2008: 123)

Bury distinguishes between two aspects of the meaning of illness: the practical *consequences* which symptoms and illness management may have for everyday life; and the wider issue of the *significance* of illness, for example the fear of future pain and deformity which may result from a diagnosis of rheumatoid arthritis, or mixed feelings when multiple sclerosis is diagnosed, an element of which may be relief that diffuse symptoms now have a name. In Bury's view, biographical disruption can be partially mitigated by trying to construct an explanation for why the illness has occurred, and by trying to establish its legitimacy in the patient's life, by re-establishing daily life and social networks.

Coping is a widely used term in the self-management of long-term illness, and Bury warns us against its evaluative use, whereby people are 'successful' or not in coping. Radley (1994) differentiates 'emotion-based coping' from 'problem-based coping'; the former concerns the ways in which people maintain or recover their sense of self-worth during long-term illness, whereas the latter refers to the strategies that people adopt and the resources they are able to mobilise, not only in terms of their own physical resources, for example by pacing themselves in undertaking tasks, but also in terms of social support and social networks. In Williams' (1993) study, as in many others about long-term illness, the social network – where it existed – provided little support, and spouses provided most of the day-to-day support. With respect to 'styles' of managing chronic illness, Bury observes that people's actions will be influenced by their level of confidence in managing their situation. Corbin and Strauss (1991) consider that with sufficient material resources and a supportive social network, it is possible to shift from 'the disabled self' to 'the capable self'. This involves experimentation and requires a sense of humour.

Carel (2008: 81) argues that health can be found within illness, if researchers (and perhaps clinicians) ask the right questions. For example, lung function tests are presented as percentage of the normal, but clinicians may not enquire what the person can actually *do* with their reduced lung capacity. She also proposes a wide concept of adaptability, which is not just psychological adjustment, but physical, social and temporal. 'It is not a smooth process but a series of dialectic encounters of a body with an environment, of a demand with failure, and of failure with the need for modification.'

An important theme in sociology, which overlaps both with the sociology of health and illness and the phenomenology drawn on by Carel (2008), is the sociology of the body. This has been used by nursing writers, most notably Lawler (1991), to examine the hidden aspects of bodily care. Twigg (2000) uses this work to examine care work in older people's homes, including the management of disgust, and balancing intimacy and distance, primarily from the viewpoint of the care workers. However, a related paper on the 'social bath' (Twigg, 1997) also examines the importance of the setting in which the care occurs, i.e. the home. Twigg (1997) states that the ideology of the home as a private place became accentuated in the nineteenth century, and has come to epitomise the values of privacy, security, independence, self-expression and identity. Visitors enter the home only by invitation; privacy is lost when the person has to accept help. Also in situations of physical decline, the person is able to manage for longer in a familiar environment, although they may be upset by the decline in their housekeeping skills. Home may also embody the presence of a lost partner. This is contrasted with the ward environment, where there is little personal space and few possessions and no boundary between the social and the medical, so that food becomes 'nutrition' and visits become 'social support'.

The experience of long-term illness

Anderson and Bury (1988) examine the experience of chronic illness in relation to environmental conditions, material resources and the demands of contemporary society. The individually authored chapters cover stroke, multiple sclerosis, Parkinson's disease, arthritis, heart attack, diabetes, epilepsy, rectal cancer, renal failure and psoriasis; common themes include stigmatisation, the impact of the illness on family life and employment, its effect on personal identity and the use of health services, including the problems which treatment may create. Jobling's chapter on living with the treatment of psoriasis has graphic data on the problems caused by showers of skin scales in shops and other public settings, and the exhausting routines needed to stay in hotels, including brushing the carpets and protecting the sheets from staining ointments. Jobling (1988: 229) comments:

'The psoriasis sufferer must cope not simply with the "biological entity" but psoriasis under particular forms of treatment. While undoubtedly part of the "solution", therapeutic regimes are equally undeniably part of the "problem". This simple but fundamental insight is ignored, or at best taken for granted by many dermatologists.'

Also, in relation to the problems which treatment may create, MacDonald's chapter on living with the aftermath of rectal cancer contains worrying data from patients who felt that they had not been properly informed about what the surgery would entail, and were horrified to find that they had a colostomy; it is to be hoped that the greater emphasis on properly informed consent in the last twenty years would reduce such findings in a study undertaken today. Although patients with a higher income were protected from the uncertainties of poverty, which other cancer patients may experience, they were no less likely to feel stigmatised; 'the felt stigma of cancer and a mutilated body was powerful enough to overcome the protection of privileged social position' (MacDonald, 1988: 197). Feelings of stigma did not prevent individuals from working, but they were much more likely to cut themselves off socially than those who did not feel stigma.

Kelly (1992) explores the identity of people who have had radical surgery for ulcerative colitis, resulting in an ileostomy. The sociological concept used is that of the self (Mead, 1934), summarised by Kelly as the imaginative view of ego by ego, which is constantly rehearsed, constructed and reconstructed. As in MacDonald's study, several respondents were shocked by the extent of the surgical mutilation and also by the post-operative pain, even though they had had extended periods of sub-acute pain due to their colitis. Kelly considered that many had mixed feelings, since the major surgery had provided a cure, but at the cost of considerable body disfigurement. People may, however, put on a brave face, since 'on the surface the person has, may feel obliged, or may simply want, to present to the world, an ordinary front' (Kelly, 1992: 400). Skills of managing the appliance had to be learnt, and Kelly (1992: 400, 401) points out that the taken-for-granted nature of the body no longer exists. 'The shared meanings concerning body, body functioning and body shape are visibly demonstrated to be violated or altered ... Attending to the bag is a permanent feature of self because incontinence is a permanent feature of self.' That constant attention is generally a private matter, but it can become very public if the appliance fails and leaks.

Changes in body structure were also a considerable barrier and source of anxiety in sexual relationships.

'At the heart of the concerns are fears that the legitimacy of self as a sexual being will be denied. Thus, despite the conventional wisdom espoused by counsellors and doctors – that people with an ileostomy can have a normal sex life ... The identity which ... may be assigned by others is that of sick person, non-normal and not a legitimate sex partner.'

(Kelly, 1992: 405, 406)

Kelly concludes that although patients are generally offered plenty of information and advice before surgery, the critical issues on which counsellors should focus are the management of anxiety, managing social interaction, and in particular talking through how to manage sexual interaction.

Patients as experts

As people become familiar with their illness, they may become expert, comparing notes with other patients, or gaining information from the media. In particular, accounts of serious and terminal illness in book form, as blogs, and in the general news have become a recent feature, the most notable and controversial being the 2009 account of the demise of the reality TV personality Jade Goody (McVeigh, 2009), leading to debates about how widely details of illness should be discussed. One argument is that the information, if accurate, can be helpful to other people with the same illness, or could prompt people at risk to go for screening. In illnesses such as multiple sclerosis, 'careful experimentation' (Robinson, 1988) with medication may take place. Robinson also suggests that a 'pooling of expertise' between the patient and the practitioner is more useful than concern about whether the patient is 'compliant'. This phrase, which has generally been replaced by the term concordant, may be particularly inappropriate in long-term illness, as compliance implies that there is a simple problem and a simple solution, whereas treatments may be complex and intrusive, as discussed above and elsewhere in this book.

Williams (1993) found that patients with chronic obstructive pulmonary disease used several criteria to assess their treatment. First, the degree of symptom relief; second, the extent to which they were able to manage activities of daily living better; third, the acceptability of side effects; fourth, the amount of time taken up with treatment, and any difficulties or restrictions it imposed; and fifth, any intrusion or embarrassment caused by the treatment. When hospitalisation was necessary, it was often viewed with a mix of relief and apprehension. Relief, since exacerbations of respiratory illness may lead to acute anxiety, which in turn may exacerbate dyspnoea, but apprehension, since the hospital environment may result in the loss of a hard-won sense of control over the illness.

The recognition that patients are often well informed, and that the successful management of LTCs is dependent on self-management, has grown in tandem with the wider issue of consumerism in health care and other public services. Consumerism as a social movement has developed gradually from the 1960s. Walsh (1994) states that there was mounting criticism of public services in the United Kingdom from the mid 1970s, which accelerated in the 1980s. This led to the importation of business practices and vocabulary by the Conservative government. By the early 1990s, the debate had broadened to include the concept of the citizen as customer. There is however a greater problem in defining the quality of services than there is the quality of goods, since the former is more intangible and in health care the patient is a 'co-producer' of his or her health. 'Voice' (i.e. complaint) and 'exit' are two means by which the customer may make his or her views known; in the public sector, the voice of the user may be muted, and their exit from the service provided may be limited by the lack of alternatives. Lupton *et al.* (1991) argue that the consumerist approach to health care depends on the patient having bargaining power, freedom of choice, the knowledge and motivation to choose a particular option, and the power to challenge medical authority. At the point of consultation, many patients will be worried and vulnerable (Warde, 1994). Haug and Lavin (1983) in a large scale study undertaken in the United States in the late 1970s found that although a substantial segment of the population had a consumerist approach to health care, this did not necessarily lead to consumerist behaviour. The possession of health knowledge was more important in developing consumerist behaviour than either age or level of education, as were poor health and the experience of medical error.

Consumerism cannot however be equated with whether or not a patient complies with treatment (Haug and Lavin, 1983). Marland (1998) states that adherence to medical treatment is considerably lower in LTCs. It is then difficult for the clinician to assess how effective the treatment is. Interventions which solely attempt to educate or to persuade are unlikely to succeed, and the patient may simply suppress their disagreement and not disclose how they use their medication. Holm (1993) argues that doctors often prescribe standard treatment, without discussing how appropriate that is to the patient's situation. A systematic review (Haynes *et al.,* 1996) found greater success with more complex combinations, including more convenient care, counselling, reminders, and family therapy, although the improvement was not great. A study comparing mental health patients' and nurses' views (Lund and Frank, 1991) found that nurses were generally aware when patients were not adhering to their treatment, but often were not aware of the reasons, and so did not always address the issue effectively. Concordance may be particularly problematic in adolescence, since at that life-stage it may be more important to be like one's peers, despite the risk of serious complications from non-adherence to treatment (Atkin and Ahmad, 2000). It may also be an issue when the patient does not accept the 'label' of their diagnosis, as Adams *et al.* (1997) argue in their study of people diagnosed with asthma. These issues are discussed further in the Self Management and Medicines Management chapters.

Person-centred care

Research by the King's Fund (Corben and Rosen, 2005) highlights the importance of shared decision making between clinicians and patients in person-centred care. However, studies have shown that both doctors and nurses may set limits on this. Although nurses are seen in English policy documents as having a key role in the management of LTCs (Department of Health, 2005), Wilson *et al.* (2006) in their study of nurses, GPs and physiotherapists found that the majority of non-specialist nurses whom they spoke to in focus groups and interviews were anxious about expert patients, and thought that they would be held liable if the patient followed their own treatment plan which then had adverse effects. Although Wilson *et al.* (2006) do not pick up on this, three quarters of the nurses had a secondary care background, and may therefore have been less attuned to the autonomy which care in the patient's own home confers (see Twigg, 1997). All the professionals in the study relied on physical measures to assess how expert the patient was; both the nurses and physiotherapists portrayed patients as appearing to know more than they actually did. The nurse specialists, like the GPs and physiotherapists, saw spending time with the patient early on as a worthwhile investment. The generalist nurses did not, and were concerned that the time pressure in clinics did not allow them to spend time answering patients' questions; they generally did not seem to have control over their workload. These nurses also did not convey confidence in their own knowledge base, and felt that it 'counted for nothing' and was being challenged by expert patients. Their role in giving emotional support, which was valued by patients, was generally not articulated, and not greatly valued, by the non-specialist nurses. The authors considered that the majority of the nurses were too imbued with bureaucracy to exercise independent judgement. 'Far from being expanded, the restrictive nature of their role appeared to cause feelings of resentment that was [*sic*] quite frequently directed at expert patients' (Wilson *et al.*, 2006: 811). Overall, these nurses did not trust the patients' capacity to self-manage their illness, and also construed the patients' questioning as lack of trust in the nurse.

Rogers *et al.* (2005) in their evaluation of a self-management programme for people with inflammatory bowel disease found little evidence of a shift to shared decision making; the consultants considered that they were already sufficiently patient-centred and interpreted self-management narrowly as compliance with medical instructions. In particular, although both doctors and patients recognised the importance of medication, doctors largely ignored wider issues such as diet. There were also organisational constraints such as poor continuity of care, lack of privacy due to the presence of medical students, and lack of thought on the timing of clinics. As one respondent stated with some irritation, it was 'stupid that all these people with bowel disorders' had to go to morning clinics, when many of them might need several hours in the bathroom in the morning. Rogers *et al.* (2005: 236) comment that 'although the individual consultations might have been patient centered, nothing else about the organization of NHS outpatient clinics was', highlighting the need for a person-centred approach discussed elsewhere in this book.

Conclusion

This chapter has discussed the sociological literature on the doctor–patient relationship, deviance and stigma, help seeking, illness as biographical disruption and consumerism in health care, relating these topics to the care of people with LTCs. In particular, it has provided powerful personal accounts from the literature which augment those provided elsewhere in this book, in order to illuminate the lived experience of having a long-term illness, and the 'biographical disruption' which may often accompany it.

References

Adams, S., Pill, R. & Jones, A. (1997) Medication, chronic illness and identity: the perspective of people with asthma, *Social Science & Medicine*, 45(2), pp. 189–201.

Anderson, R. & Bury, M. (1988) *Living with Chronic Illness.* Unwin Hyman, London.

Arksey, H. (1994) Expert and lay participation in the construction of medical knowledge, *Sociology of Health and Illness*, 16(4), pp. 448–468.

Arksey, H. & Sloper, P. (1999) Disputed diagnoses: the cases of RSI and childhood cancer, *Social Science & Medicine*, 49, pp. 483–497.

Atkin, K. & Ahmad, W. I. U. (2000) Pumping iron: compliance with chelation therapy among young people who have thalassaemia major, *Sociology of Health and Illness*, 22(4), pp. 500–524.

Bajekal, M., Osborne, V., Yar, M. & Meltzer, H. (eds) (2006) *Focus on Health. National Statistics*. Palgrave Macmillan. Available at: www.statistics.gov.uk.

Bambra, C., Whitehead, E. & Hamilton, V. (2005) Does 'welfare-to-work' work? A systematic review of the effectiveness of the UK's welfare-to-work programmes for people with a disability or chronic illness, *Social Science and Medicine*, 60, 1905–1918.

Becker, H. S. (1963) *Outsiders: Studies in the Sociology of Deviance*. Free Press, New York.

Black, C. (2008) *Working for a Healthier Tomorrow*. The Stationery Office, London. Available at: www.workingforhealth.gov.uk.

Bloor, M. & Horobin, G. (1975) Conflict and conflict resolution in doctor–patient relationships. In: *A Sociology of Medical Practice*, (eds C. Cox & A. Mead). Collier Macmillan, London.

Bury, M. (1982) Chronic illness as biographical disruption, *Sociology of Health and Illness*, 4(2), pp. 167–182.

Bury, M. (1997) *Health and Illness in a Changing Society*. Routledge, London.

Carel, H. (2008) Illness. *Acumen*, Stocksfield, Northumberland.

Corben, S. & Rosen, R. (2005) *Self-Management for Long-Term Conditions. Patients' Perspectives on the Way Ahead*. King's Fund, London.

Corbin, J. & Strauss, A. (1991) Comeback: the process of overcoming disability. In: *Advances in Medical Sociology*, (eds G.L. Albrecht & J.A. Levy), vol. 2. JAI Press, Greenwich, CT.

Davis, F. (1964) Deviance disavowal: the management of strained interaction by the visibly handicapped. In: *The Other Side* (ed H. Becker). Free Press, Glencoe, IL.

Department of Health (2005) NHS hospital and community health services non-medical staff in England: 1994–2004, *Statistical Bulletin*, March. Available at: www.dh.gov.uk.

Dingwall, R., Fenn, P. & Quam, L. (1991) *Medical Negligence: a Review and Bibliography*. Centre for Socio-Legal Studies, Wolfson College, Oxford.

Fabrega, H. & Manning, P. K. (1972) Disease, illness and deviant careers. In: *Theoretical Perspectives on Deviance* (eds R. A. Scott & J. D. Douglas). Basis Books, New York.

Field, D. (1976) The social definition of illness. In: *An Introduction to Medical Sociology* (ed D. Tuckett). Tavistock, London.

Freidson, E. (1970) [and 1988] *Profession of Medicine: a Study of the Sociology of Applied Knowledge*. University of Chicago Press, Chicago.

Freidson, E. (1972) Disability as social deviance. In: *Deviant Behaviour and Social Reaction* (eds C. L. Boydell, C. F. Grindstaff & P. C. Whitehead). Holt Rinehart and Winston, Toronto, pp. 4–23.

Gerhardt, U. (1987) Parsons, role theory and health interaction. In: *Sociological Theory and Medical Sociology* (ed G. Scambler). Tavistock, London.

Goffman, E. (1961) *Fun in Games*. Bobbs-Merrill, New York.

Goffman, E. (1968a) *Asylums: Essays on the Social Situation of Mental Patients and Other Inmates*. Penguin, Harmondsworth.

Goffman, E. (1968b) *Stigma: Notes on the Management of Spoiled Identity*. Penguin, Harmondsworth.

Goffman, E. (1969) *The Presentation of Self in Everyday Life*. Penguin, Harmondsworth.

Gove, W. (1970) Societal reaction as an explanation of mental illness: an evaluation, *American Sociological Review*, 35, pp. 873–884.

Grewal, S., Joy, S., Lewis, J., *et al.* (2006) *'Disabled for Life?' Attitudes Towards, and Experiences of, Disability in Britain*. DWP Research Report 173, Leeds.

Haug, M. & Lavin, B. (1983) *Consumerism in Medicine: Challenging Physician Authority*. Sage, Beverly Hills.

Haynes, R.B., McKibbon, K.A. & Kanani, R. (1996) Systematic review of randomised trials of interventions to assist patients to follow prescriptions for medications, *The Lancet*, 348(9024), pp. 383–386.

Hiscock, J. and Ritchie, J. (2005) *The Role of GPs in Sickness Certification*. Department for Work and Pensions Research Report no. 148.

Holm, S. (1993) What is wrong with compliance? *Journal of Medical Ethics*, 19(2), pp. 108–110.

Hughes, B. & Paterson, K. (1997) The social model of disability and the disappearing body: towards a sociology of impairment, *Disability & Society*, 12(3), pp. 25–40.

Illich, I. (1975) *Medical Nemesis*. Calder & Boyars, London.

Jobling, R (1988) The experience of psoriasis under treatment. In: *Living with Chronic Illness* (eds R. Anderson & M. Bury). Unwin Hyman, London.

Kelly, M. (1992) Self, identity and radical surgery, *Sociology of Health and Illness*, 14(3), pp. 390–415.

Lawler, J. (1991) *Behind the Screens: Nursing, Somology and the Problem of the Body*. Churchill Livingstone, Melbourne.

Lund, V.E., & Frank, D.I. (1991) Helping the medicine go down, *Journal of Psychosocial Nursing*, 29(7), pp. 6–9.

Lupton, D., Donaldson, C. & Lloyd, P. (1991) Caveat emptor or blissful ignorance? Patients and the consumerist ethos, *Social Science and Medicine*, 33(5), pp. 559–568.

MacDonald, L. (1988) The experience of stigma: living with rectal cancer. In: *Living with Chronic Illness* (eds R. Anderson & M. Bury). Unwin Hyman, London.

Marland, G. (1998) Partnership encourages patients to comply with treatment, *Nursing Times*, 8 July, 94(27), pp. 58–59.

McKeown, T. (1976) *The Role of Medicine: Dream, Mirage or Nemesis?* Nuffield Provincial Hospitals Trust, London.

McVeigh, T. (2009) 'Why Jade's struggle for life is a tale of our times', *The Observer*, 8 February, p. 30.

Mead, G. (1934) *Mind, Self and Society*. University of Chicago Press, Chicago.

Meerabeau, E. (1998) Consumerism and health care: the example of fertility treatment, *Journal of Advanced Nursing*, 27, pp. 721–729.

Mowlam, A. & Lewis, J. (2005) *Exploring How General Practitioners Work with Patients on Sick Leave*. Department for Work and Pensions Research Report no. 257, ISBN 1 84123 840 6. Available at http://research.dwp.gov.uk/asd/asd5/rports2005-2006/rrep257.pdf.

Nettleton, S. & Hanlon, G. (2006) "Pathways to the doctor" in the information age: the role of ICTs in contemporary lay referral systems. In: *New Technologies in Health Care. Challenges, Changes and Innovation* (ed A. Webster). Palgrave Macmillan, London.

Oakley, A. (1980) *Women Confined: Towards a Sociology of Childbirth*. Martin Robertson, Oxford.

Oliver, M. (1996) *Understanding Disability: from Theory to Practice*. Macmillan, London.

Parsons, T. (1951) *The Social System*. Free Press, Glencoe, IL.

Parsons, T. (1964) *Social Structure and Personality*. Free Press, Glencoe, IL.

Parsons, T. (1978) The sick role and the role of the physician reconsidered. In: *Action Theory and the Human Condition*. Free Press, New York.

Radley, A. (1994) *Making Sense of Illness: the Social Psychology of Health and Disease*. Sage, London.

Robinson, I. (1988*) Multiple Sclerosis*. Routledge, London.

Rogers, A., Kennedy, A., Nelson, E. & Robinson, A. (2005) Uncovering the limits of patient-centeredness: implementing a self-management trial for chronic illness, *Qualitative Health Research*, 15, pp. 224–239.

Scambler, G. (1984) Perceiving and coping with stigmatizing illness. In: *The Experience of Illness* (eds R. Fitzpatrick, J. Hinton, S. Newman, G. Scambler, & J. Thompson). Tavistock, London.

Scambler, G. (2006) Sociology, social structure and health-related stigma, *Psychology, Health and Medicine*, 11, pp. 288–295.

Scambler, G. (2009) Health-related stigma, *Sociology of Health and Illness*, 31(3), pp. 441–455.

Scheff, T. (1966) *Being Mentally Ill: a Sociological Theory*. Aldine, Chicago.

Schneider, J. and Conrad, P. (1981) Medical and sociological typologies: the case of epilepsy, *Social Science and Medicine*, 15(a), pp. 211–219.

Silverman, D. (1987) *Communication and Medical Practice: Social Relations in the Clinic*. Sage, London.

Shakespeare, T. (1993) Disabled people's self-organisation: a new social movement? *Disability, Handicap and Society*, 8(3), pp. 249–264.

Shaw, M., Dorling, D., Gordon, D. & Davey-Smith, G. (1999) *The Widening Gap. Health Inequalities and Policy in Britain*. Policy Press, Bristol.

Stimson, G. (1976) General practitioners: trouble and types of patients. In: *The Sociology of the NHS, Sociological Review Monograph no. 22* (ed M. Stacey). University of Keele, Keele.

Stimson, G. & Webb, B. (1975) *Going to See the Doctor: the Consultation Process in General Practice*. Routledge and Kegan Paul, London.

Strauss, A. (1975) *Chronic Illness and the Quality of Life*. Mosby, St. Louis.

Strong, P. & Davis, A. (1977) Role, role formats and medical encounters: a cross-cultural analysis of staff/client relationships in children's clinics, *Sociological Review*, 25(4), pp. 775–800.

Strong, P. (1979) *The Ceremonial Order of the Clinic: Parents, Doctors and Medical Bureaucracies*. Routledge and Kegan Paul, London.

Topping, J. (2009) Staff wellbeing. Fitter, happier, *Health Service Journal*, 22 January 2009, pp. 26–27.

Tuckett, D., Boulton, M., Olson, C. & Williams, A. (1985) *Meetings Between Experts*. Tavistock, London.

Twigg, J. (1997) Deconstructing the 'social bath': help with bathing at home for older and disabled People, *Journal of Social Policy*, 26(2), pp. 211–232.

Twigg, J. (2000) Carework as a form of bodywork, *Ageing and Society*, 20, pp. 389–411.

Waitzkin, H. (1979) Medicine, superstructure and micropolitics, *Social Science and Medicine*, 13A, pp. 601–609.

Walsh, K. (1994) Citizens, charters and contracts. In: *The Authority of the Consumer* (eds R. Keat, N. Whiteley & N. Abercrombie). Routledge, London, pp. 189–206.

Warde, A. (1994) Consumers, identity and belonging: reflections on some theses of Zygmunt Bauman. In: *The Authority of the Consumer* (eds R. Keat, N. Whiteley & N. Abercrombie). Routledge, London, pp. 58–74.

Williams, S. (1987) Goffman, interactionism, and the management of stigma in everyday life. In: *Sociological Theory and Medical Sociology* (ed G. Scambler). Tavistock Publications, London, chapter 6, pp. 134–164.

Williams, S.J. (1993) *Chronic Respiratory Disorder*. Routledge, London.

Wilson, P. M., Kendall, S. & Brooks, F. (2006) Nurses' responses to expert patients: the rhetoric and reality of self-management in long-term conditions: a grounded theory study, *International Journal of Nursing Studies*, 43, pp. 803–818.

Zola, I. K. (1973) Pathways to the doctor: from person to patient, *Social Science and Medicine*, 7, pp. 667–689.

Chapter 5

Psychological effects of long-term conditions

Ben Bruneau

School of Health and Social Care, University of Greenwich, Eltham, London, UK

Introduction

Long-term conditions (LTCs) are known to be associated with a reduced state of psychological well-being. The quality of life of individuals is significantly curtailed when they have these conditions and this quality of life diminishes further in the presence of psychological ill-effects. Psychological impairment subsequently impedes medical interventions for individuals and their efforts to rehabilitate and self-manage their condition.

Living with an LTC can result in many changes and adaptations to a person's life. LTCs may involve a degree of disability brought about by some pathological change, which can prove difficult or almost impossible to reverse. The management of this disability can be quite demanding for the individual as well as for those who may have the responsibility for supporting and providing care. It often requires training and a new approach for the one being cared for and, sometimes, for the carer. A high degree of motivation would be necessary on the part of these people. An LTC also includes all the difficulties and remedial efforts that come with an acute condition. For example, the initial difficulties encountered by a person when first diagnosed with arthritis, such as the experience of pain and restricted mobility, would tend to linger because of permanent damage to joints. The use of analgesics and physiotherapy would continue, with the possibility of these being supplemented by the wearing of orthoses, such as rigid joint supports, with the affected individual relying more on others for personal daily activities of living. The experience of living with an LTC may, therefore, require that the person has to make alterations and adaptations to their life and how they choose to live (see Chapters 4, 8 and 6 for more discussion on experiences of living with an LTC).

On being ill long-term

As discussed in the previous chapters, people with LTCs have, first of all, to make sense of their experience. They then have to view their 'impaired' or failing bodies in ways that enable some form of emotional and social resolution, including acceptance and adaptation (Charmaz, 1995). An LTC may give rise to a number of challenges for the individual.

Long-Term Conditions: Nursing Care and Management, First Edition. Edited by Liz Meerabeau and Kerri Wright.
© 2011 Blackwell Publishing Ltd. Published 2011 by Blackwell Publishing Ltd.

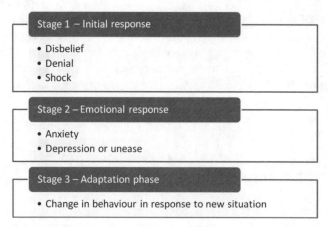

Figure 5.1 A three-stage model of LTC and response (adapted from Holland and Gooen-Piels, 2003).

Using Holland and Gooen-Piels' (2003) three-stage response (see Figure 5.1), Lethborg *et al.* (2008) argue that this model is appropriate not only for cancer care, but also for other conditions such as diabetes and coronary heart disease.

The first stage is the person's initial response to the knowledge of their LTC. The person refuses or is reluctant to believe that the condition exists (disbelief), refuses to acknowledge painful realities, thoughts or feeling (denial) and displays a disturbance of function, equilibrium or mental faculties (shock).

The second stage is an emotional phase characterised by anxiety, depression or unease (dysphoria). The person is distressed and displays the related symptoms of distress such as insomnia, reduced appetite and poor concentration.

The third stage involves a change in the person's behaviour in response to the new situation (adaptation).

People with LTCs are thought to progress from stage 1 to stage 3 in a spiral rather than a linear fashion. That is while in stage 2, they can show the features of stage 1 and while in stage 3 they may still display the features of either stage 1 or stage 2. Thus, they move across the stages more than once. This set of responses resembles the stress response in that they mimic responses seen in stressful situations (Lazarus and Folkman, 1984). Indeed the diagnosis of an LTC may be a stressful event, and may well induce a stress reaction in the individual.

Stress is a transaction between an individual and a stressor or stressful event (Lazarus, 1999) and results in a physiological response to a perceived threat (see Chapter 9 for further discussion of this response). Stress is known to be associated with long-term ill-health such as asthma, cancer, irritable bowel syndrome and ulcerative colitis (Alexander, 2002; Ferguson, 2002; Greenberg, 2002; Morrison and Bennett, 2006; Redwood and Pollak, 2007; Warwick *et al.*, 2008). It is recognised that once a relationship between the LTC and stress is established, the situation can further affect the individual's quality of life, and the subsequent management of the situation may become more complex and difficult for the person concerned.

The individual has to find a way of including their condition into their daily life, and this is not an easy task. On the whole, however, most people cope and they tend to adapt to the situation and, to some extent, adopt new roles or new strategies. As they lose their old 'self' and identity, they need to use new approaches to adapt and develop a new self-identity. Charmaz (1991) suggests that when the effects of a condition are overwhelming there is a danger that a person's self-identify becomes so embedded with their LTC that they can start to redefine themselves according to their condition rather than as a person (see also Smith and Osborn, 2007).

Psychological consequences of an LTC

Many people living with LTCs experience poor mental health and psychological impairment. Repeated correlational studies have demonstrated clear links between a number of LTCs and impaired mental health. Further, comparative studies have shown a higher incidence of psychological impairment among individuals with LTCs than those without. This impairment often manifests itself in affective disorders, with depression the most common disorder. However, psychological impairment is not necessarily accounted for just by depression. Anxiety, hopelessness, loss of self, or low self-esteem can be either present on their own or linked with one or more of these psychological effects. Table 5.1 summarises the research findings linking psychological impairment to LTCs.

Depression, however, does not always occur by itself; it is often preceded by a deep sense of anxiety, which can then linger throughout the individual's remaining lifespan. Chapman *et al.* (2007) suggest that generally most people would be anxious when faced with the possibility of a diagnosis of coronary heart disease and even more so once they have been given such a diagnosis. Anxiety, according to Chapman *et al.* (2007) could contribute to a possible long-term depressive state. Folkman and Greer (2000) also suggest a similar establishment of a continuous anxiety state with people who are quadriplegic.

Table 5.1 Relationship between long-term conditions and psychological effects: the research evidence.

Authors	Date	Findings
McVeigh, Mostashari & Thorpe Anderson *et al.*	2004 2001	Higher rates of depression in those with diabetes
Shih *et al.* Shih & Simon	2006 2008	Higher prevalence of serious psychological distress among people with long-term medical conditions than those without those conditions
Smith *et al.* Chapman *et al.*	2006 2007	Link between depressive symptoms and asthma Link between coronary heart disease and depression
Evans *et al.* Shih & Simon	2005 2008	Link between hypertension and depression
Shih & Simon	2008	Increase in rates of depression when long-term conditions co-occur

The coexistence of anxiety and depression or the presence of each state on its own also changes the way affected individuals view the future. Shih and Simon (2008) demonstrate that depression or anxiety, and even just the LTC on its own, can lead to an individual feeling a sense of hopelessness, whilst Charmaz (1995) argues that an LTC can lead to the loss of self-identity or individuality. Folkman and Greer (2000) further affirm that such a condition can result in low self-esteem. These findings demonstrate an important relationship between an LTC and detrimental psychological effects. This relationship is examined in the next section.

The nature of the relationship between an LTC and psychological effects

The presence of an LTC compels the individual to think long and hard about the implications of having the condition. Their thinking is focused on both the present and the future, especially in terms of the ways to manage the condition and whether this could lead to a satisfactory life. These feelings can affect an individual's thinking and can result in actions to try to avoid this unease. In this attempt to cope with the emotional and mental challenges of the LTC, the individual can experience detrimental effects to their psychological well-being as they may find the whole experience overwhelming. Such a development is based on an association of factors which can be explained in three ways.

First, there is the causal relationship where the experience of the LTC is seen to be the reason for the mental impairment. Such impairment is new and is not noticeable prior to the condition. Second, a person's own psychological make-up can be contributory to the emergence of an LTC, in that the person can be predisposed to psychological effects. For example, an individual's personality and more specifically his or her personality type, such as a type A personality (Rosenberg, 1975), may give rise to coronary heart disease in that person. Third, psychological make-up can itself have an effect on an individual's management of an LTC. Figure 5.2 displays that relationship.

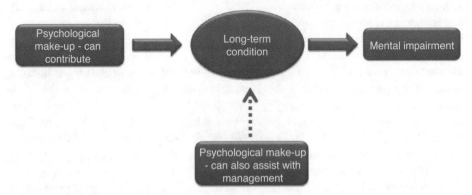

Figure 5.2 The relationship between psychological make-up, long-tem condition and mental impairment.

The experience of an LTC

Psychological reactions to some LTCs can be complex. This complexity was postulated by Veenstra *et al.* (2005) when they demonstrated the intricate relationship that existed between psychological effects and diabetes and between these effects and hypertension. However, there is an adequate explanation as to what happens when someone is faced with an LTC. Bury (1997) suggests that the LTC changes the whole aspect of how the individual sees himself or herself, how they relate to others and how they view the future. The individual can see this future as bleak, which, in turn, may have a detrimental effect on their mood (Conrad, 1987). Further, in their study of women with breast cancer, Carver *et al.* (1994) found, for instance, that a sense of pessimism, as opposed to one of optimism, was related to the women's poorer adjustment over time.

The condition can become a threat to the individual's self and identity in that it permeates all aspects of this individual's life. The individual can become depersonalised and is recognised by others more for their LTC than for their individuality. Ultimately, the person can be seen, by health care workers, for example, as a condition and as an array of regimens that are set to manage the condition (Veenstra *et al.,* 2005). Finally, an LTC introduces uncertainty in the individual's life, a factor which can have an effect on the individual's behaviour, emotions and thinking (BET). These three aspects are considered one at a time. However, they are not seen to happen independently of each other. They are intertwined and the presence of one factor is often related to or is influenced by the existence of either two remaining factors.

Behavioural aspects of an LTC

There are common immediate reactions to the diagnosis of an LTC. The affected individual can take the news of a diagnosis with disbelief and in some cases may even deny that the diagnosis of a condition is true. Others may show anger, either towards themselves as, for example, when they blame themselves for having the condition or towards others.

However, by far the most obvious changes in behaviour are those that are related to depression, anxiety state and the reactions to stress. The individual with an LTC may display one or many of the following behaviours related to depression: disturbance in sleep pattern that manifests itself in the inability to fall asleep, agitated sleep, waking up many times during the night or getting up very early in the morning after having fallen asleep. There could also be other signs such as becoming withdrawn and preferring to be alone rather than mixing with people. They could overeat or undereat, and might show signs of irritability. An anxiety state may show itself in the individual appearing nervous and agitated, with affected speech or visible shaking. As for the signs of reactions to stress, these may be similar to those responses found in depression and, to some extent, the anxiety state, plus further agitation and even overt emotional expressions such as tearfulness or anxious laughter.

However, it should be noted that the sign of withdrawing from the company of others could be due to depression or could also occur as a specific reaction to a condition (Link and Phelan, 2006). For example, in their study of individuals with multiple sclerosis and in people with the disabling consequence of incontinence, Mitterness and Barker (1995) found that affected individuals often withdrew from the company of others and chose to be alone in their homes. These individuals also avoided such things as shopping trips, going out to work or even the company of their spouses. Nicolson and Anderson (2001) later explained that such behaviour could be accounted for, for example, when some individuals with multiple sclerosis feel embarrassed, and at times intensely so by their incontinence.

A change in behaviour is also demonstrated in some phases of another LTC: rheumatoid arthritis. This condition is characterised by periods of flare and remissions that tend to be unpredictable. During periods of flare, a significant number of individuals have reported that they often chose not to mix with others. Danoff-Borg and Revenson (2000) have demonstrated that this behaviour would be more apparent when pain, fatigue or physical disability interferes with their ability to participate in activities.

Emotional aspects of an LTC

The emotional aspect of an LTC is by far the most common and perhaps the most debilitating psychological development. Serious Psychological Distress (SPD) (Shih and Simon, 2008) has been found to be higher among adults with LTCs than those without. Chapman *et al.* (2007) and Evans *et al.* (2005) argued that SPD could in turn contribute to mental ill-health in these adults. There were clear links between an LTC, SPD and impaired mental health. But by far the greatest problem that may be associated with an LTC and/or managing it is the pathologically low mood that may accompany any of the stages of the condition. Affective disorders, including depression, are potentially present and their symptoms can often be resistant to treatment whilst exerting a detrimental effect on the general well-being of the individual with the LTC.

In addition, affective disorders have been found to be implicated in specific LTCs. Anderson *et al.* (2001), Golden *et al.* (2004), McVeigh *et al.* (2002), Shih *et al.* (2006) and Smith *et al* (2006) have demonstrated that people with heart disease, diabetes, arthritis, asthma and hypertension have all been found to have higher rates of depression, depressive symptoms and/or psychological distress. Krueger *et al.* (2001) have further found that depression is a significant disability in many people. More evidence for depression has emerged in organic brain diseases such as dementia (Heun *et al.*, 2002, 2003) and Siegel *et al.* (2004) have additionally postulated that depression and depressive symptomatology are concordant among spouses when at least one partner has an LTC. Finally, in a study by Dickens *et al.* (2002) depression was found to be more common in people with rheumatoid arthritis than healthy individuals.

Depression is also known to significantly and negatively affect the quality of life of someone living with an LTC. Jonkman and De Weerd (2001) found that the person's quality of life was highly and adversely affected a year after a disease-related depression and that there was no doubt that depression correlated with low quality of life. House *et al.* (2001), Lewis *et al.* (2001) and Jones (2006) demonstrated a link between stroke, mood disorder and life dissatisfaction. Further, social constraints were seen to be associated with lower well-being and greater depression among women with breast cancer (Cordova *et al.*, 2001).

This is supported by Jones' (2006) findings that mood disorders, of which depression is the most significant and common disorder, and life dissatisfaction are interrelated. Two reasons are usually given for such a relationship. Firstly, a person with an LTC deals with disappointment on a daily basis, simply by knowing that the situation is here to stay, and that recovery is most unlikely. Secondly, the situation is worsened by the fact that many of the LTCs, for example rheumatoid arthritis and stroke, are conditions which are more commonly found in the older adult and that advancing age and a reduction in cognitive abilities may well add further burdens (Jones, 2006). However, some LTCs may occur in younger populations; for example, psoriasis is a long-term skin disease that manifests itself in late adolescence and early adulthood, and sometimes even earlier. The clinical symptoms of this psoriasis can be debilitating, in particular long-term skin irritation (de Korte *et al.*, 2004) and can have serious psychological effects on the individual with depression often a long-term consequence of living with this condition (de Korte *et al.*, 2004; Stern *et al.*, 2004; Tying *et al.*, 2006).

Cognitive aspects of an LTC

Whilst it has earlier been suggested that when people are first faced with an LTC they tend to experience a sense of uncertainty, they also have to begin to make sense of their new condition. They have to understand the condition, to the extent of knowing what aspects of their lives it can affect, what restrictions it places on them and how best to cope with current and future difficulties. Charmaz (1995) posits that people view their bodies in a new light, which inevitably alters their self-perceptions and self-concept. For example, incontinence, and the risk and fear of incontinence, as in the case of multiple sclerosis, can have far-reaching consequences for both the management and the progress of the condition. A person may perceive the situation to be hopeless, a self-assessment which would affect their general well-being. They may as a result, withdraw from ordinary daily activities and isolate themselves from the company of others (Link and Phelan, 2006; Mitterness and Barker, 1995). Nicolson and Anderson (2001) demonstrated that patients considered their incontinence was a source of great embarrassment. This personal assessment can, however, be erroneous and distorted by age as ageing brings with it some declining cognitive function (Skarupski *et al.*, 2006). Also, they have to place that condition within their daily lives, and commonly, the condition and its management take priority over and influence all actions of the day. The ensuing loss of confidence and loss of belief that the action they take might make a difference to their health (British Medical Association, 2008) can adversely affect their psychological well-being. This point of view is well supported by the work of Meyer *et al.* (1985), Weinman and Petrie (1997) and Williams (1997), who find that cognitive representations, where people create their own models or representations of their condition, are important factors that contribute to their adaptive actions. Leventhal *et al.* (1984) and Leventhal and Diefenbach (1991) had earlier proposed the basis for this concept when they proposed a self-regulated model, where people's representations of their condition are based around distinct components which can then determine their coping with the condition (see Chapter 8 for further discussion on this model). Cognitive behaviour therapy (CBT) is used as a popular intervention to help people understand their condition, appraise their situation and thereby cope better with its various, and at times very demanding, facets. CBT is the form of treatment which considers the role of thinking in how an individual feels and behaves. It was originated by Ellis (1980) and is referred to in Chapter 6.

Personality and its role in LTCs

In the search for an explanation as to why psychological effects are sequels of LTCs, numerous studies have focused upon the possible influence personality might have on the long-term unwell person. Personality has subsequently been argued as particularly implicated both in the development and establishment of an LTC. For instance, Ouellette and Di Placido (2001) have suggested that personality can influence health outcomes through mediating and moderating variables. Personality is seen as potentially able to affect health and influence a condition. This belief can be traced back more than 2,000 years to Hippocrates (*ca.* 460 BC to *ca.* 370 BC). People's attitudes and habits, which form part of the characteristics that make up their individuality and, therefore, personality, are considered to be fairly stable over time. They have long-lasting beliefs, likes and dislikes, views towards objects, ideas or concepts and they tend to do things in a consistent and particular way (Sanderman and Ranchor, 1997). In addition, their personality traits are also said to be stable over time (Ranchor *et al.,* 1996). Examples of personality traits are extraversion, denoting the extent to which a person is comfortable in the presence of others; introversion as to how stable a person's emotions are; and openness, which refers to how open an individual is to experiencing new things. These traits are seen as unique characteristics that distinguish one person from another. Altogether these personality characteristics may potentially form a significant factor that predicts the onset of a condition as well as its progression.

When examining the relationship between personality and a long-term physical condition two approaches are usually considered: the specificity approach and the generality approach (Cohen, 1979; Hawkins, 1982; Sanderman and Ranchor, 1997).

The specificity approach

The specificity approach refers to the person's personality traits that relate to a specific LTC. For example, it is suggested that there is a coronary-prone personality and a cancer-prone personality. People with type A personality, who display such features as hostility, competitiveness, impatience, time-urgency and aggression, are more prone to heart disease than people with type B personality, a trait characterised by patience, ability to relax easily and slowness to anger (Suls and Sanders, 1989). Individuals with type C personality are viewed as apologetic and of an acquiescent disposition, sensitive, overly cooperative and passive. With such a personality they are said to be cancer-prone (Sanderman and Ranchor, 1997).

The generality approach

The generality approach refers to when a person's general susceptibility to an LTC is influenced by personality factors which either facilitate or hinder the onset of a condition. For example, a resilient personality consisting of personal high self-esteem, optimism and perceived control may buffer the deleterious effects of stress on a person, allowing him or her not to develop hypertension and its possible consequence. However, in recent research, the specificity approach is given more attention, whilst the generality approach is viewed as being less important.

Further, there are three approaches which examine how personality influences the development and, particularly the progression of a condition (Krantz and Hedges, 1987). These are the etiologic trait approach, the stress-moderator approach and the illness behaviour approach. In the first, the etiologic trait approach, personality is viewed as a risk factor for a condition, regardless of the existence of any other risk factors. It is, therefore, seen as a predisposition to the condition. The overanxious person may be predisposed to colitis, asthma or arthritis, for example. In the second, the stress-moderator approach, personality is considered as a moderator in the relationship between stress and the condition (Nandino *et al.*, 2003). In the transactional theory regarding stress and the individual, the individual mediates the impact of the environmental stimulus and their response to this, for example, through remaining calm. In addition, the perceptual cognitive and physiological characteristics of the individual also have an effect and become a significant component of the environment (Lazarus, 1976, 1981). The person's personal attributes are, therefore, important in how a stressful event is received by the individual and how it is managed, which then may result in the development of an LTC or not.

In the third, the illness behaviour approach, personality is regarded as affecting the health and illness behaviour of the individual. The illness and personality factors combine in the individual's perception and attentiveness to symptoms and in the individual's likelihood of using health care facilities and seeking medical care. Individual differences are seen to be particularly influential. Depending on these differences, for example, a diabetic person who is predisposed to an anxiety state may see their condition as particularly serious and life threatening and may become extremely meticulous about every aspect of their style of living. Such a situation would add to the demands on this person (see Figure 5.3).

Personality also plays a part in a person's adjustment to an LTC and to the condition's outcome, which either refers to death, relapse or aspects of quality of life. It is argued that the same set of personality factors may not necessarily be responsible for both the onset and the effects of a condition (Nandino *et al.*, 2003). In the study by Nandino *et al.* (2003), the trait of neuroticism was found to be correlated with a slower adjustment to and slower improvement of hypertension.

LTCs and their influence on personality

Whilst there is a predictive role of personality in the onset of coronary heart disease (type A personality) and cancer (type C personality) there is also evidence to suggest that there

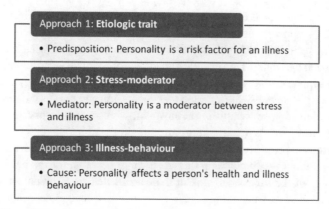

Figure 5.3   The relationship between personality and condition.

could be changes in personality itself as the affected individual experiences the LTC and its effects. Nelson *et al.* (2003), for example, showed that a significant number of people with multiple sclerosis displayed a change in personality after as short a time as 3 years and that this change was not only apparent, but was often accompanied by an effect on an individual's emotional functioning.

A similar argument is made by Sanderman and Ranchor (1997) for a change of personality in those with long-term cardiovascular disorders, although the association between the disorders and personality change was weak and is still undergoing further assessment. Hostility, as a reaction to a condition is, however, consistently observed in some persons with coronary heart disease (Sanderman and Ranchor, 1997). In their study of cardiac artery disease, Helmers *et al.* (1993) found that hostility scores were positively related to ischaemia. Such findings support or confirm the characteristics identified within the type A personality concept, suggesting that indeed this personality type could either precede the onset or accentuate coronary heart disease. Further, Sundin *et al.* (1994) showed that type A personality, based both on self-report and observations by the spouse, changed from pre- to post-test, in an experimental group. They also found some changes in some of the cardiovascular parameters, which illustrated a possible link between change in personality and long-term outcome.

Further, the existence of type C personality becomes more noticeable in the progression of an LTC. Women who have had cancer for some time tend to repress their emotions, especially negative emotions such as anger, and they have a tendency not to make personal demands (Amelang *et al.,* 1996). Additionally, irrespective of gender, Quander-Blaznik (1991) found an association of low expression of anxiety and unfulfilled need for closeness in individuals with a type C personality who had lung cancer.

Interventions in LTCs

Once an LTC is firmly diagnosed, it becomes paramount to lessen its impact on the person's general health and, in particular, his or her psychological well-being. The person's quality of life could, as mentioned earlier, be threatened and in some cases greatly diminished. Whilst health care practitioners can consider what can be done for the person, the onus for ensuring that psychological health is preserved remains firmly in what the person does, feels and, especially, thinks. However, health care professionals have an important part to play and can support people in these three domains. In the case of personal action-taking, for instance, Garcia *et al.* (1994) reported that depression and non-use of problem-solving strategies, while people were still in the hospital, were related to psychiatric morbidity in the longer term – the psychiatric morbidity might be an indication of a poor recovery process. Therefore, people require support to assess their condition and what they can do to make a situation less difficult and, therefore, more bearable for them. For example, in the initial stage of the illness, such as in the case of diabetes, the person can be given information on what is happening to them, the way to manage the condition and what other ongoing services are available to them. This approach can reassure them and even help with their general well-being, including psychological well-being. A meaningful conversation could take place between the person and the professional, where the person would start to think through their situation and ask questions to gain answers that would be most valuable to them in the management of the condition.

The adaptations to life and the attempts to create meaning with an LTC are influential periods which can affect the ongoing welfare of the individual. Bandura (1982) sees the onset of an LTC as an occasion where the person is undergoing intense appraisal of their life and the meaning of their illness within this. Bandura (1977) argues that cognitive appraisals are important mediators of action, affect and thought, and are the ways that a person interprets an encounter in its entirety, and its relevance to their well-being (Lazarus and Folkman, 1984). Cognitive appraisals can affect a person's outcomes by increasing their self-efficacy and their belief that they can control and manage the situation they are in. The concept of self-efficacy encapsulates the view that in an adverse situation, the affected person plays the most important part of appraising how well they can execute the course of action required to deal with that situation. In other words, the person's own judgment of self-efficacy will influence or determine the choice of activity, amount of effort to be expended and perseverance with a solution for an obstacle. This judgment may also determine how successful they are with coping with the emotions attached to their condition. Bandura (1982) proposed that if the person perceived that they would be inefficacious in dealing with their condition, the condition itself would become anxiety provoking for them. So, helping the person to clearly think through a condition and its various aspects would be an important way to help them manage that condition.

In order to manage a situation, Bandura (1977) proposes that interventions should help people set alternative sub-goals to guide longer term behaviour and smaller goals instead of big ones. The person's small but sustained achievement would then increase their self-efficacy. By simply encouraging their self-belief, people with an LTC can increase their self-esteem and provide themselves with some hope for the future. Helping them to think positively about the management of their condition would be an effective addition to their behaviour change as well (Sanderson, 2004).

The aim is to develop a strong sense of self-efficacy behaviour in the person. Low self-efficacy suggests that the person may give up persevering with the management of their condition and see everything in a negative way. They will also have a greater physiological response to the condition, a situation which would present itself as stressful to them. People with high self-efficacy may also be more prepared to use their knowledge and help themselves more, especially in their behaviour. However, knowledge of the condition may not change the behaviour of the person altogether. Clark and Gong (2000), Holman and Lorig (2000), and Von Korff *et al.* (2005) postulate that knowledge of the disease does not necessarily change the behaviour of the affected person and that a more active self-management approach is desirable both for people and their families.

Consequences to the person of having an LTC

LTCs have known detrimental effects on the person who has an established LTC. Although Cassileth *et al.* (1985) did not find a relationship between psychological variables (such as anxiety, worry and low mood) and survival rate among those with LTCs there is now adequate up-to-date evidence to suggest the existence of such a relationship. Conrad (1987), Bury (1997) and Veenstra *et al.* (2005) confirm that an LTC almost inevitably introduces uncertainty in the life of the person, a threat to their life and identity and the way they manage their regimens. Greer (1994) also points out that passive and helpless or hopeless responses are related to poor outcome but a fighting spirit can lead to a favourable outcome. Quality of life and psychological well-being will both be at risk. Further, Carver *et al.* (1994) demonstrated that a sense of pessimism was related to a poorer adjustment over time, among women with breast cancer. People's coping styles played a great part in those who displayed a better outcome. For example, lower depression and anxiety was found in those who actively sought ways to cope with their condition, than those who just accepted they had a new situation to deal with. Also, those with better outcomes had acted quite swiftly to deal with their condition as soon as diagnosis was made and showed improvement at follow-up sessions. However, in some conditions, this improvement or indeed the positive outcome may be difficult to establish. In the case of the person with multiple sclerosis, for example cognitive dysfunction may well exist; it is known that up to 60% of people with this condition will show this impairment, which could, in many cases, make it difficult for the person to deal with their regime (Lyon-Caen *et al.*, 1986; Rao *et al.*, 1991; Benedict *et al.*, 2001; Chiaravalloti and De Luca, 2003; Lima *et al.*, 2007).

Implications for the professional of caring for someone with an LTC

When planning and providing care for the person with an LTC the health practitioner has various aspects to consider. The affected person should be encouraged to be more involved in their care. This will encourage autonomy, reduce the psychological ill-effects on them and increase their sense of self-efficacy and ultimately their quality of life and general well-being. Practitioners must be on the lookout for any abnormal behaviour, unclear expressions of thoughts and extreme variations in mood in the persons they look after.

Particular attention should be paid to those individuals who have a tendency to isolate themselves from others, indulge in as little social interaction as possible, express ideas of frustration and feelings of distress. Hauenstein (1990) and Kuster and Merkle (2004) suggest that these are signs for taking some sort of action.

Developing therapeutic relationships between the person and the professional, or encouraging such a relationship between the person and their carer is also beneficial and is a strong predictor of adaptation to an LTC (Sarason *et al.*, 2001; Schmaling and Sher, 2000). In contrast difficult or unhelpful relationships can have a detrimental effect on the psychological well-being of people with an LTC. Revenson *et al.* (1991) argue that strained relationships, for example those involving criticism, absence of support or unwanted support, are associated with poor psychological adjustment to LTCs, including rheumatoid arthritis.

Finally, the professional must keep in mind that a type A personality can be modified (Helmers *et al.*, 1993). So, although people with type A personality are predisposed to cardiac conditions and such a personality may still prevail after they have had a long-term heart condition diagnosed and dealt with, it may still be possible to help them improve their quality of life.

Supporting the psychological well-being of people with LTCs

The availability of support is seen as pivotal in helping people with LTCs. The onset of a condition, be it an acute or long-term one, carries with it a certain amount of stress (Greenberg, 2002). In order to cope with such stress, individuals find benefit in seeking support from others or in receiving support without asking. It is useful for the professional to be alert to providing support, especially to those who may be reluctant to seek assistance because, for example, they think they have no future left or there is nothing anyone can do to help them. They should be made aware that assistance through informational and emotional support does exist, is vital for their well-being and is associated with better psychological adjustment (Wills and Fegan, 2001).

Additionally, Lepore (2001) finds that people facing LTCs who perceive that others are willing to help and support them are likely to experience enhancement in feelings of self-worth, sense of control and cognitive adaptations such as the ability to find benefits in the experience. Thus, they will be in a position not only to receive and keep to their regimen, but also to enhance their quality of life.

Furthermore, support can be more effective and long lasting if it is complemented with some sort of counselling approach where the person is allowed to express their views, problems and fears. Enabling a person with an LTC to disclose his or her difficulties or fears may help them to regulate their emotions by changing their focus of attention, increasing their habituation to negative emotions and facilitating positive cognitive reappraisals of threats they perceive (Stanton and Danoff-Borg, 2002). Sturgeon *et al.* (2005) state in their study on the usefulness of counselling in disease that it improves the psychological well-being of frequent attendees and people with asthma, diabetes and hypertension.

Assessment of mental health

It is vital that a psychological assessment of a person with an LTC is carried out as part of the initial assessment and ongoing work with that person. A number of psychometric tools exist for that purpose. Two simple, easy to use and non-invasive ones are the General Health Questionnaire (GHQ-12) (Goldberg and Williams, 1992) and the Psychological General Well-Being Index (PGWBI) (Dupuy, 1984). The GHQ-12 can be supplemented by the use of the PGWBI. A combination of both would be useful in the care situation.

The general health questionnaire

The GHQ-12 (Goldberg and Williams, 1992) is designed to detect non-psychotic psychiatric disorders in people using a self-report approach. Its purpose is to identify cases as well as the degree of the disorders (see Table 5.2).

The GHQ-12 aims to identify two main types of problems: (1) inability of a person to carry out normal 'healthy' functions and (2) the appearance of new phenomena of a distressing nature in a person. Thus, the questionnaire focuses on breaks in normal functioning. It measures personality disorders or patterns of adjustment, and is designed to measure four identifiable elements of distress: depression, anxiety, social impairment (not able to function with and around people) and hypochondriasis (the feigning of illness). Table 5.3 shows the first three items of the questionnaire, which correspond to the first three aspects referred to in Table 5.2 earlier. This questionnaire must be used by someone who is conversant with the purpose of the tool, skilled in the interpretation of its score and knowledgeable about how to use the data that it elicits

Scoring of GHQ-12

The measure consists of 12 items (see Table 5.3), each of which refers to the experience of a particular symptom or item of behaviour in the recent past, using a four-point Likert scale: 0 = 'less than usual', 1 = 'no more than usual', 2 = 'rather more than usual' or 3 = 'much more than usual'. Respondents simply have to underline one of these statements for each item. A total score for a respondent, obtained by the sum of their ratings on the scale

Table 5.2   Aspects of the GHQ-12 Questionnaire.

Ability to concentrate
Managed amount of daily sleep
Feeling of usefulness
Capability to make decisions
Perceived intensity of strain
Management of difficulties
Ability to enjoy normal day-to-day activities
Ability to face problems
Feeling of unhappiness and depression
Loss of personal confidence
Thought of worthlessness
Degree of feeling of happiness, all things considered

Table 5.3   The GHQ-12 questionnaire (extract).

We should like to know if you have had any medical complaints and how your health has been in general, over the last few weeks. Please answer the following questions simply by underlining the answer which you think most nearly applies to you. Remember that we want to know about the present and recent complaints, not those that you had in the past.

Have you recently . . .

1.	been able to concentrate on whatever you're doing?	Better than usual	Same as usual	Less than usual	Much less than usual
2.	lost much sleep over worry?	Not at all	No more than usual	Rather more than usual	Much more than usual
3.	felt that you are playing a useful part in things?	More so than usual	Same as usual	Less useful than usual	Much less useful

can, therefore, range from 0 to 12. Either of the first two ratings on the scales receives a zero value. Equally, either of the other two ratings receives a value of 1. Scores are useful for comparing degrees of disorder and higher scores indicate a greater probability of a psychological problem, with scores of 4 or above being indicative of a psychiatric disorder (Goldberg and Williams, 1992).

The psychological general well-being index

The PGWBI (Dupuy, 1984) is a health-related quality of life questionnaire developed to produce a self-perceived evaluation of psychological well-being expressed by a summary (see Table 5.4). In its original format it consists of 22 items. However, in its shortened format, the one recommended here, it consists of only six items that relate to the domain of anxiety (question 1), vitality (questions 2 and 6), depressed mood (question 3), self-control (question 4) and positive well-being (question 5). Each item is rated on a six-point scale, from 0 to 5. A score of 30 points would indicate a maximum level of well-being and one of 0, the minimum level of well-being. The PGWBI has been validated and used in many countries on large samples of the general population and on specific population groups (see, for example, Barlesi *et al.,* 2006; Grossi *et al.,* 2006).

Conclusion

The presence of an LTC usually compels individuals to appraise their life situation both for now and the future. This appraisal, influenced by personality factors, often leads to a changed emotional state characterised by the symptoms and behaviour seen in depression. Depression and a lowered mood add to the problems of these individuals and diminish their quality of life. Health and lay care workers should learn to recognise the signs of psychological difficulties and mental impairment. This particularly applies to health workers who can also use valid and reliable tools to assess psychological effects in people

Table 5.4   The Psychological General Well-Being Index (PGWBI).

Please read: The following questions ask you about how you feel and how things have been going with you. For each question check ☐ the answer which best applies to you.

1. **Have you been bothered by nervousness or your 'nerves' during the past month?**
   (Check one box)

   Extremely so – to the point where I could not work or take care of things . . . . . .   ☐ 0

   Very much so   ☐ 1

   . . . .

   Quite a bit   ☐ 2

   . . . .

   Some – enough to bother me   ☐ 3

   . . . .

   A little   ☐ 4

   . . . .

   Not at all   ☐ 5

   . . . .

2. **How much energy, pep or vitality did you have or feel during the past month?**
   (Check one box)

   Very full of energy – lots of pep   ☐ 5

   . . . .

   Fairly energetic most of the time   ☐ 4

   . . . .

   My energy level varied quite a bit   ☐ 3

   . . . .

   Generally low in energy or pep   ☐ 2

   . . . .

   Very low in energy or pep most of the time   ☐ 1

   . . . .

   No energy or pep at all – I felt drained, sapped   ☐ 0

   . . . .

3. **I felt downhearted and blue during the past month.**
   (Check one box)

   None of the time   ☐ 5

   . . . .

   A little of the time   ☐ 4

   . . . .

(Continued)

Table 5.4   The Psychological General Well-Being Index (PGWBI). (*Continued*)

Some of the time	☐ 3
A good bit of the time	☐ 2
Most of the time	☐ 1
All of the time	☐ 0
4. **I was emotionally stable and sure of myself during the past month.** (Check one box) None of the time	☐ 0
A little of the time	☐ 1
Some of the time	☐ 2
A good bit of the time	☐ 3
Most of the time ,	☐ 4
All of the time	☐ 5
5. **I felt cheerful and light hearted during the past month.** (Check one box) None of the time	☐ 0
A little of the time	☐ 1
Some of the time	☐ 2
A good bit of the time	☐ 3
Most of the time	☐ 4
All of the time	☐ 5

Table 5.4   The Psychological General Well-Being Index (PGWBI). (*Continued*)

6. I felt tired, worn out, used up or exhausted during the past month. (Check one box)	
None of the time	☐ 5
A little of the time	☐ 4
Some of the time	☐ 3
A good bit of the time	☐ 2
Most of the time	☐ 1
All of the time	☐ 0

and think of appropriate interventions such as counselling and CBT that are known to improve individuals' affect by making them think through their situation. A reappraisal can raise the individual's perception of their condition, increase their level of self-efficacy, control and optimism and in this way enable them to manage or tolerate their condition better. Consequently, there will be an improvement in their quality of life.

References

Alexander, T. (2002) *A Bright Future for all: Promoting Mental Health in Education*. The Mental Health Foundation, London.

Amelang, M., Schmidt-Rathjens, C. & Matthews, G. (1996) Personality, cancer and coronary heart disease: further evidence on a controversial issue, *British Journal of Health Psychology*, 1, pp. 191–205.

Anderson, R.J., Freedland, K.E., Clouse, R.E. & Lustman, P.J. (2001) The prevalence of comorbid depression in adults with diabetes: a meta-analysis, *Diabetes Care*, 24, pp. 1069–1078.

Bandura, A. (1977) Self-efficacy: toward a unifying theory of behavioral change, *Psychology Review*, 84, pp. 191–215.

Bandura, A. (1982) Self-efficacy mechanism in human agency, *American Psychologist*, 37, pp. 122–147.

Barlesi, F., Doddoli, C., Loundou, A., Pillet, E., Thomas, P. & Auquier, P (2006) Preoperative psychological global well being index (PGWBI) predicts postoperative quality of life for persons with non-small cell lung cancer managed with thoracic surgery, *European Journal of Cardio-Thoracic Surgery*, 30(3), pp. 548–553.

Benedict, R. H. B., Prore, R. L., Miller, C., Munschauer, F. & Jacobs, L. (2001) Personality disorder in multiple sclerosis correlates with cognitive impairment, *Journal of Neuropsychiatry and Clinical Neuroscience*, 13(1), pp. 70–76.

British Medical Association (2008) *Caring for the NHS @ 60, 1948–2008*. British Medical Association. Available at: http://www.bma.org.uk/ (accessed on August 22, 2008).

Bury, M. (1997) *Health and Illness in a Changing Society*. Routledge, London.

Carver, C. S., Pozo-Kaderman, C., Harris, S. D. *et al.* (1994) Optimism versus pessimism predicts the quality of woman's adjustment to early stage breast cancer, *Cancer*, 73, pp. 1213–1220.

Cassileth, B. R., Lusk, E. J., Miller, D. S., Brown, L. L. & Miller, C. (1985) Psychological correlates of survival in advanced malignant disease, *New England Journal of Medicine*, 312, pp. 1551–1555.

Chapman, D. P., Perry, G. S. & Strine, T. W. (2007) The Vital Link Between Chronic Disease and Depressive Disorders. Preventing Chronic Disease. Available at: http://www.cdc.gov/pcd/issues/2005/jan/04_0066.htm (accessed on 10 July 2009).

Charmaz, K. (1991) *Good Days, Bad Days: The self in Chronic Illness and Time*. Rutgers University Press, New Brunswick, NJ.

Charmaz, K. (1995) The body, identity, and self: Adapting to impairment. *The Sociological Quarterly*, 36(4), pp. 657–680.

Chiaravalloti, N.D. & De Luca, J. (2003) Assessing the behavioral consequences of multiple sclerosis: an application of the frontal systems behavior scale (FrSBe), *Cognitive and Behavioral Neurology*, 16(1), pp. 54–67.

Clark, N. M. & Gong, M. (2000) Management of long-term disease by practitioners and patients: are we teaching the wrong things? *British Medical Journal*, 320, pp. 572–575.

Cohen, F. (1979) Personality, stress and the development of illness. In: *Health Psychology: A Handbook, Theories, Applications and Challenges of a Psychological Approach to the Healthcare System* (eds G. C. Stone, F. Cohen, N. E. Adler & associates), New York, Guildford, pp. 77–111.

Conrad, P. (1987) The experience of illness: recent and new directions. In: *The Experience and Management of Chronic Illness* (eds J. A. Roth & P. Conrad), JAI Press, Greenwich, Connecticut, pp. 1–31.

Cordova, M. J., Cunningham, L. L., Lauren, L. C., Carlson, C. R., Charles, R. & Andrykowski, M. A. (2001) *Journal of Consulting and Clinical Psychology*, 69(4), pp. 706–711.

Danoff-Borg, S. & Revenson, T. A. (2000) Rheumatic illness and relationships: coping as a joint venture. In: *The psychology of couples and illness* (eds K. B. Schmaling & T. G. Sher), American Psychological Association, Washington, DC, pp. 105–133.

Dickens, C., McGowan, L., Clark, C. D. & Creed, F. (2002) Depression in rheumatoid arthritis, *Psychosomatic Medicine*, 64, pp. 52–60.

Dupuy, H. J. (1984) Psychological General Well-Being (PGWB) index. In: *Assessment of Quality of Life in Clinical Trials of Cardiovascular Therapies* (eds N. K. Wegner, M. E. Mattison, C. D. Furberg & J. Ellinson), Le Jacq, New York, pp. 170–183.

Ellis, A. (1980) Rational-emotive therapy and cognitive behavior therapy: similarities and differences, *Cognitive Therapy and Research*, 4(4), pp. 325–340.

Evans, D. L., Charney, D. S. & Lewis, L. (2005) Mood disorders in the medically ill: scientific review and recommendations, *Biological Psychiatry*, 58, pp. 175–189.

Ferguson, S. (2002) *Student Mental Health: Planning, Guidance and Training*. Lancaster, Lancaster University. Available at: http://www.studentmentalhealth.org.uk (accessed on February 2, 2010).

Folkman, S. & Greer, S. (2000) Promoting psychological well-being in the face of serious illness when theory, research and practice inform each other, *Psycho-Oncology*, 9, pp. 11–19.

Garcia, L., Valdes, M., Jodar, I., Riesco, N. & Deflores, T. (1994) Psychological factors and vulnerability to psychiatric morbidity after myocardial infarction, *Psychotherapy and Psychosomatics*, 61, pp. 187–194.

Goldberg, D.P. & Williams, P. (1992) *A User's guide to the General Health Questionnaire*. NFER-Nelson, London.

Golden, S. H., Williams, J. E., Ford, D. E., *et al.* (2004) Depressive symptoms and the risk of type 2 diabetes: the atherosclerosis risk in communities study, *Diabetes Care*, 27, pp. 329–435.

Greenberg, J. S. (2002) *Comprehensive Stress Management* (8th edn). McGraw-Hill, Boston.

Greer, S. (1994) Psychological response to cancer and survival, *Psychological Medicine*, 21, pp. 43–49.

Grossi, E., Groth, N., Mosconi, P., *et al.* (2006) Development and validation of the short version of the Psychological General Well-Being Index (PGWB-S), *Health & Quality of Life Outcomes*, 4, pp. 88–96.

Hawkins, D.R. (1982) Specificity revisited: personality profiles and behavioural issues, *Psychotherapy Psychosomatics*, 38, pp. 54–63.

Hauenstein, E. J. (1990) The experience of distress in parents of chronically ill children. Potential or likely outcome? *Journal of Clinical Child Psychology*, 19, pp. 356–364.

Helmers, K. F., Krantz, D. S., Howell, R. H., Klein, J., Bairey, N. & Rozanski, A. (1993) Hostility and myocardial ischaemia in coronary artery disease patients: evaluation by gender and ischaemic index. *Psychosomatic Medicine*, 55, pp. 29-36.

Heun, R., Papassotiropoulos, A., Jessen, F., Maier, W. & Breitner, J. C. (2002) A family study of Alzheimer's disease and early- and late-onset depression in elderly patients, *Archives of General Psychiatry*, 58(2), pp. 190–196.

Heun, R. & Kockler, M. (2003) Gender differences in the cognitive impairment of Alzheimer's disease, *Archives of Women's Mental Health*, 4(4), pp. 129–137.

Holland, J. C. & Gooen-Piels, J. (2003) Principles of psycho-oncology. In: *Cancer Medicine* (eds J. F. Holland *et al.*) (6th edn). B.C. Decker, Ontario.

Holman, H. & Lorig, K. (2000) Patients as partners in managing chronic diseases, *British Medical Journal*, 320, pp. 526–27.

House, A., Hackett, M. & Anderson, C. (2001) *Effects of Antidepressants and Psychological Therapies for Reducing the Emotional Impact of Stroke*. Royal College of Physicians, Edinburgh.

Jones, F. (2006) Strategies to enhance chronic disease self-management: how can we apply this to stroke? *Disability and Rehabilitation*, 28, pp. 13–14, 841–847.

Jonkman, E. & De Weerd, A. (2001) Quality of life after a first ischaemic stroke: long term developments and correlations with changes in neurological deficit, mood and cognitive impairment, *Acta Neurologica Scandinavia*, 98, pp. 169–175.

de Korte, J., Sprangers, M. A., Mombers, F. M. & Bos, J. D. (2004) Quality of life in patients with psoriasis: a systematic literature review, *Journal of Investigative Dermatology Symposium Proceedings*, 9, pp. 140–147.

Krantz, D. S. & Hedges, S. M. (1987) Some cautions for research on personality and health, *Journal of Personality*, 55, pp. 351–357.

Krueger, G., Koo, J., Lebwohl, M., Menter, A., Stern, R.S. & Rolstad, T. (2001) The impact of psoriasis on quality of life: results of a 1998 National Psoriasis Foundation patient-membership survey, *Archives of Dermatology*, 137, pp. 280–284.

Kuster, P. A. & Merkle, C. J. (2004) Caregiving stress, immune function, and health: implications for research with patients of medically fragile children, *Issues in Comprehensive Pediatric Nursing*, 27, pp. 257–276.

Lazarus, R. S. (1976) *Patterns of Adjustment*. McGraw-Hill, New York.

Lazarus, R. S. (1981) The stress and coping paradigm. In: *Models for clinical psychopathology* (eds C. Eisdorfer, D. Cohen, A. Kleinman & P. Maxim). Spectrum, New York.

Lazarus, R. S. (1999) *Stress and Emotion: A New Synthesis*. Free Association Books, London.

Lazarus, R. S. & Folkman, S. (1984) *Stress, Appraisal and Coping.* Springer, New York.

Lepore, S. J. (2001) A social-cognitive processing model of emotional adjustment to cancer. In: *Psychosocial interventions for Cancer* (ed B. Anderson). American Psychological Association, Washington, DC, pp. 99–118.

Lethborg, C., Aranda, S. & Kissane, D. (2008) Meaning in adjustment to cancer: a model of care. *Palliative and Supportive Care,* 6(1), pp. 61–70.

Leventhal, H., Nerenz, D. R. & Steele, D. J. (1984) Illness representations and coping with health threats. In: *Handbook of Psychology and Health: Social Psychological Aspects of health* (eds A. Baum, S. E. Taylor & J. E. Singer), vol. 4. Earlbaum, Hillsdale, New York, pp. 219–252.

Leventhal, H. & Diefenbach, M. (1991) The active side of illness cognition. In: *Mental Representation in Health and Illness* (eds J.A. Skelton & R.T. Croyle). Springer, New York, pp. 219–252.

Lewis, S., Dennis, M., O'Rourke, S. & Sharpe, M. (2001) Negative attitudes among short term stroke survivors predict worse long-term survival, *Stroke,* 31, pp. 1640–1645.

Lima, F. S., Simioni, S., Broggimann, L., *et al.* (2007) Perceived behavioral changes in early multiple sclerosis, *Behavioural Neurology,* 18, pp. 81–90.

Link, B. G. & Phelan, J. C. (2006) Stigma and its public health implications, *Lancet,* 367(9509), pp. 528–529.

Lyon-Caen, O., Jouvent, R., Hauser, S., Chaunu, M. P., Benoit, N., Widlocher, D. & Lhermitte, F. (1986) Cognitive function in recent onset demyelinating diseases, *Archives of Neurology,* 43, pp. 1138–1141.

McVeigh, K. H., Mostashari, F. & Thorpe, L. E. (2002) Serious psychological distress among persons with diabetes – New York City, MMWR. *Morbidity and Mortality Weekly Report,* 53, pp. 1089–1092.

Meyer, D., Leventhal, H. & Gutmann, M. (1985) Common-sense models of illness: the example of hypertension, *Health Psychology,* 4, pp. 115–135.

Mitterness, L. S. & Barker, J. C. (1995) Stigmatising a normal condition: urinary incontinence in late life, *Medical Anthropology Quarterly,* 9(1), pp. 188–210.

Morrison, V. & Bennett, P. (2006) *An Introduction to Health Psychology.* Pearson/Prentice-Hall, Harlow.

Nandino, J. L., Reveillère, C., Sailly, F., Moreel, V. & Beaume, D. (2003) Sensibilité aux tracas quotidiens et personalité des étudiants. Importance du facteur Nevrosisme, *Revue Européenne de Psychologie Appliquée,* 53(3-4), pp. 239–244.

Nelson, L. D., Elder, J. T., Tehrani, P. & Groot, J. (2003) Measuring personality and emotional functioning in multiple sclerosis: a cautionary note, *Archives of Clinical Neuropsychology,* 18, pp. 419–429.

Nicolson, P. & Anderson, P. (2001) The psychological impact of spasticity-related problems for people with multiple sclerosis: a focus study group. *Journal of Health Psychology,* 6(5), pp. 551–568.

Ouellette, S. C. & Di Placido, J. (2001) Personality's role in the protection and enhancement of health: where the research has been, where it is stuck, how it might move. In: *Handbook of Health Psychology* (eds A, Baum, T.A. Revenson, & J.E. Singer). Lawrence Erlbaum Associates, Mahwah, NJ, pp. 175–193.

Quander-Blaznik, J. (1991) Personality as a predictor of lung cancer: a replication, *Personality and Individual Differences,* 12, pp. 125–130.

Ranchor, A. V., Bouma, J. & Sanderman, R. (1996) Vulnerability and social class: differential patterns of personality and social support over the social classes, *Personality and Individual Differences,* 20, pp. 229–237.

Rao, S. M., Leo, G. C., Bernardin, L. & Unverzagt, F. (1991) Cognitive dysfunction in multiple sclerosis 1. Frequency, patterns, and prediction, *Neurology*, 41, pp. 685–691.

Redwood, S. K. & Pollak, M. H. (2007) Student-led stress management programme for first-year medical students, *Teaching and Learning in Medicine*, 19, pp. 1, 42–46.

Revenson, T. A., Schiaffino, K. M., Majerovitz, S. D. & Gibofsky, A. (1991) Social support as a double-edged sword: the relation of positive and problematic support to depression among rheumatoid arthritis patients, *Social Science and Medicine*, 33, pp. 807–813.

Rosenberg, M. (1975) *Society and the Adolescent Self-Image*. Princeton University Press, Princeton, N.J.

Sanderman, R. & Ranchor, A. V. (1997) The predictor status of personality variables: etiological significance and their role in the course of disease, *European Journal of Personality*, 11, pp. 359–382.

Sanderson, C. A. (2004) *Health Psychology*. John Wiley & Sons, Inc., New York.

Sarason, B. R., Sarason, I. G. & Gurung, R. A. R. (2001) Close personal relationships and health outcomes: a key to the role of social support. In: *Personal Relationships: Implications for Clinical and Communit Psychology* (eds B.R. Sarason & S. Duck). John Wiley & Sons, Inc., Chichester, pp. 15–41.

Schmaling, K. B. & Sher, T. G. (2000) (eds) *The Psychology of Couples and Illness*. American Psychological Association, Washington, DC.

Shih, M. & Simon, P. A. (2008) Health-related quality of life among adults with serious psychological distress and chronic medical conditions, *Quality of Life Research*, 17, pp. 521–528.

Shih, M., Hootman, J. M., Strine, T. W., Chapman, D. P. & Brady, T. J. (2006) Serious psychological distress in US adults with arthritis, *Journal of General Internal Medicine*, 21, pp. 1160–1166.

Siegel, M. J., Bradley, E. H., Gallo, W. T. & Kasl, S. V. (2004) The effect of spousal mental and physical health on husbands' and wives' depressive symptoms, among older adults: longitudinal evidence from the health and retirement survey, *Journal of Aging and Health*, 16, pp. 398–425.

Skarupski, K. A., Mendes De Leon, C. F., McCann, J. J. *et al.* (2006) Is lower cognitive function in one spouse associated with depressive symptoms in the other spouse? *Aging & Mental Health*, 10(6), pp. 621–630.

Smith, A., Krishnan, J. A., Bilderback, A., Riekert, K. A., Rand, C. S. & Bartlett, S. J. (2006) Depressive symptoms and adherence to asthma therapy after hospital discharge, *Chest*, 130, pp. 1034–1038.

Smith, J. A. & Osborn, M. (2007) Pain as an attempt on the self: an interpretative phenomenological analysis of the psychological impact of chronic benign low back pain, *Psychology and Health*, 22, pp. 517–534.

Stanton, A. L., Danoff-Borg, S., Sworowski, L. A., Collins, C. A., Branstetter, A., Rodriguez-Hamley, A. *et al.* (2002) Randomized controlled trials of written emotional expression and benefit finding in breast cancer patients, *Journal of Clinical Oncology*, 20, pp. 4160–4168.

Stanton, A. L. & Danoff-Borg, S. (2002) Emotional expression, expressive writing, and cancer. In: *The writing cure* (eds S. J. Lepore & J. M. Smyth). American Psychological Association, Washington, DC, pp. 31–51.

Stern, R. S., Nijsten, T., Feldman, R. S., Margolis, D. J. & Rolstad, T. (2004) Psoriasis is common, carries a substantial burden even when not extensive, and is associated with widespread treatment dissatisfaction, *Journal of Investigative Dermatology Symposium Proceedings*, 9, pp. 136–139.

Sturgeon, P., Hicks, C., Barwell, F., Walton, I. & Spurgeon, T. (2005) Counselling in primary care: a study of the psychological impact and cost benefits for four chronic conditions, European Journal of Psychotherapy, *Counselling and Health*, 7(4), pp. 269–290.

Suls, J. & Sanders, G. S. (1989) ' Why do some behavioral styles place people at higher risk?' In: *In search of coronary-prone behavior* (eds A. W. Siegman & T. M. Dembroski). Erlbaum, Hillsdale, NJ, pp. 1–20.

Sundin, O., Ohman, A., Burrell, G., Palm, T. & Strom, G. (1994) Psychophysiological effects of cardiac rehabilitation in post-myocardial infarction patients, *International Journal of Behavioral Medicine*, 1, pp. 55–75.

Tying, S., Gottlieb, A., Papp, K., *et al.* (2006) Etanercept and clinical outcomes, fatigue, and depression in psoriasis: double-blind placebo-controlled randomized phase 111 trial, *The Lancet*, 367, pp. 29–35.

Veenstra, M, Moum, T. & Roysamb, E. (2005) Relationship between health domains and sense of coherence: a two-year cross-lagged study in patients with chronic illness, *Quality of Life Research*, 14, pp. 455–465.

Von Korff, M., Glasgow, R. E. & Sharpe, M. (2005) Organising care for chronic illness, *British Medical Journal*, 325, p. 94.

Warwick, I., Maxwell, C., Statham, J., Aggleton, P. & Simon, A. (2008) Supporting mental health and emotional well-being among younger students in further education, *Journal of Further and Higher Education*, 32(1), pp. 1–13.

Weinman, J. & Petrie, K. L. (1997) Illness perceptions: a new paradigm for psychosomatics? *Journal of Psychosomatic Research*, 2, pp. 133–116.

Williams, C. (1997) A cognitive model of dysfunctional illness behavior, British *Journal of Health Psychology*, 2, pp. 153–165.

Wills, T. A. & Fegan, M. F. (2001). Social networks and social support. In: *Handbook of Health Psychology* (eds A. Baum, T. A. Revenson & J. E. Singer). Lawrence Erlbaum Associates, Mahwah, NJ, pp. 139–173.

Chapter 6

Counselling skills

Val Sanders
School of Health and Social Care, University of Greenwich, Eltham, London, UK

Introduction

This chapter offers health care practitioners a contextualised discussion of how counselling skills may enhance their practice. In recognising the many elements of loss which face the patient coming to terms with a long-term condition (LTC), I start by considering elements of grief theory, to help the practitioner recognise these phenomena, and particularly how they might manifest with this patient group. To help understand people's responses to LTCs, I move on to look at three principal perspectives of counselling theory from the person-centred, psychodynamic and cognitive behavioural schools, in each case with examples of how these might provide helpful insight and be used to support patients as they adjust to living with an LTC.

Grief theory and adapting to change

Loss is a feature of LTCs. Whatever the nature of the condition, whether progressively degenerative or more static in symptoms, implicit in the experience are elements of loss. For this reason, I start the chapter by discussing in some depth aspects of grief theory. This discussion explores what happens psychologically when an individual suffers a loss and describes, from the perspective of various theorists, how that individual goes about accommodating the loss into his or her lifestyle. An understanding of the process of adjustment to an LTC will help the health care professional to recognise and respond more effectively to her patients' needs.

In this section, we will illustrate the experience of loss of health or mobility, and then go on to consider in particular the work of three theorists (Kübler-Ross, Parkes and Worden) who have written extensively on grief work, all having worked as practitioners and researchers in the field. Although much has been added to the literature on this subject, with some notable contributions by Leader (2008) and Machin (2009), the work of these three is seminal and has great relevance for today. The health care professional who understands the principles discussed in this section will be well placed to provide a sympathetic and valuable service to her patients.

Long-Term Conditions: Nursing Care and Management, First Edition. Edited by Liz Meerabeau and Kerri Wright.
© 2011 Blackwell Publishing Ltd. Published 2011 by Blackwell Publishing Ltd.

Though not in the context of extraterrestrial life forms, the now immortalised (though misquoted) words of Mr Spock might well bear out the experience of those who develop a long-term life-limiting condition: 'It's life, Jim, but not as we know it!' From the point of confirmed diagnosis, there is a commonly felt sense that life will never be the same again, and the journey of ongoing adjustment begins.

Whatever experiences and circumstances the past has brought, the salient point is that life has been 'as we know it', and there has been a sense of familiarity and, therefore, security in that knowledge. Whatever surprises or traumas have occurred have been faced from a position of acquaintance with one's body and a presumption of, and reliance upon, the sustainability of its functions and capacities, part of what Colin Murray Parkes designates as our 'assumptive world' (Parkes, 2006). With the diagnosis of an LTC slowly dawns a sense of not knowing, of wondering what the body will do/not do, and how one will adapt, and how close friends and family will manage with a sometimes seemingly cataclysmic change of circumstance. The psychological process of working through and adapting to a one-off, or continuing series of changes (as in the case of a degenerative condition), is analogous to that of bereavement and the course of adapting to the loss of a loved one. Bereavement is normally accompanied by a series of expressions and behaviours that typify grief. Albom's poignant chronicling of the failing health of his erstwhile professor, Morrie Schwartz, who contracted Lou Gehrig's disease (otherwise known as amyotrophic lateral sclerosis, or motor neurone disease) recognises this phenomenon:

'As my old professor searched for answers, the disease took him over, day by day, week by week. He backed the car out of the garage one morning and could barely push the brakes. That was the end of his driving. He kept tripping, so he purchased a cane. That was the end of his walking free. He went for his regular swim . . . and found he could no longer undress himself. So he hired his first home care worker . . . who helped him in and out of the pool, and in and out of his bathing suit. In the locker room, the other swimmers pretended not to stare. They stared anyhow. That was the end of his privacy'.

(Albom, 2003: 8, 9)

Before considering the specifics of grief theory, it may be helpful to keep in mind the existential perspective on death: that an awareness of the certainty and inevitability of death gives meaning to life (May, 1975; Yalom, 1980). Again, Morrie Schwartz's perspective in the face of his degenerative condition illustrates this: 'It's only horrible if you see it that way', Morrie said. 'It's horrible to watch my body slowly wilt away to nothing. But it's also wonderful because of all the time I get to say good-bye' (Albom, 2003: 57).

Many of us, however, live our lives as if we were immortal and take no cognisance of the fragility of our existence – until, that is, something happens to draw it to our attention. Perhaps a loved one dies, and we are suddenly confronted with the reality that our assumptive world is subject to change and the certainties we believed in are based upon a false belief of immortality. Or we may receive a diagnosis of a terminal or debilitating condition, which reminds us of the vulnerability of our health and, in a stark and unkind way, that we are going to die (whether sooner or later).

And so begins a process of adjustment and accommodation, coming to terms with a finite loss, and/or the loss of a faculty or lifestyle which, heretofore, we had not even questioned. The ease and manner in which we adapt are determined by the interplay of a myriad of historical, psychological, personality and situational factors. But work through the process we must if we are to manage the rest of our lives successfully. Whether the grief process follows a bereavement by death, or the loss of health (or job, location, etc.), theorists agree that there are two major areas which need to be successfully negotiated to ensure ongoing psychological health. These relate to coming to an intellectual and emotional acknowledgement of the loss and working through the accompanying affect on the one hand and making physical, emotional and practical adjustments to life on the other, in order to face a different future without the lost object. These have been defined in the dual process model of bereavement as the 'loss orientation' and the 'restoration orientation' (Stroebe and Schut, 1999).

Proponents of various theories offer models of stages (Kübler-Ross, 1970), phases (Parkes, 1972) and tasks (Worden, 2003), but each recognises that coming to terms with loss is a process involving both these orientations, which has recognisable characteristics, as well as individual degrees of deviance.

The theory of Elizabeth Kübler-Ross

Kübler-Ross originally worked with dying patients, and identified a staged model of working through terminal diagnosis. This model has, equally, been applied to the process of bereavement. There are five stages to her model: (1) denial, (2) anger, (3) bargaining, (4) depression and (5) acceptance (see Figure 6.1).

Initially, Kübler-Ross recognises that a normal response to being told of a life-limiting condition is 'denial and isolation' (Kübler-Ross, 1972: 34–43), and this is a commonly recognised coping mechanism which protects the patient from the full impact of the bad news. At a particularly vulnerable point in life, having suffered or been told of a significant loss, a patient may not have the psychological resources to face the reality of this immediately, and so denial serves to cushion the blow in the initial stages.

The second stage of Kübler-Ross's model is 'anger' (Kübler-Ross, 1972: 44–71) where the patient responds to his sense of powerlessness over this thing which has invaded his body by feelings of rage, much as a cornered animal would do. The anger serves no real purpose, but gives a spurious sense of power in a situation which feels disempowering. It is most frequently directed at loved ones or health care professionals, but viewing it as a normal part of the grief process may make it easier not to take such attacks personally.

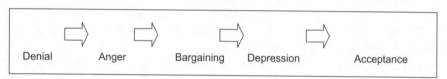

Figure 6.1   Stages of grief (Kübler-Ross, 1970).

Kübler-Ross's third stage – 'bargaining' (Kübler-Ross, 1972: 72–74) – is one which has received less attention from later writers, and she was of course writing 40 years ago, at a time when the United Kingdom was less multicultural than it is today. Developing the theme of seeking to combat the sense of powerlessness experienced by loss, she notes a time where anger dissipates and gives way to bargaining, usually with God. If there is no change in the situation from an angry outburst, perhaps we can reason with the Almighty to twist his arm for at least a little more time? With the increasing secularisation of society, less is heard today of this concept, although there may be elements of bargaining with medical staff, for example in wishing to delay the inception of treatment programmes until after an important life event like a daughter's wedding.

Moving on through anger and bargaining, Kübler-Ross then identifies a stage where the patient hits 'depression' (Kübler-Ross, 1972: 75–98). This is where he realises that attempts to counter the illness are fruitless. There may be financial and emotional pressures surfacing as time passes, and the illness affects not only the patient, but also his loved ones. The situation feels bleak, so spirits flag and depression sets in.

In the final stage of Kübler-Ross's model, depression gives way to 'acceptance' (Kübler-Ross, 1972: 99–121). The time of struggling against the diagnosis is over and, coupled with the dawning realisation of the inevitability of the disease process taking its course, comes an acceptance of this, and a sense of preparedness, having mourned the past. I well remember working with a middle-aged Iraqi gentleman, Mr Y, referred to me for counselling through the NHS, whose surgery for bowel resection had met with complications and left him to live with a colostomy. He seemed stuck in the 'anger' stage of the grief process when I first met him and spent much of our time together railing against the doctors, the NHS, this country and God. He was consumed with the unfairness of his predicament. The 'bargaining' phase for Mr Y took the form more of regrets and 'if onlys', many of which were very poignant, as he had left his two daughters in Iraq when he fled the country, and feared he would never see them again. One morning, however, he arrived at the surgery bearing a letter from his daughter, announcing her pregnancy and writing fondly of what she would tell her child of its grandfather. He told me of this with tears in his eyes, and appeared finally at peace, as if this knowledge enabled him to accept the reality of his physical limitations and impending death with a serenity I had not witnessed before. I believe he had reached stage 5.

The work of Colin Murray Parkes

Building on the work of Kübler-Ross, and resulting from his various research projects – principally the London study, the Bethlem study and the Harvard study – Parkes (1998) identified differing categories of complicated responses to bereavement (chronic, inhibited and delayed), as well as synthesising the common elements of 'normal' grief behaviour and affect disturbance, into his phased model.

Clearly discernible to Parkes were four phases to the outworking of grief: (1) numbness, (2) pining, (3) disorganisation and despair and (4) reorganisation and recovery (see Figure 6.2).

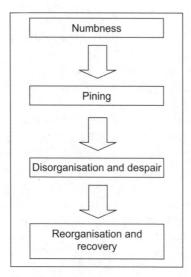

Figure 6.2 Phases of grief (Parkes, 1998).

Although the phases of grief are not presented as linear, and Parkes recognised fluidity between them, it is common that the bereaved person's initial response to loss is characterised by shock and disbelief – a seeming inability to comprehend or assimilate what has happened (phase 1). In much the same way as the body goes into shock following physical trauma, which to some extent anaesthetises the sufferer in the early stages, so Parkes saw that the trauma of psychological loss usually resulted in an initial sense of shock and numbness for the bereaved person, even if the death was expected. The bereaved person may seem in a daze and feel slightly removed from reality for a while – a protective mechanism to mitigate the full impact of the pain of loss, equating to Kübler-Ross's first stage.

Numbness, Parkes observed, gave way to pining and searching behaviour (phase 2) after a while. His theory links here particularly with Bowlby's work on attachment and loss, and the protest which Bowlby associated with the first response to separation anxiety (Parkes *et al.*, 1996), may be demonstrated very clearly through the pining phase of grief. Emotional pining and longing is often accompanied by tears and sobbing, but also outbursts of anger and rage. Physical searching behaviour may frequently be witnessed, for example visiting places associated with the deceased.

The progression from protest to despair, which Bowlby (1998) identifies as separation behaviour, links to Parkes' third phase of grief: disorganisation and despair. The searching ceases, and the truth begins to dawn that death is final and the deceased will not be returning (or in our case, the recognition that a specific faculty or aspect of healthy functioning is over). The world of the bereaved person is turned upside down, and despair and apathy may set in. Life, as it was known previously, has come to an end, and psychologically giving that up can be very painful and disorientating, particularly where there has been a dependent relationship.

The final recovery phase happens when the bereaved person begins to reinvest in life and look to the future, finding interest in other things and a new identity, rather than being focused on the deceased. Parkes' later emphasis on psychosocial transition theory (Parkes in Stroebe *et al.*, 2006; Parkes, 2008) highlights the restoration orientation, which will be more familiar to medical and nursing practitioners as the natural focus of their clinical practice. However, awareness of the need for grieving and paying attention to the loss orientation is essential for health workers accompanying those with chronic and debilitating conditions upon their journey. Parkes cites the example of a patient with severe arterial disease who was informed that he needed to have his leg amputated. The patient's initial response was denial and a refusal to agree to the surgery. Parkes recognises that the consultant's first impulse was to underline to the patient the seriousness of his condition and inform him that without the surgery he would die. This would, however, be a counter-productive strategy at this stage, as it would serve to raise the patient's level of fear and thus seriously impair his capacity for rational thought. With an understanding of grief theory and the process of bereavement, clinicians can provide containment by offering patients time to talk through the situation, both with themselves and their families, and allow them time to begin the process of adjustment rather than prematurely being forced to sign a consent form (Parkes, 2008).

The contribution of J. William Worden

Like Parkes, William Worden bases much of his work on grief on the seminal work of John Bowlby on attachment and loss, and the content of his discussion on responses to grief overlaps with Parkes' views. Where Worden differs from Parkes is in the focus of his work. His most famous book, *Grief Counselling and Grief Therapy* (Worden, 2003), is written primarily for the clinician and those therapeutically accompanying the bereaved person on their journey. Rather than just describing the phases or stages of grief, Worden defines four tasks which he believes typify the activity involved in resolving grief. In the description of each task, factors which might inhibit its successful completion are identified which may help the clinician recognise where remedial work needs to be focused (see Figure 6.3).

The four tasks may be achieved and worked on in any order, and/or concurrently, and may be revisited at many points in the grief cycle. The first task is to 'accept the reality of the loss' (Worden, 2003: 27), and its antithesis 'denial' is the focus of therapeutic

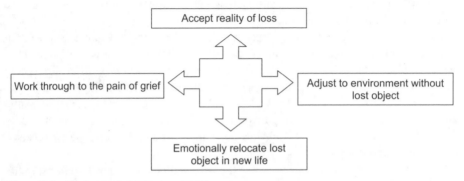

Figure 6.3   Tasks of grief (Worden, 2003).

work at this stage. Like Kübler-Ross and Parkes, Worden recognises the numbness which frequently accompanies the shock of bereavement, and he elaborates further to consider the psychological numbness which is often sought when the bereaved seeks to minimise the impact of the loss in a variety of ways, such as denying it has happened, denying its importance, denying its finality. In the same way as Parkes underlined the fluidity of his stages of grief, Worden notes that his tasks may not be accomplished in order, though normally it is necessary at least to have made some progress on task one before task two can be engaged in.

Task two is about the importance of expressing emotional affect. Worden calls it 'working through to the pain of grief' (Worden, 2003: 30). Again, this is reminiscent of Bowlby's attachment theory, where appropriate emotional responses need to be linked with autobiographical competence in order for psychological healing to take place (Holmes, 1993). A patient who becomes fixated at this point will be cut off from his emotions. Thus, the practitioner's task will be to encourage and facilitate the patient in accessing these feelings, and opportunity may be given for this in a GP surgery, at the bedside, in a formal counselling setting, or at home/with friends and family. The point of relevance for health care professionals particularly is to allow space for feelings to be expressed, where there might be a tendency to focus exclusively on practical matters.

Task three links Parkes' third and fourth phases, which Worden refers to as 'adjusting to an environment in which the deceased is missing' (Worden, 2003: 32). This necessarily involves disorganisation and breaking down of the old way of life which included the deceased (or elements of health which are being lost through an LTC), and making appropriate changes which will allow the person to continue living, but living a different life. Worden notes that this involves both internal and external adjustments (e.g. having to move home, or having adjustments made like the installation of handrails or a downstairs shower room). Where people struggle or fail to achieve this task will be when they find it difficult to adapt; for example, the person with diabetes who ignores exhortations to limit sugar intake and make dietary adjustments, the smoker who refuses to stop even though he develops chronic obstructive pulmonary disease (COPD), or the person with arthritis who disregards the need to follow an exercise regime. Whilst putting strong pressure on a patient to adhere to such medical advice may be counter-productive in these instances, by understanding non-compliance as a part of the grieving process, the health care professional will be better equipped to explore with the patient what underlies his behaviour (probably a struggle to accept the diagnosis), and seek to find ways of working through this, either together or by putting in place specific psychological support.

Worden's final task is about 'emotionally relocating the deceased and moving on with life' (Worden, 2003: 35). In earlier editions of his book, he wrote of 'withdrawing emotional energy from the deceased and reinvesting it in another relationship' (Worden, 2003: 35), but later felt that 'relocating' was a more accurate verb, concurring with the sentiments of continuing bonds with the person who has died, but memorialising him or her in such a way that it does not interfere with ongoing life (as might happen in the early stages of bereavement). For patients with LTCs, 'emotionally relocating' their loss would involve a recognition of the aspect of themselves that they have lost, and incorporating this into their ongoing sense of self, rather than resorting to a tendency to define the self in terms of their current restrictions and lack of abilities. This might be much in the same way as a middle-aged woman might wistfully pick up an old photograph of herself, with a youthful figure, dark hair and unlined complexion, but rather than simply bemoaning the fact that those days are gone and she is now fat, grey-haired and wrinkled, she might recognise that the image in the photograph is one and the same person, and the experiences of youth have made her who she is today.

Different factors affect the bereavement journey, such as the nature and circumstances of the death and the relationship with the deceased, and are crucial determinants of the complexity of the grieving process. Similarly, it is helpful to give cognisance to a range of socio-economic and ethnographic considerations which will affect the patient's ability to adapt to living with an LTC, including the following: general personality traits such as intrinsic disposition to optimism/pessimism; levels and mechanisms of support; the nature of the condition and whether it is degenerative, or requires drastic change, such as adherence to a dietary regime; dependency upon and frequency of hospital visits/inpatient episodes; marital and family status; and financial situation.

For health care practitioners, supporting patients through the grief process, whatever the loss, can be challenging. This can sometimes lead to a focus on 'tasks'. Given that the resolution of grief is a process, and accompanying the bereaved can be a difficult, if not harrowing, experience for the helper, it could be argued that the notion of having 'tasks' to accomplish stems from wishing to mitigate the discomfort of the helplessness which professionals so often feel. If we can tell ourselves that we are 'doing' something, rather than just 'being with' our patients, maybe we feel less uneasy and more effective as practitioners.

As will be apparent, although these various theorists have been able to identify common patterns in people's responses to loss and bereavement, each individual's experience is unique and will demonstrate distinctive nuances of feelings, thoughts and behaviour. Each patient undertaking the journey of living with an LTC will wish to process and express his experience in his own way, so, whilst a general theoretical understanding of the nature of bereavement will be helpful for practitioners in recognising the manifestations of symptoms of stages in the process, careful listening skills and attitudes are of paramount importance to understand the distinctive experience of each person.

A knowledge of grief theory is, thus, a helpful framework from which to start to understand patients' experiences of coming to terms with an LTC. Building on this, we turn now to bring insights to bear from specific counselling theories, and will consider person-centred, psychodynamic and cognitive behavioural perspectives. Common to these, and, indeed, to all theories of counselling, is a belief in the centrality of the relationship between therapist and client, though the emphasis and nature of this relationship may vary depending upon the theoretical underpinning. We will start our exploration with a consideration of the person-centred approach, because the relationship pertaining in this model is the most appropriate for nursing and medical practitioners, and their patients.

Counselling theory: Person-centred perspectives

We turn here to the work of Carl Rogers who identified three prevailing attitudes which are necessary for good relationships in general, and also for the professional helper seeking to establish a therapeutic relationship with her patient. These 'core conditions' are generally referred to as: empathy, unconditional positive regard (also called 'acceptance', 'respect', 'non-possessive warmth' or 'prizing') and congruence (also called 'transparency', 'genuineness' or 'authenticity') (Rogers, 2001; Mearns, 1994; Mearns and Thorne, 1996).

Empathy

Much has been written about 'emotional intelligence' (Goleman, 1997) and the capacity to empathise with another (Klein, 1975) as an important milestone in psychological development. An individual completely devoid of this ability would be deemed sociopathic, and yet cultivating an attitude of real empathy towards another is a rigorous, self-abstinent discipline which few naturally attain. The process of fostering an empathic attitude necessarily means suspending our own assumptions – which are usually tainted either by our own experience of similar situations or our acquired theoretical knowledge. In seeking to practise truly empathic responses, we need to listen without preconceived ideas to the communication of our patient, not only his expressed words, but his non-verbal cues. Our aim is to achieve an understanding of what his experience is like for him. 'Such an understanding involves on the therapist's part a willingness and an ability to enter the private perceptual world of the client without fear and to become thoroughly conversant with it' (Thorne, 1994: 38).

Aspiring to this empathic ideal is only half the challenge, as we then need to find a way to communicate this understanding back to our patient. Rogers, reflecting upon research carried out by Heine, notes: 'The therapist procedure which they [the participants] had found most helpful was that the therapist clarified and openly stated feelings which the client had been approaching hazily and hesitantly' (Heine, 1950 cited in Rogers, 2001: 43). One day, whilst telling me of having heard news of his elderly mother's diagnosis of Parkinson's disease, my client, Mr P, struggled to articulate his thoughts. I heard the fear underneath his broken sentences '...wondering how she'll manage ... I'm not able to get over there very frequently ... what if she falls? ... she's very independent ... it would break her heart ...' and softly suggested to him that he seemed afraid of her having to go into residential accommodation, whereupon he broke into huge sobs. He had not been able to voice his fear, but when it was recognised and I communicated to him that I understood what he was trying to tell me, it was a great relief. Specific skills related to this process are discussed below.

For nursing and medical practitioners, an empathic attitude also extends to an openness to recognise and interpret a patient's signals as to when he might desire time to talk through his feelings and fears, which may present a great challenge, and generate additional stress, should this occur in the middle of a busy working day. It might be that a later appointment needs to be made, or another professional on the multidisciplinary team needs to be brought in for the purpose, but the importance of maintaining an empathic attitude to the patient throughout is paramount, even if simply to acknowledge the need.

Unconditional positive regard

The second of Rogers' core conditions is unconditional positive regard. This requires of the practitioner an ability to recognise her own judgments, prejudices and agendas as well as her preconceived ideas and expectations of how patients 'should' be responding. If a patient remains stuck in the 'denial' phase of bereavement and stoutly refuses to accept. his diagnosis, and therefore the treatment to be administered, the practitioner may struggle to respect his position as it interferes with her ability to do her job.

Rogers articulates some very self-searching questions in this regard: 'Can I permit him [the patient/client] to be what he is – honest or deceitful, infantile or adult, despairing or overconfident? Can I give him the freedom to be? Or do I feel that he should follow my advice, or remain somewhat dependent on me, or mould himself after me?' (Rogers, 2001: 53). Cultivating an accepting attitude may be aided by seeking deliberately to empathise with the patient, and trying to imagine life from his point of view; thus, empathy and unconditional positive regard are mutually complementary attitudes. Working with an elderly Indian gentleman who had suffered a mild heart attack, I was aware that I strongly disagreed with his avowed intention not to tell his wife and family of the seriousness of his condition. I struggled to accept his decision, and respected his right to it, as I deemed it ultimately unhelpful for his wife and family. What enabled me to move closer to a position of unconditional positive regard was to seek to empathise with his perspective, and try to imagine what it would be like from his cultural position, where it was anathema for the male of the household to demonstrate weakness, and where he had to maintain dignity at all times (even to the point of seeking to hide his feelings in the session). The more I was able to appreciate his values, the easier it became.

Congruence

The third aspect of the core conditions trilogy is congruence. This is best described as the practitioner genuinely being herself in her dealings with her patients; in other words, the feelings and thoughts that she has on the inside are matched by those expressed on the outside. Congruence might also be apparent in our willingness to be honest with a patient about life expectancy or expected difficulties ahead, rather than offering false hope and colluding with denial. There may also be occasions where judicious use of self-disclosure may feel appropriate, and a practitioner may wish to share with a patient something of her own personal or professional experience, though there needs to be careful consideration of the likely effect of any personal revelations upon the patient, and the practitioner needs to ensure that whatever might be shared is done so for the patient's benefit and not as a self-indulgence. Congruence is more about not withholding the self than being self-revealing. Mearns and Thorne (1996: 82) elaborate on this distinction: '[C]ongruence is not the same as self-disclosure. . . . Our own view is that clients differ on this matter; for some the counsellor's self-disclosure is a relevant dimension in that it helps the client to trust. For other clients, however, it is equally obvious that the last thing they want to do is listen to the counsellor's experience.'

Being congruent can, at times, be challenging, but when offered in the context of a trusting relationship, can also be very powerful. I well remember a session with a middle-aged English woman who presented as rather austere, and by whom I felt slightly intimidated. She was bemoaning the fact that her grandchildren had not been to see her for weeks and she believed her daughter kept away deliberately. She had been referred to me because she was lonely and her worsening asthma made getting out increasingly difficult.

We had explored her experiences in childhood and recognised a pattern of behaviour which pushed others away by her prickliness. With my heart in my mouth, I was able to reflect back to her my own experience of her and talk about my own sense of feeling a little intimidated by her demeanour as an immediate way in to this issue. Slowly, we were able to explore the reasons for her prickliness along with its impact upon others, and take a perspective on its long-term result of achieving exactly the opposite of what she needed, which was friendships and comfort.

Blocks in the practitioner

The core conditions may be construed as attitudes to which we aspire, but there are several obstacles along the way which may block any one of them. Blocks to empathy may take the form of straightforward practical concerns, such as physical tiredness and the stresses of pressurised workloads. It is not without reason that the British Association for Counselling and Psychotherapy (BACP) includes self-respect as a principle in its ethical guidelines (BACP, 2002), and places emphasis on the practitioner's need to care for herself and ensure that she is equipped in this way to undertake her role. Medical and nursing professionals are all too familiar with working under pressure, and self-care may take second place to the exigencies of the workload. The pressures of twenty-first century living can thus militate against maintaining an empathic attitude to patients.

Personal identification with the experience of a patient may also make it difficult to empathise, as there might be unconscious assumptions that this person's experience will necessarily be the same as our own, whereas in practice, although it might bear some resemblance, it might also be very different. We need to be vigilant that we are aware of this possibility.

Issues of cultural, religious, socio-economic or other types of difference may also preclude empathic understanding, either because the practitioner is not taking difference into account at all, or because she might hold stereotypical beliefs about certain religions, cultures, etc., which may not apply to her patient. There is a need to be cautious about presumptions around diversity, and to be willing to enquire and check these out with the individual concerned.

A further area which might complicate and hamper the understanding and expression of empathy is where the practitioner earnestly desires to find a solution to the patient's anguish or difficulty. Particularly for nursing and medical staff, where the thrust of the profession is geared towards making better and treating symptoms, it can be difficult for the practitioner to stay with the patient's distress, appreciating the therapeutic value of empathising. As recognised above, working through diagnoses and coming to terms with living with chronic complaints is a process which can be protracted, and some of the most vital help which a caring professional can offer is to be willing to stay with uncomfortable feelings without seeking to cure them. Solutions detract from empathy.

Blocks to unconditional positive regard come in the form of the practitioner's own prejudices and biases and fixed ideas as to what is 'right' and 'appropriate'. Suspension of individual opinions and judgments can only be achieved once the practitioner becomes aware of them, so self-reflexiveness is an important skill to learn in this regard.

There may be many reasons why a helping professional abstains from being congruent with her patient, principally connected with fear of exposure, embarrassment, a desire 'not to hurt' the other party, or a consideration of the patient's family – who may, for example, have expressed a wish that their loved one not be informed of the severity of his condition, and it may well be appropriate not to be congruent at certain times. The deciding factor needs to be the welfare of the patient, and as practitioners we need to make the decision based upon his best interests.

Thus, the core conditions describe succinctly the prevailing attitudes to which the professional helper may aspire as a basis for her listening work. Attitudes alone, however therapeutic they may be, are not enough. As mentioned above, for instance, actually feeling empathy towards another is, per se, insufficient to help the person. It needs to be communicated in an appropriate manner.

Communication skills

Before examining the nature of specific interventions, it needs to be noted that communication happens on a variety of levels by diverse overt and covert signals. It is well known that only 7% of the impact of any message is determined by the actual words spoken. More significant is the tone of voice used (36% of the impact) and the accompanying body language (57% of the impact) (Mehrabian, 1971). In this section, we review these aspects of communication, and consider specific verbal and non-verbal counselling skills.

Non-verbal communication

Nursing and medical staff are receiving a plethora of messages from, and communicating as many to, their patients, in addition to the verbal signals consciously given. The smallest cue indicating care or disinterest, attention or distraction, openness or hostility is likely to be picked up unconsciously, and affect the response and disposition of the recipient. Whilst we are training ourselves to be vigilant in reading the body language of our patients, and respond to the whole message rather than just the spoken language, we may be sure that they, too, will be reading us and will be susceptible to our nuances of vocal inflexion, eye movement and gesture.

Of crucial importance in building a relationship of trust with a patient is an attitude of attentiveness and non-verbal communication which gives the message: 'I am concerned that you hear what I have to tell you clearly, and I am listening to you. I am interested in what you have to say and how you are feeling. I want to understand you'. Imparting difficult news of an unwelcome diagnosis or shocking prognosis may evoke feelings in the practitioner, which would propel her to avoid eye contact, or taking time with a patient, as it is such a distasteful thing to do. At these times more than ever, nevertheless, it is important to seek to suspend our own discomfort and be attentive and available to our patient.

A 30-year-old Ugandan called Dominic recounts his experience of discovering his diagnosis:

> 'The attitude of these people was strange. . . . He never answered [when I asked what was wrong with me], but told the nurse to put my name in the foreigners register. . .

The nurse brings the register and puts it on the table and there is this big sticker – AIDS. So that's how I came to know.'

(Richardson and Bolle, 1992: 26)

Although it is unlikely that the doctor or nurse were gratuitously callous and uncaring about the patient, a greater awareness of their non-verbal communication and a recognition of the impact of this on the patient would have enhanced the encounter and imparted a greater sense of worth to Dominic, already reeling from the shocking discovery of his condition. At times such as this, there is an even greater need to be treated with respect and dignity as a human being, and it may take a supreme effort on the part of the practitioner to look beyond the disease and the treatment programme to the individual who is facing a life crisis. Davis Phinney, an American Olympic cyclist, was diagnosed with Parkinson's disease in 2000. He writes of his difficulty adjusting and getting on with life in these words: 'I think what happens quite frequently when you have a disabling disease is that you stop being able to see the forest because the tree is right in your face all the time. . . . All you see are the shadows of the disease and its effects on you' (Carley, 2007: 6). It may also be appropriate to offer time and space, and silence, to give the patient time to absorb the news he has heard, but showing by our continued presence and attention to him that we are supporting and seeking to understand what is happening for him as a person.

Much has been written about body language and postures viewed as 'open' or 'closed' (Fast, 1971; Cohen, 1992; Pease, 1993). A traditionally viewed 'open' body stance of unclenched hands, uncrossed legs and sitting squarely in one's chair may, however, appear a little stilted and unnatural, and the perpetrator may end up feeling uncomfortable and self-conscious, and therefore, not fully receptive to the other. Each individual needs to find his own balance, and be aware of the signals being communicated by, for example, holding a document tightly across the chest with arms folded defensively over it, or fidgeting with a pen, or tossing/attending to his hair. On the other hand, caricaturing conventionally acceptable 'open' body language appears artificial, and thus not congruent.

Offering focused concentration on the patient and not being sidetracked by external distractions conveys a clear message that the patient is important and top priority at that moment. We have probably all had experiences where a spouse, or friend, or GP, or tutor makes affirmative noises to indicate understanding whilst, at the same time, attending to a computer screen or other diversion. The net result is a sense of feeling sidelined and unimportant, and may inspire anger or resentment, and certainly will do little to further the relationship.

In some cultures, prolonged steadfast eye contact may be viewed as challenging and even insolent, and some individuals feel more comfortable than others sustaining another's gaze. It is incumbent upon us to be sensitive to the individual preferences of our patient, and to try to gauge from his response whether we have hit the right balance for that particular person. Whether looking directly at someone or looking away out of respect, what is important is that our attention stays fully with the patient, and our concentration is not usurped by other concerns.

Certain people need more encouragement to talk than others, and it may be appropriate to give a non-verbal signal from time to time to indicate we are still listening, even though we may not be responding with words 'mmm', 'uh-huh', etc. Such wordless noises can be helpful in conveying empathy, as they replicate early communication with the primary caregiver at a pre-verbal time, and so can engage the listener comfortingly at that deeply unconscious level.

Tone of voice and pace of speech is another consideration. A distressed patient may talk in a very rapid and rushed manner, and we can help to slow things down for him by responding more deliberately and unhurriedly, conveying a sense of containment. In the course of a difficult conversation, patients may become distressed, and level and pitch of voice may drop to a whisper, or be broken. In responding to this, the practitioner will best also lower her inflection and allow space for the patient to talk, even if it means remaining in silence for some time.

When communicating difficult diagnoses and prognoses, there may be a tendency for doctors and nurses to hide behind technical terminology, simply because it feels less emotive and more clinical, and therefore less threatening for them. The patient, however, may prefer to hear, and have a better chance of understanding if the words used are in vernacular English, and we need to be prepared to explain things several times, as it may be difficult for the patient to absorb first time around.

Kate Carr recalls her visit to the hospital where she was told of her cancer diagnosis:

'I can see the X-ray clearly now as I write, even though I only saw it that once. What's harder for me to remember is what Mr Sinnett said to me, because, as he started to speak, I started to float away. His voice became muffled. I seemed to be looking down at him, at myself, from somehwere near the ceiling. The nurse I hardly registered. One look at her face, full of barely concealed pity, and I turned away from her. . . . I kept asking him to repeat himself. I couldn't take in anything.'

(Carr, 2004: 16)

The other aspect which Kate describes as difficult here is the 'barely concealed pity', and we need to make a very clear distinction between empathy and sympathy. Patients will be comforted and reassured somewhat by empathic responses and vocal inflections, but not by sympathy and pity. We may feel genuine pity for an individual in this position, but it is not likely to be helpful to him if we communicate this. Patients need to feel held and have mirrored for them a sense of containment. So, here is another balance to be achieved between being pragmatic and empathic, as opposed to cold/clinical and sympathetic/pitying.

Specific counselling skills

And so we come to a brief look at some specific interventions which may be helpful for practitioners to master. As mentioned above, the nature of the helplessness engendered in both patient and professional when faced with an LTC may mean that communication is clumsy, uncomfortable or even avoided. Having explicit guidance in this skill may make a world of difference.

Much of the content of conversations between nursing and medical staff and patients is factual – giving and eliciting information about physical considerations and ascertaining specific areas for practical support. Counselling skills can aid us in maintaining a helpful attitude to patients (particularly empathy and unconditional positive regard) and may also enable a deeper exploration of the psychological aspects of living with an LTC. Reflecting skills are the bedrock of many counselling approaches and the health practitioner who is versed in judicious use of these will be able to enhance her therapeutic relationship with her patients.

Reflecting skills

As cited above, in order for empathy to be effective, it needs to be communicated, and the health care professional can, with the simplest of interventions, offer a greater depth of understanding and relationship to this vulnerable group of patients.

Nodding and saying 'yes' every now and then in conversation goes some way to acknowledging what a patient is telling us; however, the patient will really know that he has been understood if he has opportunity to hear the helper quoting his words back to him: 'So, you're feeling quite confused by all this . . .'; 'you've been coping quite well, but now are starting to feel quite depressed about the future . . .'; 'you're telling me it's been hard these last few months and you are concerned about your family as you become less able to care for your children'. Reflecting back to a patient his own words in this way provides him with an opportunity to hear what he has said, and clarify whether this is, in fact, what he feels; it will show him that he has been heard and acknowledged and respected as a whole person, and may encourage him to say more and share more deeply other things which are bothering him, because we have shown that we understand thus far.

Using reflecting skills also serves the purpose of slowing down a conversation, and allowing time for reflection to let the import be absorbed. If a patient talks uninterruptedly for long stretches, the likelihood is that salient points will be missed or glossed over, so by picking up certain words and phrases, the listener helps the speaker to engage more fully with his material. Picking up on significant words and phrases is a skill which may be used to good effect. For example, a patient may make a statement such as: 'When I was first diagnosed with COPD, I was really scared and didn't know how I'd manage, but my family were very kind and the neighbours have been good at looking out for me. . . .' Here he has given an indication of some strong feelings, and yet almost negated them by going on to focus on the kindness of others, a common coping strategy. This may feel more comfortable for the practitioner also, and so the conversation could move on to discussing the level and nature of support received. However, a simple intervention like repeating back the word 'scared' or saying 'you say you felt scared . . .?' might enable the patient to talk about it further, and thus provide a valuable space where these feelings may be explored. Indeed, it may be the only place where the patient has this opportunity, with family and friends wanting to focus on positive, helping messages and not to hear of the underlying fears, as this, in turn, makes them feel helpless or uncomfortable. As something of a leitmotif, reflecting skills may also be overdone, where the helper's responses resemble a parrot's mimicry. However, when undertaken selectively and in an attitude of caring and attentiveness, they can be a very powerful tool to build rapport, enhance the relationship and provide support.

Probing skills

Some patients may benefit from more gentle probing to reach this deeper level understanding, and here tentative questioning may be useful. Bearing in mind the already existing power dynamic in nurse–patient/doctor–patient relationships, any attempt to probe into a patient's emotional life needs particularly to be undertaken with sensitivity and gentleness as an invitation to share more, rather than a directive. For this reason, it may be good to employ softeners such as: 'I'm wondering if you'd like to tell me more about . . .'; 'would it be helpful to explore that a little more?'; 'It sounds as if this has been painful for you. Shall we think about what is at the heart of your distress.' This way the patient has an opportunity to decline further exploration if he is not ready, or is unwilling, to expose his feelings more without seeming to offend the professional.

Once rapport has been built and trust established, it may be possible to go on to probe more obviously: 'and how did that affect you?'; 'what was it like for you when . . .?' In order for the patient not to feel interrogated or bombarded by questions, it is helpful to be clear and ask one question at a time, rather than a multiple of questions, and ask open questions, which invite a full response, rather than closed questions, which invariably lead to further questions, and put the questioner in control of the conversation rather than allowing the patient to determine the direction the dialogue takes by his answers.

The majority of patients welcome an opportunity to talk through their symptoms, fears and other emotions with a congenial listener, and respond willingly when sensitively questioned about their experience and concerns. Many, however, are defensive and unwilling to engage in conversation, at least initially, and may take time to trust a professional sufficiently to open up.

Challenging skills

Although medical and nursing staff are not counsellors, and the deeper, more challenging work of psychotherapy is best left to those trained in the discipline, there may be occasions where gentle challenges are appropriate and, indeed, a nurse or doctor may be well placed to offer these tentatively to their patients. For example, the patient who asserts that he is managing his condition well whilst, at the same time, shaking his head, or affirms his ability to cope in a hesitant or panicky manner, may benefit from having the incongruity brought to his attention: 'Your words are telling me you're doing well, but your head is saying otherwise'; 'You say that you're coping well, but I hear your voice breaking and you don't sound so convincing'. Most patients will be grateful to have been seen in this way provided that they are challenged sensitively and kindly.

Counselling theory: Psychodynamic perspectives

The health care practitioner, thus, appreciates that her patient's non-verbal and covert communication is out of synchronicity with his overt verbal message. Freud's (1962,

1991) discovery of the unconscious offers a plausible explanation for this phenomenon as a mechanism to remove from consciousness unbearable anxiety. Where a patient is exhibiting contradictory behaviour or giving an ambiguous message, we would do well to reflect upon the fact that there is likely to be some anxiety he is seeking to banish from consciousness. A range of psychological defence mechanisms have been identified, and there follows some discussion of some of these: denial, regression, displacement and projection, and how they might manifest in patients with LTCs. The purpose of each defence is to protect the individual from a grim or painful reality. Thus, each operates as a form of denial of the truth.

Denial

As noted earlier when discussing aspects of grief and bereavement theory, denial is a common feature of the early experience of those facing losses of various kinds. Its function is to seek to avoid pain, and it may be a necessary coping mechanism in the early stages of diagnosis or awareness of degenerative conditions, when the full impact of the news may be unable to be assimilated, such as Danny's initial response to being given news of a diagnosis of HIV: 'Hang on a second, they got my test mixed up with somebody else' (Richardson and Bolle, 1992: 20).

However, if denial is protracted, the patient will remain psychologically stuck, and will not be able to move on or make the necessary adaptations to his lifestyle. The most direct form of denial is manifested in a patient's refusal to believe his prognosis, and dismissal of medical advice for ongoing care of his condition, like the morbidly obese patient diagnosed with unacceptably high cholesterol levels, who does not monitor his diet or modify his sugar intake.

There may also be elements of denial demonstrated in a patient's stoicism in the company of his loved ones: an 'I'll be fine' attitude, intended to reassure others as well as himself. Alternatively, the patient may minimise the importance of the loss of faculty by convincing himself that curtailing his physical activities and taking more time to rest would not make much difference to his life, as he prefers a sedentary lifestyle anyway. An appreciation of these natural phenomena of defence is essential for the health practitioner, whose role may include enabling the patient to accept his diagnosis.

Regression

Denial may also appear in more subtle and less easily recognisable ways. Regression and regressive behaviour may indicate a refusal to engage with reality and make the necessary adjustments, seen perhaps in a patient who becomes overidentified with his diagnosis. Reverting to a childlike state of helplessness obviates the need to accept the reality of having to learn new skills and adapt to a new life. The natural position of any patient, particularly an inpatient, is, to some extent, one of regression, by virtue of his being dependent upon others for treatment and care. The fear and anxiety which many patients with LTCs may experience serve to exacerbate this feeling of vulnerability and dependence. The wise practitioner will, however, be alert to patients who might prolong their regressive behaviour as an avoidance of facing reality.

Displacement

Displacement is another psychological defence which is frequently in evidence. The natural feelings evoked, when coming to terms with unpalatable news, frequently include anger and frustration, in response to the sense of powerlessness over a physical condition which has control of the body. Daisy recalls her feelings: 'Well, you know what it is, don't you – "she's got AIDS" that's how we were told. I wanted to punch her. I've never felt so angry in all my life' (Richardson and Bolle, 1992: 38).

Frequently, rather than acknowledging and expressing anger at the situation directly, it is displaced and directed towards others: family, carers and medical staff. A patient who is frustrated because his hands will not stop shaking, or his breathlessness prevents him walking upstairs, may become angry with the care assistant who forgot to take his tea tray away, or the doctor who cannot offer him an appointment for three days, or the nurse who keeps him waiting for ten minutes.

Much of my own work dealing with complaints for the cancer services directorate at a large London teaching hospital, frequently necessitated an understanding of the operation of this defence, and that making a formal complaint was part of the mechanism for expressing anger about the implications of a surgical complication, or death of a loved one which left the instigators feeling powerless and angry. Clinical practitioners may expect to be the recipients of displaced anger, and at times it can be very challenging not to respond defensively or take these attacks personally.

Projection

The phenomenon of projection may be another defence mechanism employed. Rather than admit his own fears for the future, a patient may attribute them to his spouse or his children: 'My wife is very worried about me', or 'I'm concerned about how my wife will cope with my disability'. On the surface, the difficulty lies with the third party; however, underlying these expressions may well be a projection of his own anxiety and apprehension, which he struggles to own or articulate.

The skill for the practitioner is to recognise these defence mechanisms at work. However, rather than trying to dismantle them, it is important, first, to understand what it is they are shielding the patient from, and to help him articulate the anxiety which is being avoided. A huge amount of psychological energy is expended defending the self against anxiety in this way, and the therapeutic value of being able to acknowledge this can be vast. Once the anxiety is named and faced, the patient will almost certainly feel relief, even though it may mean he then has to move on to face distressing reality. Bill Commans, diagnosed with Parkinson's disease, describes how initially he felt 'very sorry for myself. ... I felt defeated', but 'concluded that there was no use in denying that I had it – the disease was not going to disappear. I chose to announce my ailment rather than hide it and I also learned to accept assistance from others' (Carley, 2007: 45). Having come to a place of acceptance, the patient is then enabled to adapt to his situation, and be open to help from others.

Counselling theory: Cognitive behavioural perspectives

Another theoretical perspective through which to construe some of the psychological difficulties which confront people living with LTCs is the cognitive behavioural slant, which views problems largely as the result of distorted thinking, which may be challenged and reality-tested to good effect. The fundamental principle of cognitive behavioural therapies is that events and circumstances are not what cause us distress, but our perception of these which dictates how we feel and behave.

Thus, our attitudes, and what we believe about a given issue, will be the determinant of how well we cope with it. If a person believes, for example, that a diagnosis of renal failure means that he will never be able to engage in normal exercise again, and that being physically active is essential to being happy, he is likely to become depressed and withdraw from physical activities. His depression and withdrawal would be seen, from a cognitive behavioural point of view, as stemming not from his diagnosis per se, but from his irrational beliefs (a) that in order to be happy he must engage in physical activity, and (b) that the malfunctioning of his kidneys precludes him from exercising (whereas, in fact, the reverse may be medically recommended).

In identifying these erroneous beliefs, a medical practitioner may well be able to challenge their validity on factual grounds, and help the patient recognise where he is operating from a position of unrealistic assumptions. This, in turn, may help him see that, although he may have to modify his sports pursuits to some extent, he may be able to engage in other less strenuous activities which can be equally enjoyable.

Cognitive behavioural therapy aims to identify an individual's faulty thinking patterns at various levels – from the more superficial 'negative automatic thoughts' (or NATS) through to deep-seated core beliefs (Westbrook *et al.*, 2008). The process is achieved by working backwards from experiences which have been painful or problematic, by a process of Socratic questioning, to recognising the belief which generates the distress. For instance, a patient may adopt a depressive and fatalistic attitude to his failing health, making comments such as: 'It's just my luck!'; 'I was never going to amount to much anyway and now my chances of success are scuppered'; 'No-one's going to want to marry someone who's going to end up in a wheelchair by the age of 40'. These are NATS, whose foundation may be an underlying core belief that 'I am a bad person', or 'I don't count'. It is this core belief which is generating the patient's distress, and therapeutic change can ultimately only be achieved by challenging the distorted thinking. Feelings and behavioural responses will be remedied consequentially.

This level of therapeutic work may be beyond the scope of medical and nursing practitioners. They may, however, become attuned to recognising distorted thinking by the things patients say, and gently challenge these, thus opening the way to the possibility of change. There are various categories of cognitive distortions which may be discerned, as discussed below.

Dichotomous thinking

Situations are viewed in black-and-white terms, with no middle ground. For example, our patient may be telling himself: 'Because my multiple sclerosis precludes me from becoming an Olympic athlete, my sporting days are over forever; I'm a failure; my life is not worth living.' This type of thinking is often accompanied by unrealistically high expectations of self and others, and thought patterns riddled with extreme demands, which translate as 'shoulds', 'oughts' and 'musts' – what Albert Ellis termed 'musturbation' (Ellis, 1998, 1999). The insistence that things be a certain way leaves no room for compromise or negotiation, and a concomitant sense of failure and despair when things are unable to conform to expectation. A patient needing to undergo a hospitalised treatment procedure, which may preclude her from attending her son's graduation, may torture herself with guilty feelings and negative beliefs about herself as a mother if she has an inflexible, demanding mindset. If she can be helped to recognise that her belief is unrealistic and idealised, she may be helped to a more appropriate emotional response of disappointment. Gentle challenges such as: 'Who says you must?'; 'What would it mean if you didn't?'; 'What would you think of me if I were in your position?' can be helpful to open up other avenues of thinking.

'Catastrophising'/'awfulising'

These distortions are other forms of extreme thinking which can be psychologically very debilitating (Dryden, 2001; Ellis, 1998). This is where a person develops a mindset which always assumes the worst and uses its imagination to fantasise all manner of tragedies, above and beyond the real. Stephen's reaction to being told his HIV+ status could be seen in this category: 'When the news was disclosed to me, I thought of committing suicide straight away' (Richardson and Bolle, 1992: 61). He believed that all was lost, and life was over. A sensitive practitioner may be able to reality check this type of thinking by supplying information about the condition and likely prognosis, and taking time to go over the effects with the patient (possibly several times).

Selective abstractions

Other types of cognitive distortions come under the category of selective abstractions (Westbrook *et al.*, 2008) – where individuals focus on a part of the truth, and either overgeneralise this or filter out other contra-indicatory information. Here, the role of the practitioner may be to draw attention to the twisted thinking, and indicate contrary evidence, or question how it follows that, for example, because there has been one setback, the path is downhill from now on. Depending on the relationship with the patient, this may even be done with humour, as way to help restore perspective to the situation.

Mind-reading/jumping to conclusions

Another category of dysfunctional cognition incorporates those beliefs which rely on the individual's intuition (Westbrook *et al.*, 2008). On these occasions, a person will jump to conclusions about others' beliefs about him, or base his logic upon a feeling. For example, a patient may attend a consultation in a low mood, and convince himself that the outcome will bring bad news because he is feeling down. He will be less likely to hear the reality of the clinician's words, interpreting what he hears in the light of his emotions.

Personalisation and labelling

Habitual patterns of faulty thinking also occur around people's tendency to take things personally, label themselves and criticise themselves. One patient's, Sarah's, reaction to her HIV diagnosis illustrates this: 'I hated myself, I felt dreadful. I felt I must have deserved this, it was like it was my punishment. You hadn't been good enough in your life. It was like the wrath of God' (Richardson and Bolle, 1992: 63). This type of rationale may be seen as a spurious attempt to take some power in a situation which feels out of control. If Sarah believed it was her fault, then it meant she had some influence over the situation, which might have seemed preferable to being a victim of circumstance. Such cognitive distortions may also need to be challenged by practitioners in order to help patients come to a more realistic appraisal of their situation.

Nursing and medical practitioners are unlikely to have the luxury of extended or repeated interviews with their patients in which to engage in intense psychotherapeutic techniques; thus, wisdom and sensitivity is needed to judge what can and can't be achieved in the course of an interaction towards addressing faulty thinking patterns. Simple prompts, which challenge the validity of irrational statements, and seek to establish any evidence for the belief might be all that can be achieved, but may have the effect at least of beginning to help the patient acknowledge alternative ways of viewing things. Such interventions as 'I wonder what makes you say that?', 'Where did that idea come from?' and 'Who told you . . .?' might enable dialogue and exploration to begin.

There is also the possibility that a practitioner may identify patients, who need specific input from psychological therapies, as part of their treatment plan, either through the NHS or on a private basis (perhaps by contacting the BACP). However, nursing and medical practitioners may usefully become skilful in recognising cognitive distortions, and by bringing these to the patient's attention, sow the seeds that there is another perspective, and that the patient has a distorted view of his life or condition which exacerbates his distress.

Conclusion

In conclusion, we have seen how there is a theoretical underpinning to explain some of the psychological difficulties encountered by patients diagnosed and living with LTCs. We have recognised that the processes involved in coming to terms with losing a limb or a faculty, or having to modify an aspect of 'normal' healthy living, is analogous to that of bereavement and losing a loved one, and traced some of the phases of normal grief reactions. The need to contain and accommodate the loss orientation as well as the restoration orientation is a key factor for medical and nursing practitioners in caring for their patients, and empathic, accepting and congruent attitudes and responses are vital in effecting this. The importance of communicating empathy not just in words but also by vocal inflection, facial expression and body language has also been explored.

We have discussed a variety of unconscious psychological defence mechanisms frequently encountered in patients coming to terms with life-limiting and life-threatening conditions, and how an understanding of the underlying anxiety, from which these strategies are designed to protect, is paramount in dealing sensitively with them, and how acknowledging the anxiety and painful feelings, rather than increasing distress, can be a way to open the door to deeper understanding and acceptance.

Cognitive behavioural perspectives have also been highlighted, and awareness drawn to recognising a plethora of types of dysfunctional thinking, and how these might also gently be challenged, in order to help patients embrace a more realistic view of their situation.

Whilst it has only been possible to scratch the surface of this vast and significant aspect of patient care, it is hoped that the insights gained will be of use to enhance the experience of both practitioner and patient.

References

Albom, M. (2003) *Tuesdays with Morrie: An Old Man, a Young Man and Life's Greatest Lesson.* Time Warner, London.

Bowlby, J. (1998) *Loss, Sadness and Depression, Attachment and Loss,* Vol. 3. Hogarth, London.

British Association for Counselling and Psychotherapy (BACP) (2002) Ethical framework for good practice in counselling and psychotherapy (revised edn). BACP.

Carley, G. (2007) *Surviving Adversity: Living with Parkinson's Disease.* Macmillan, London.

Carr, K. (2004). *It's Not Like That, Actually: A Memoir of Surviving Cancer – and Beyond.* Vermilion, London.

Cohen, D. (1992) *Body Language in Relationships.* Sheldon Press, London.

Dryden, W. (2001) *How to Make Yourself Miserable.* Sheldon Press, London.

Ellis, A. (1998) *How to Control Your Anxiety Before It Controls You.* Citadel, New York.

Ellis, A. (1999) *How to Make Yourself Happy and Remarkably less Disturbable.* Impact, California.

Fast, J. (1971) *Body Language.* Pan, London.

Freud, S. (1962) *Sigmund Freud: Two Short Accounts of Psychoanalysis.* Penguin, London,

Freud, S. (1991) *Sigmund Freud: Introductory Lectures on Psychoanalysis.* Penguin, London.

Goleman, D. P. (1997) *Emotional Intelligence: Why It can Matter More Than IQ.* Thorsons Audio, London.

Heine, R. W. (1950) A Comparison of Patients' Reports on Psychotherapeutic Experience with Psychoanalytic, Non-directive, and Adlerian Therapists. Unpublished doctoral dissertation, University of Chicago, Chicago.

Holmes, J. (1993) *John Bowlby & Attachment Theory.* Routledge, London.

Klein, M. (1975) *Love, Guilt and Reparation and Other Works 1921–1945.* Free Press, New York.

Kübler-Ross, E. (1970) *On Death and Dying.* Routledge, Oxford.

Leader, D. (2008) *The New Black: Mourning, Melancholia and Depression.* Hamish Hamilton, London.

Machin, L. (2009) *Working with Loss and Grief.* Sage, London.

May, R. (1975) The Courage to Create. Norton, New York.

Mearns, D. (1994) *Developing Person-Centred Counselling.* Sage, London.

Mearns, D. & Thorne, B. (1996) *Person-Centred Counselling in Action.* Sage, London.

Mehrabian, A. (1971) *Silent Messages.* Wadsworth, Belmont.

Parkes, C. M. (1972) *Bereavement: Studies of Grief in Adult Life.* Penguin, Harmondsworth.

Parkes, C. M. (1998) *Bereavement: Studies of Grief in Adult Life.* Penguin, London.

Parkes, C. M. (2006) *Love and Loss: The Roots of Grief and Its Complications.* Routledge, London.

Parkes, C. M. (2008) *Dr Colin Murray Parkes Presents: Bereavement, Loss and Change,* Vol. 1 [DVD]. Available at: www.mentalhealth.tv.

Parkes, C. M., Stevenson-Hinde, J. & Marris, P. (eds) (1996) *Attachment Across the Life Cycle.* Routledge, London.

Pease, A. (1993) *Body Language: How to Read Others' Thoughts by Their Gestures.* Sheldon Press, London.

Richardson, A. & Bolle, D. (1992) *Wise Before Their Time: People with AIDS and HIV Talk About Their Lives*. Harper Collins, London.

Rogers, C. R. (2001). *First published 1967. On Becoming a Person: A Therapist's View of Psychotherapy*. Constable, London.

Stroebe, M. & Schut, H. (1999) *Death Studies 23:3*. Routledge, London.

Stroebe, M., Stroebe, W. & Hansson, R. O. (eds) (2006) *Handbook of Bereavement: Theory Research and Intervention*. Cambridge University Press, Cambridge.

Thorne, B. (1994) *Carl Rogers*. Sage, London.

Westbrook, D., Kennerley, H. & Kirk, J. (2008) *An Introduction to Cognitive Behaviour Therapy: Skills and Application*. Sage, London.

Worden, J. W. (2003) *Grief Counselling and Grief Therapy: A Handbook for the Mental Health Practitioner* (3rd edn). Routledge, London.

Yalom, I. D. (1980) Existential Psychotherapy. Basic Books, New York.

Chapter 7

Living with long-term conditions: Tommy's story

Tommy Magee

Foreword by Kerri Wright

This chapter is Tommy's story of his life and his long-term conditions (LTCs) told in his own words through a series of interviews. This book contains a large amount of information and theories about LTCs and how these can affect people's lives. It is important though that throughout this emphasis on theory and knowledge, we do not lose sight of the person. Tommy's story shows how LTCs are entwined within the person's life and how these are tied up with the totality of our life experiences. You cannot separate out the LTCs from Tommy or his life. We need to view Tommy as a whole. Many themes in the chapters within this book are touched on in Tommy's story; for example, the psychological effect and social implications of living with LTCs, the importance of self-management and empowerment, the role of medication in supporting Tommy to manage his symptoms, the cognitive behavioural approaches used by Tommy which he learnt within the Expert Patients Programme (EPP).

The theories and insights presented in the different chapters are powerful when they are reflected in a real life context as they are so clearly in Tommy's story. But I am anxious that Tommy's narrative should not be reduced down solely to these applied theories. Tommy's story is vital and important because it is just that; his story. As Dame Cicely Saunders, the founder of the hospice movement said, 'You are important, because you are you' (Clark, 2002). We must remember that the patient or client that sits in front of us with LTCs is first and foremost a person and as a person should be valued for who they are. One of the most powerful ways of developing respect and understanding for a person is through listening to their story.

I am grateful to Tommy for taking the time to share his story and for the insights and reflections that he has offered into his life and health. I am especially grateful to Tommy for sharing his experiences with me, and through this work with the readers of this chapter too.

'I have spread my dreams under your feet;
Tread carefully because you tread on my dreams'
                                    W D Yeats

Long-Term Conditions: Nursing Care and Management, First Edition. Edited by Liz Meerabeau and Kerri Wright.
© 2011 Blackwell Publishing Ltd. Published 2011 by Blackwell Publishing Ltd.

Tommy's story

My name's Tommy and I currently live with a number of LTCs. I was born in Ireland, of a very large family, and am the third eldest. I left home when I was 15 and started work. I worked for over 30 years and eventually retired on health grounds in my late forties. I am currently an expert patient leader and also a member of several steering groups at local hospitals. I am also regularly asked to talk to student nurses at my local university and share my experiences of living with LTCs with them. This is my story.

Long-term conditions

My LTCs basically started in 1984. I had one prior illness to that, which was a burst duodenal ulcer at the age of 26 and I had a lot of complications with it afterwards, particularly with my bowels which became very, very loose. For the next fourteen years, I had diarrhoea. And that was every day, even to the fact of going to work, I'd get on the bus and I'd have to get off the bus at the next stop. And it was panicky. It took some 14 years of constant bowel movements, before I had an operation which sorted this.

I have emphysema, which was COPD until the doctor sent me to the hospital lung thing, and I had all these machines, and it came out that I have emphysema. I also have a heart condition, and I also have angina. Thankfully now, after three major operations on my stomach and my bowels, the only problem I have is what probably every woman would want – I never get hungry! If I didn't eat during the day, I would have to think at night, have I eaten anything? Because there's nothing in there that would tell me. So my stomach's alright. I have also what the specialist called dumping diabetes. I haven't got diabetes, I've got dumping diabetes, and apparently that is when I eat, because of the operation on my stomach, it just sends all the insulin out, and then I get woozy and the runs and things. But thankfully I'm on top of that now. But worst of all is chronic depression. Unfortunately I've never got rid of that, or it never went away from all of the things I'm doing, so whether it's in me or not I don't know. I still see a psychiatrist for this.

Personal story

Around about 1981, after having been made twice redundant, I moved from the Northeast down to Hertfordshire, and it was a fantastic place, with fantastic people. I worked as a caretaker of a secondary school. But about two or three years after I'd started there I was starting to cough a lot, and particularly of a morning, my throat was getting very sticky with phlegm, very hard to clear. I went around to the doctors, and the doctor told me it was asthma. So I was a 34 year old, and I was told I had asthma. I'd never had it before.

Within the working of that job was a very, very large boiler house, with two large boilers. What I didn't realise at the time was that the whole block inside the boiler house was actually made of asbestos. Never been painted, and in hindsight I know this, but not at the time. We had to rake the boilers, which meant long steel bars into the boiler, and then pulling them back out, which very often hit the asbestos shapings around the boiler house. We had a lot of problems with ceiling pipes going along the ceilings, underneath all asbestos. Unfortunately every time a problem occurred with the boiler, I was the one that was called.

My cough was getting worse and worse. I went back to the doctors who sent me up to Harefield, to get it checked through. They had me in for a few days, checked me through and told me I had COPD. They let me out, and told me to always keep steroids at home, which you can't do because doctors don't always see things the same way . . . if the consultant said keep hold of a prescription of steroids, and I go to the doctor and say can I have a prescription for steroids, I'm just told where to go, you know, he decides when I'm going to have steroids, and no-one else!

But it was just gradually getting worse and worse, and I was starting to get very, very tired. My body was getting tired as well, and I found that by the time the end of the evening came, I was having to do another hour or two hours work just to do the same work as what I was doing a year before.

The other side, which I found very hard to talk to anybody about, was actually the way I was feeling personally about what was happening. And it was hard to say, I can't understand why I'm coughing and this is making me feel . . . it was like a circle, it just seemed to go one with the other. My chest would be clear, then I'd find I started having chest pains, which the doctor in the hospital said was COPD, but then I'm told it was angina as well and the depression was coming in then, into me.

I found this very hard to talk to anyone about, because I was brought up in Ireland, at the age of 15 I could have gone to college but I had to go away and work because there was no work within Belfast itself. And I'd got a job in the Isle of Man, which meant moving. So I'd been, from the age of 15, very, very independent, and a little bit of this stubbornness comes in when you're trying to say to someone, well, not say to someone 'oh yes, I'm alright, this is alright'. Yet I was actually getting weaker and my breathing was getting worse and worse.

Well up to this stage I'd managed another ten years. During this time I'd moved to be a manager of a teacher's training centre, and then towards the 90's they'd moved me up as site manager of a conference centre and teacher's training centre. I was very happy with it, it was like a promotion, I was very, very glad that, after being made redundant twice and then the school I was caretaker at closing, I was very glad that the state wanted to give me work. To me it made me feel I'm a young man, I've got my two hands, I should always work. But anyhow, between '84 to '94, my chest, bowels, breathing they were getting me down more and more, and I've got to admit, I started drinking. And believe it or not, alcohol does let you breathe more easily, provided you don't take too much of it! So I was alright for a while, just one or two pints seemed to put more fluid into me for some reason. But it then started worrying me where I wasn't sleeping, because I knew I was having great problems with the job and I felt pressurised because it was me that had brought my wife down from Middlesbrough and my two daughters, so I had to make it work.

So I think the depression was definitely getting to me, and the drinking got stronger and stronger. I got into the habit that if I had a few drinks, just so I could sleep properly.

It was just a spiral really I'd maybe have a bit too much on the night, a bit too much in morning, and over a period of years, it got to where I was feeling very bad in the morning. So in between trying to cough out my chest, vomit up because of the drink, they were all part of the same thing; I got to the point where I just couldn't take it anymore.

The firm could see what was happening. I got in touch with my local shop steward and accepted early retirement on the grounds of health. When I left them, I found it harder still. I was out of work; I was on the sick, so I couldn't actually go to work anyway.

I'd had a change within that year of my marriage, my wife, the children split up. I had re-married again, and my wife was an accountant. She was working away and I was minding three step-children. But the chest was getting worse and worse. It just keeps getting back to that, and if I didn't get the chest, right, the heart would be out, or the stomach would be out. I was never feeling really good with one of them. But I was fine. I'd left my second wife, after ten years. I was married to my first wife twenty years, and the second one was ten years. Well, my second wife died in '92. And I was there. I found her lying on the settee, stark naked, just lying there. She'd overdosed on tablets and alcohol. It was a kick in the teeth, actually.

It was a terrible, terrible year for me, because over the eighteen months prior, my mother had died, my younger brother died, my wife had committed suicide, and my mother's sister, my aunt Mary had died as well and it was just . . . I was in a . . . well I don't know what I was in, I was just in a daze going around.

After that I moved down here to my sister Eileen's, and I was going down, I think I was going crazy. I'd been drinking for thirty years, I got near the end and I couldn't stop. I tried and I tried, I went through AA, everywhere, and I actually ended up living rough at King's Cross for a bit, because I just couldn't live with the alcohol, let alone the depression, let alone the way I was feeling.

I honestly at that time could not understand why anybody thought I had a problem with drinking. I'd think 'I like a drink, what's the matter with them?' But I think I drunk for the effect, not the pleasure. I think I'd got to the stage that my own life was in a mess, but it was the realisation that the family's going to be affected, no matter what I am. Even now, if something happens. I didn't seem to think that my daughters they would have to worry. If I'd kick the bucket, they'd get on with their lives. And I'd honestly see it that way. I had no fear of dying, I hope and prayed, sometimes I used to wake in the morning and think 'oh God, not again'.

Anyhow, it came to the end when my body just couldn't take it and I decided that was it, once and for all. I think I also came to the realisation that alcohol was destroying other people's lives. This was November 2002, and with the help of friends, nurses and family as well, so much the family, I managed to give up the drink. I owe my family my undying love, because none of them gave up, and I was just as welcome in any one of their doors, you know. They made sure I was nowhere near alcohol. So now I've had nothing to drink since 2002, just over seven and a half years.

I'd got into a local mental health hospital to get off alcohol, because I was becoming suicidal, and I had attempted in two or three cases to do that. And it was a genuine intention in the manner that the way my mental state was, I just couldn't go on. . . . you know, wife gone, you've got to house share, can't eat right, can't go out drinking, not supposed to be smoking. That was the way it was going through my mind.

It felt like I'd given everything up and I hadn't prepared for anything else to take up the time on the mental thing. So it kept going round and round my head. Then I heard about a local alcohol programme or project, or whatever it's called, and I got in with that, and that was, I would say, the making of me from the alcohol side, because I never felt under pressure, and I had a phone.... which of course, is the same in all the others, but they set it up so it seemed so easy to do. It's like the consultant says to me, when my depression comes on very bad, right, give us a ring, ring up the day team. So I'd go and see him the next time and he'd say 'have you rung them yet?' No. For me, the way I was brought up in Ireland, it's very hard to ring somebody and say 'help'. I would give the world to go the other way, I'd help anybody. But doing it yourself is very terrible. But anyway, thankfully I've never had a drink from that.

Once I came off the alcohol that was when I'd gone back to the doctor because I was sick. If it wasn't my chest it was pains in my chest. If it wasn't asthma, I was feeling awful. My bowels, stomach wouldn't be right. So I'd gone to the doctor and I said to him, I'm going down, told him all about feeling low, still not drinking or anything like that, and I said 'well this is absolutely stupid. I didn't have all these other things when I was drinking all the alcohol', I said, 'I didn't have anything wrong with me'. And he said, 'woah, woah, woah'. And I said, 'well I didn't come down here, I didn't suffer', and he said 'no, you were anaesthetised. So your chest cough would only become a throat cough, aches would become less, because with the drinking, you're numbing it'. That's when he brought me back to the hospital and diagnosed me with recurrent depression.

And the first three, two and a half years, it went fantastic, well fantastic as it goes with depression. I did get better and better, and then about six months ago it was, you know, hard. My daughter was unwell, she'd had one of her knees done and I'd had the car crash, the car written off. Anyhow, I think that started off the depression, the last depressive episode, and when they'd been like that before, they were serious. But because I wasn't drinking and I knew a bit about what I was doing and what way I was feeling, well you can sort of say, you've got to expect that feeling instead of saying 'what's that feeling?' You know, oh, that's part of the other one, you know you're not getting yourself high and worried sick.

Then I got a new GP and for the first time, this doctor, he seemed to want to put things together. I would only go in with one thing, I would only tell him about my lungs, and I wouldn't mention how good the other or how bad the other. But this is the first time I've been at a doctors that everything was collated together – my heart, my lungs, the depression, it was all there, and he was asking me about all of them, not just the one I went in with.

Anyway, he sent me to see his nurse, and that was Ann. I didn't want that, because she was a stickler, no, not say stickler, she was an absolutely lovely woman, and a very attractive woman, but when she wanted you to do something, she would remember that next week and ask you straight up, have you done it? Why haven't you done it? And she was a bit of a stickler that way. So she was dealing with my lungs and my chest and she mentioned about the Expert Patients, which I had no idea what it was. So this Ann booked me down for a go at this Expert Patients, and I knew I had to go because I knew she was going to ask me, and I knew I wouldn't get out of it. So I went.

Expert Patients Programme (EPP)

The first day of the Expert Patients Programme, the first day seemed OK, you know, I felt at home, I didn't feel as if, oh, they've got their illness and I've got my illness and that. After the second week and third week, my toes were buzzing, because I knew there was something there, and I hadn't got it yet, but I knew it was going to help me. Because I'd actually got to the stage where, if I wanted a cup of tea I would not have the energy to go in to the kitchen to make a pot of tea. I was just convinced mentally that I couldn't do it. So that meant my shopping wasn't done. I had sisters running up and down all over for me. So for the other four weeks of the EPP, I put my heart into it. And I reaped the benefits of being able to get from this house to that very end shop and back up here with a loaf of bread, because I couldn't, before the EPP, I was at the stage where I couldn't move. If I got up, I was absolutely shattered, if I went round to the shops, I was shattered. Yet, when I'd done the walk and come back, I wasn't more tired, I was less tired. 'If you don't walk around there, you'll never walk around. If you get up and do it, you'll feel better when you get back'. And I kept telling this to myself. I'd be down feeling, and my chest had been bad all day, or the breathing, I was breathing damp, clammy, very cold weather, coughing, coughing, and yet for some reason it just seemed . . . click, click, click – this is it. And I've never, ever looked back.

When we talked about this at the Expert Patients it all come together, and this is what I was very, very excited about. Most of the stuff that's in there, the vicious cycle, depression, everything, it's all there, it's the same information that I've been through in other places, but this came out in a certain way, in the manner of, you sort of dealt with one, but it gave you ideas of starting on the next problem, so to speak. And it actually changed my opinion around to me thinking; well maybe I have got a bit of fatigue or tiredness, or maybe this depression isn't really me sitting here, you know, and over the next two to three weeks, my life changed at the Expert Patients. And it didn't change in the manner that my illnesses didn't actually get any less, but I knew all about them. And I think that was the greatest thing, was that it gave me a belief to do something.

Since I've been to Expert Patients, I've been to hospital once and that was because of a car crash. And that's in three and a half years. Before EPP I would be in hospital twice, three times a year. But it's not just that, my medication is less. I was the first person to say I always took my medication, and I was a liar! I honestly got up in the morning sometimes and forgot to take them. And you know, i've got a fair few tablets. And it would be coming on to the night-time and I was like, oh, I can't take them now, I'll take them in the morning. But the EPP helped me see how important medication is, and how important it is to take what you're getting, from your doctor, the way that he wants you to take it, rather than the way you want to take them.

I'm also having to see the doctor and the nurse less. Now my visits to the doctor have been cut by two thirds. In the past I've been a regular weekly visitor to the doctors. Now I might see my own doctor eight times a year. And that's just for the check-up and things. It's very important that I do see them, to keep up on track. But I do feel in hindsight that I wasn't doing the bit that the National Health had hoped that I would do to make me better. I was taking their tablets, they would tell me what was the matter with me, but I wasn't doing anything, I was just saying; 'that's what a doctor's for'.

I've no fear of my illness now. Emphysema, that for me, in particular with my mother having it frightened the life out of me. The way she was at the end. With depression, trying to get any knowledge and trying to put any belief into myself, I couldn't really do it until I'd done the EPP. The small amount of knowledge took away the fear of the illness. And by the fear of the illness being away, I was more inclined to, not say mess with my medicine or anything, but see the doctor and say, well this is happening, can I do that, would it be a good idea?

I also learnt to tell people how I am. I'd get up in the morning, and I'd sit here, and I could have a really bad day and not contact anybody. Whereas now I'll ring up Eileen and say 'Hi love, how are you feeling love? Oh, my chest is killing me today. Oh you want me to bring a bit of dinner? Oh thanks love', and I'd get a dinner out of it. And that was just by communicating. You know, we are the worst, particularly men, anyway – you don't like to say to another man, oh, this is hurting. You know, it's that bravado stupidity, really, I say to it. So I've learnt that, and to ask for help, or when you're bad just say you're bad.

And I found that all of a sudden I was starting to get energy, I was starting to feel better. I was starting to go out and socialise. I took a little job, well not a job but a part-time thing in the cafe over here in the park, and I used to love that, I love associating with people, but because of the state of me for years before, the associating was either through my work, or nobody wanted to because of the alcohol. And gradually, the more and more I worked the programme, the better I felt.

It was about three months after I finished the EPP that I could see the difference it had made in me. I was feeling so well, better than I'd been for absolutely years, I just couldn't believe it. I decided, I got in contact with the EPP again, and asked them if there was a way I could join them or learn, and they were very helpful. They put me on a course, which was taught through the PCT and the National Health Service, and after I'd done so many courses I was accredited. And that was a definite achievement I never thought in my life I'd get that far, so it gave me a good pep up.

Depression

My depression is very, very deep, to the point of suicide, and has been on four occasions, which was touch and go. I've had a bad bout, which is why I've had this major change in medication, but that was only because I was telling the psychiatrist. Because, before that, for years, while I was still drinking with it, I would go to the psychiatrist and say oh, I'm feeling great. I wouldn't tell him, oh, these tablets aren't working, but now I will. And if it doesn't work, I just tell him, well can I go back on the other one? I'm more forward with the doctor now. They're not as fearsome as I thought they were!

My depression started after the asthma. That's when I started getting depressed and worked up. But it was also tied up with work, because as I say I was made redundant twice. I travelled two hundred and fifty odd miles to get another job, and within a year of getting there they said they were going to close it. After the asthma, I found myself then in the quagmire of saying, well if I don't take a few drinks I'm not going to sleep, if I don't sleep I'm not going to go to work, if I don't go to work I'm going to be made redundant, and it was a spiral. It all sounded logical to me at the time, it did, really logical. And I drank very heavy. I was lucky enough in the manner that I had to start work at half past five in the morning, and I kept my sobriety to keep my job open. It was fourteen hours a day, I was working six days a week at least, but the depression was there. The depression got worse, particularly if I was confined and I couldn't get up and do something, that really sent me down. And my mind would just sit and work, and work, and I'd find myself going deeper and deeper and deeper, you know. Well, I look at it now and I say it was idiotic, but it wasn't to me at the time, it was very, very serious. Because in the depression I could only see the dark lines, always the dark lines. And I always believed the world would be a better place without me, and that was my mind thought.

As I say, I had four bouts where they actually took me into hospital, I overdosed, I tried jumping in front of a bus, I was heading for a train and then another bus, I think it was. And even to this day I feel sorry for the poor bus driver, because he stopped and I was shouting and screaming at the top of my voice, 'you idiot, what did you stop for. Get the gears going, get it running, come on, I'm getting there'. And he's going 'ah mate', and I can see him, but at the time I was like 'what's he doing, why's he stopping?' I really thought he was in the wrong.

EPP has given me an understanding of depression. It doesn't mean I'm not going to feel that way again, but at the moment, if I get down, if things start to go wrong and you think 'uh-oh, here it comes again', and then I just look at it and think, ok, it's your time; you've got to have up and down days and if today's down, then ok. Everybody goes that way. But I learnt that at EPP.

Smoking

I still smoke. I smoke now about ten a day. I had given up, and I thought I was doing great. I've tried so many times in my life to give up smoking, and it just seems every time I give up smoking, something goes wrong. At least, I'm using that as an excuse! I stopped smoking for nearly three months, and I was on my way down to see the no smoking lady down at the hospital, and I was going down there to brag, but unfortunately a chap came out from in between cars, smashed my car, knocked me on to the Common and then drove off. I had a tumble over in Woolwich Common, the car was written off, and on my way home in the taxi, I said to the taxi driver 'buy me a packet of fags'. And I got stuck on it. I don't touch alcohol at all, not because I think there's anything wrong with alcohol, it's just me that it's not right with. And I think, I don't do any other thing, and the only thing I've got is a fag. It's like without it there's something lacking. If you wanted a drink when you got uptight, or anything went wrong you went out and had a drink – you know I'm talking about a pint, you know blokes, 'oh bugger this, I'm away'. And that's practically what I would do with a cigarette. But it's just like a longing, it's like, I've smoked for so long, I mean fifty years smoking, I'm fifty-nine now, and I'll be sixty. I've got emphysema, I've got a heart problem and I'm thinking to myself, how many years are you going to have left? And my father died at sixty-nine, so I don't know, but I know the difference in my body, breathing, is fantastic when I don't smoke.

I've paid for hypnotists, I've gone through the nasal spray, the gum, I've done the patches three times. I keep trying, and the longest I've got now is three months. So out of the last, say, year, I've had six months without smoking. But I have a fear also, you know, with stopping all the drinking and things, I always have the little fear that if I get too pressed, will I go for a drink? And that's a stupid excuse I know, and maybe I created that excuse so I could smoke. I don't think so though. Because drinking is far worse. Smoking takes thirty, forty, fifty years before you might kill yourself. With drink you can do it in a year.

At the moment, this is the way I feel. I'm not necessarily saying it's right, but the way I feel, in me, when I stop smoking, I can do it for a bit and then something builds up. It's not like a panic attack or anything, but there is a panic that what if the drink comes, because I mean with alcohol, you're not ruining your life, you're ruining everybody else's as well, and you don't even know it. And they don't even know why you're doing it. So that has got to be the first and foremost to me.

Present

My health now is good. My emphysema has never been better, my lungs have been even better; I can breathe lovely. My heart, it's gone on the quiet side, it's just sitting there. Depression is just going away, and my stomach is just starting to feel right, normal. In fact I can honestly say, over the last twenty years, thirty years, this is about the best I've felt. I mean, I can't go running or jogging around, but sitting down, happy in my own mind, that I'm getting the best out of what I've got.

Reference

Clark, D. (2002) *Cicely Saunders – Founder of the Hospice Movement: Selected letters 1959–1999.* Oxford University Press; New York.

Chapter 8

Self-management and current health care policies

Kerri Wright

School of Health and Social Care, University of Greenwich, Eltham, London, UK

Introduction

Self-management or self-care of long-term conditions (LTCs) has become an important component of health care policies (Department of Health, 2008), and aims to encourage people with LTCs to take more control and responsibility for the management of their condition. Self-management is not a new concept, however, but has been explored extensively in sociological and psychological literature through work and research with people with disabilities and those living with LTCs (e.g. Creer and Christian, 1976; Kleinman, 1988). In order to fully understand self-management and how to support and facilitate people with LTCs to self-manage, it is important that existing social knowledge and theories about people's responses to LTCs are recognised (Kendall and Rogers, 2007). This chapter draws on psychological and social theories to explore how LTCs can affect people's lives as the basis for understanding and encouraging more active self-management.

One of the difficulties with the concept 'self-management' is that it has not been conceptualised clearly (Lorig and Holman, 2003). Often the terms self-management, self-care and patient education are used interchangeably in literature when in fact they have very different meanings (Coleman and Newton, 2005) (see Box 8.1 for current definitions of these concepts). Patient education is a directive approach whereby the health care professional imparts information, skills, or knowledge to the patient with the aim of changing their behaviours (Bodenheimer *et al.*, 2002). For example, patients may be taught the importance of a healthy diet in diabetes management or the correct inhaler technique. The content of the instruction or education is often decided by the health care professional and is based on the management and control of the disease and its symptoms. The goal of patient education is to encourage the patient to comply with the behaviour changes taught which will lead to better clinical outcomes, for example better glycaemic control or higher peak flow readings. Patient education can lead to patients becoming more active in the management of their LTCs (Coster and Norman, 2009), but it is narrowly focused on the biomedical model of health and thus only acknowledges the disease and not the person or the effect the disease has on their lives (Koch *et al.*, 2004).

Box 8.1   Definitions of self-care, self-management and patient education.

Self-care

'Activities that individuals, families and communities undertake with the intention of enhancing health, preventing disease, limiting illness and restoring health' (World Health Organisation, 1983: 181)

Self-management

'individual's ability to manage the symptoms, treatment, physical and psychosocial consequences of living with a long-term disorder' (Department of Health, 2005: 6)

Patient education

'the teaching or training of patients concerning their own health needs' (Cochrane Collaboration cited in Coster and Norman, 2009: 509)

Self-management, however, refers to the 'ability to manage the symptoms, treatment, physical and psychosocial consequences and life style changes inherent in living with a chronic condition.' (Barlow *et al.*, 2002: 178). Self-management, therefore, acknowledges that the LTC cannot be separated from the person and their lives and must embrace the whole person, and how the condition affects their lives in order to be effective. A person with an LTC is responsible for their day-to-day care over the course of their condition (Lorig and Holman, 2003). Health care professionals may visit, or the person may attend hospital appointments to support the medical management of the condition, but for the rest of the person's life, they are responsible for managing their condition within their lives. In one sense, all people living with LTCs self-manage their conditions. Whatever response the person has to their condition, for example denial or actively keeping up-to-date with current research on the condition, the person is still managing their life with the condition, since it is impossible not to manage one's life (Lorig and Holman, 2003). The important point is how the person decides to manage. Self-management, therefore, is not about encouraging greater management, but focusing on how the person currently manages, and working with them to improve aspects of this management so that it enhances the quality of their life, focusing on enabling them to 'live a life' rather than 'live an illness' (Whittemore and Dixon, 2008: 184). Self-management, therefore, is more than doing, but is entwined with a sense of 'being and becoming' (Kralik *et al.*, 2004: 265).

Shattered life and self-identity

The way people manage their lives with an LTC depends in part on the meaning that it has for them in the context of their lives (Paterson, 2001; Koch *et al.*, 2004; Lundman and Jansson, 2007; Whittemore and Dixon, 2008). We all have an image or a self-identity that we have constructed over many years of what it means to be us. This self-identity is different for everyone and could depend on other people, our skills or our jobs. When a major life event happens, such as illness, this can shatter our self-identity and fragment our lives (Kralik *et al.*, 2004). For example, a person with a self-identity which is dependent on being a good mother to her children can have her life and the meaning she gains from this shattered by an illness which results in debilitating fatigue and the inability of her to mother her children in the way that she believes is necessary. LTCs can challenge individuals' self-identity by the changes that the illness demands of them to make to their lives, the dependencies which develop on other people and the continual comparison that is made to the life they led before they became unwell (Ek and Ternestedt, 2008). An LTC and the limitations this can bring to individuals' lives can bring feelings of guilt, shame and an acute sense of loss (Lundman and Jansson, 2007; Cicutto *et al.*, 2004). Understanding the meaning that the LTC has for the individual and validating the suffering experienced can help them to begin the process of reconstructing a new self-identity. This new identify is formed by integrating the LTC and the limitations it imposes on their life.

When people experience ill health, they construct narratives or stories that help them make sense of their experiences and adapt to life with an LTC (Kleinman, 1988). These stories are important to the individual and are their perceptions and beliefs about how they became unwell, when they first noticed this change, the process of being diagnosed and subsequent treatment. A person's narrative is their attempt at trying to make some 'order in the fragmentation of their life' that has occurred with the LTC (Williams, 1984: 177). Illness narratives have three main central points of reference that are considered in relation to the LTC. These reference points are: the meanings and effect the LTC has on the person's body; the effect and meaning the LTC has for their sense of self; and the way the LTC affects their role in society (Williams, 1984).

The illness narratives constructed by individuals have the same reference points as the main health care approaches to LTCs, namely biomedical, psychological and sociological approaches. These reference points are not discrete however, and narratives are constructed through a complex interaction between these three perspectives or reference points. For example, a condition that affects a biomedical function, such as blood glucose level in diabetes, requires specific behavioural management, such as insulin injections or specific dietary intake. The biomedical management of the high glucose levels affects how the person behaves socially, for example being able to drink alcohol socially, or having to inject in public places which, in turn, can have an effect on how the person views themselves as a person. Illness narratives are important in helping the individual to make sense of their experiences and serve to help them adjust and begin to construct a new self-identity (Lundman and Jansson, 2007; Koch *et al.*, 2004). The process of constructing a new self-identity is thought to be enhanced by the regular recounting and sharing of their illness narratives, and having these listened to and heard (Telford *et al.*, 2006).

People's illness narratives and the way they manage their lives with their LTC are influenced by the person's own perceptions and beliefs that they have about their illness (Leventhal *et al.*, 1984). The sense that people make of their illness forms what has been termed their 'illness representation', that is, what the illness means to them as an individual. The illness representation made by people forms as soon as they start experiencing symptoms, and is dynamic; changing and adapting with diagnosis, treatment, disease progression and how they respond to treatment. A person's illness representation is important in self-management as it has a direct effect on the way that people think and emotionally respond to their illness and as a consequence the way that they begin to cope and manage their life (Wasson *et al.*, 2008). For example, an individual who believes that depression is something only weak people develop may be reluctant to accept this diagnosis and any treatment, such as medication. People's lay beliefs about their illness need to be explored with them in order to gain a full understanding of how they think and feel about their illness and how this affects the way they manage their life. Research by Leventhal *et al.* (1984) has shown that people's overall perception of their illness includes five main components: identity, timeline, cause, consequences and cure/control. These five areas are helpful to try to understand how a person constructs their illness representation, makes sense of their LTC and how they manage this within their daily life:

1. Identity: This is the label or diagnosis of the condition and the corresponding symptoms which are believed to be common with this condition. For example, there is often an underlying belief that a cancer diagnosis will ultimately result in death, which can create greater levels of fear and anxiety in people and their families diagnosed with cancer.
2. Cause: People have their own perceptions and beliefs about the cause of their condition, which, although they may not be biologically accurate, are important to them. These beliefs are often developed from personal experience as well as discourse between health care professionals, significant others and other sources of health information, for example magazines.
3. Timeline: This is the belief about how long the illness is going to last. This belief will change and adapt over the course of the illness.
4. Consequences: These are the beliefs about how the illness will affect them physically, socially and emotionally. Again, these beliefs will change and adapt over time.
5. Cure/control: These are the beliefs about whether the condition can be cured or controlled, and the role that the individual believes they have in this.

The coping behaviours employed by individuals are directly influenced by their illness representations. Leventhal *et al.* (1984) proposed a hierarchical model, known as the self-regulatory model or common sense model, whereby people's illness representations led to the development of action plans to cope with and manage their emotional and physical response to the illness. These action plans are continually appraised and evaluated by the individuals and fed back into both the perception of their illness and subsequent action plans (see Figure 8.1). This process is identified in other studies as people using a 'trial and error' approach to managing their LTCs (Kralik *et al.*, 2004). The reappraisal of coping behaviours and their beliefs about their illness results in people's illness perceptions adapting and changing as they gain new experiences, knowledge and information, and ultimately leads to reviewing of current management strategies. For example, a person with osteoarthritis may believe that they need to exercise regularly to keep their joints

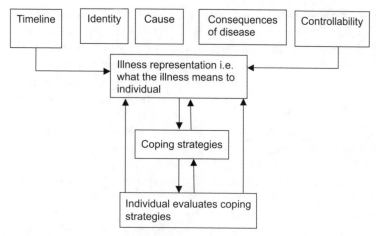

Figure 8.1 Self-regulation model (adapted from Leventhal *et al.*, 1984).

and bones strong. Regular exercise may lead to increased pain and a new belief that exercise makes their osteoarthritis worse. This can also lead to their illness representation adapting to this experience, for example that their condition will have a greater consequence for them physically and socially, and beliefs that the condition is out of their control.

> 'I realise that I am not in the driver's seat of my life anymore and that the diseases are and they control me. You know, I don't control my life. You lose control and that is the biggest issue I find.'

> (Whittemore and Dixon, 2008: 181)

The management and coping strategies adopted by individuals with LTCs are thus cumulative and evolving as people gain more knowledge and experience about their condition and how they respond to the management strategies implemented. Understanding the person's illness representation from a cognitive perspective, that is, what their thoughts are about their illness and their emotional response to this, can help to understand an individual's current management strategies (Kralik *et al.*, 2004; Lau-Walker, 2007). This provides a basis from which individual self-management can be improved, and is the premise on which many current long-term disease self-management programmes are based (Creer, 2008; Lorig *et al.*, 2001; Department of Health, 2001).

Implications for professional practice

Self-management begins with the health care professionals listening to the person's narrative about their illness and their lives. This approach assumes that we can best understand what it means to live with an LTC by listening carefully to the stories people share (Telford *et al.*, 2006; Kleinman, 1988). In order to truly understand the stories and experiences shared by people living with LTCs, health care professionals need to develop empathetic understanding, which ensures that the stories and experiences shared by the individual are viewed from the person's perspective (Rogers, 1967; Kingsbury, 2002 cited by Telford *et al.*, 2006). Empathetic understanding allows the health care professional to be sensitive to the individualistic experience of LTCs and to begin to appreciate the value of the individual's management of their condition, even if it does not fit with their own values or beliefs about how the condition should be managed. For example, listening empathetically may help to appreciate the experiences of a person with chronic obstructive pulmonary disease (COPD) who is insistent on sleeping in her armchair and is developing oedematous and ulcerated legs. The person's story may reveal the fear and panic felt at slipping down from her pillows in bed and not being able to breathe. Unless the health care professional develops the skills at listening empathetically, this person's perspective will not be heard. The health care professional will not be able to understand and appreciate the way the person is trying to self-manage their breathing difficulties at night to prevent the feelings of panic and will also not be able to work with the person at identifying other potential ways of managing her breathing at night:

> '[T]he willingness to listen and to understand what is happening for the person at the time, resisting the temptation to categorise and honouring their account will go a long way in assisting them to feel respected and truly supported. This approach is likely to foster a valued sense of self.'
>
> (Telford *et al.*, 2006: 463)

The way the person's narrative is heard and responded to is important. Empathetic listening requires the listener to demonstrate that they have heard and understand the story being told. This requires the listener to use communication skills such as non-verbal cues, paraphrasing and reflecting back what has been heard to the person. These skills are discussed in more detail in Chapter 6. Demonstrating that the story has been heard and validating the experiences the person is describing can have a positive impact on the way that they understand and are making sense of their new life with an LTC (Telford *et al.*, 2006). Stories that are not heard, however, or receive negative or dismissive reactions from the listener can result in the person feeling diminished or ashamed about themselves and their life (Kelly, 1992; Telford *et al.*, 2006). Positive reactions to a person's narrative can enhance the development of a positive self-identity, and can influence the person's coping ability (Telford *et al.*, 2006). The reactions from partners, family and friends towards the person's narrative in particular can have a significant impact on the person's developing self-identity with an LTC (Bury, 1982; Kelly, 1992; Kralik, 2002); for example, a husband who does not appreciate the degree of pain experienced by his wife and becomes frustrated by how long it takes her to get washed and dressed in the mornings. In view of this, involvement of significant others in the person's LTC management would be helpful to ensure positive support and understanding of the person's experiences and struggles. In addition to significant others, health care professionals are also influential in supporting people with LTCs, and their reactions to stories can have a significant impact on the person's developing self-identity. For example, a person whose experience of disfigurement is not listened to or is met with undisguised disgust by a health care professional can contribute to the person's sense of shame towards themselves:

'Now this young nurse had obviously never seen one of these appliances on any-body ... she walked in the door and there was me standing in all my glory, and she just went like that [grimaced and walked away] and y'know, of course I could see it' (patient with an ileostomy for management of ulcerative colitis).'

(Kelly, 1992: 461)

In order to listen to people's narratives and understand the meaning from their per-spective, health care professionals need to move away from the dominant biomedical perspective. Although nurses and doctors profess to be providing more holistic care and appreciate the need for a biopsychosocial approach to LTCs, with the biomedical, psy-chological and sociological impact of LTCs being assessed equally, research has shown that the biomedical model still dominates (Koch *et al.*, 2004; Telford *et al.*, 2006; Wilson *et al.*, 2007). Studies have indicated that when health care professionals listen to the person's narrative about their experiences of their LTC, the story heard by the health care professional is different from the actual story being told (Koch *et al.*, 2004). This is thought to be due to the health care professional actively listening for biomedical 'cues in the narrative that indicate the way that the biological organism runs down and ceases to function properly' (Telford *et al.*, 2006: 458), rather than trying to understand empatheti-cally what the illness means to the person. This has been described as 'the separate worlds of the physician and patient' (Toombs, 1992: 1). By only validating and responding to the biomedical cues that are shared by people, health care professionals can unintention-ally foster an understanding of LTCs that fits with a biomedical perspective (Hall, 1996; Lundman and Jansson, 2007). This can result in people adjusting their communication with health care professionals to reflect this and focusing solely on the medical perspective of their condition (Kralik *et al.*, 2001; Kralik, 2002).

A difficulty with the dominance of the biomedical model is that it can negate the value of other management methods for LTCs which may not fit with the biomedical perspective. For example, the person who is diagnosed as having hypertension and prescribed anti-hypertensives may decide that they wish to change their lifestyle, diet and take natural remedies to lower this, rather than take the medication. Using the biomedical model, non-adherence to medical treatment is viewed as problematic. However, if the person's narrative is listened to and the decision is understood from the individual's perspective, then this 'non-adherence' can instead be viewed as 'adaptive decision making' (Paterson *et al.*, 2001). Judging and labelling people as 'non-compliant' because they do not wish to follow the medical treatment or take the medication prescribed can further erode their self-identity. Studies have shown that people make decisions about their medication and treatment in the context of their lives, and there may be alternative explanations for the decisions made which are outside of the biomedical framework (Lundman and Jansson, 2007; Paterson *et al.*, 2001; Wasson *et al.*, 2008). Unless health care professionals listen to the person's narrative about their lives with an LTC, they will not be able to appreciate nor validate the person and the way they are managing their life. People with LTCs learn through bitter experience that the responses to their illness do not follow the patterns described or prescribed by health care professionals and 'have to find their own practice which fits with their life' (Telford *et al.*, 2006: 461).

> 'This is the thing that annoys me more than anything else . . . that nobody would listen to what I was saying. I knew what my body could do, I knew what I was capable of, but they all had their own ideas of what I ought to be doing.'
>
> (Cotterell, 2008: 669)

People with LTCs go through a process of adjustment and adaptation to their lives. This process is often referred to as the 'integration' of a person's past and present identities and roles into a new self-identity with an LTC (Kralik *et al.*, 2004). There is a feeling of reconciliation and acceptance of their new life and self-identity. The adjustment to life with an LTC varies between individuals and is influenced by the interaction between the way the person thinks and feels about their condition and the effect it has on their life:

> 'I've accepted my (illness). I don't fight it. I'm not angry about where it came from. I'm not looking for that cure so that my life can change. I'm sort of living in the between and the now . . . I think I've learned to live with myself in general . . .'
>
> (Whittemore and Dixon, 2008: 184)

LTCs can also have different disease trajectories which provide different challenges for the person managing their life with the condition, for example diabetes which can remain fairly stable with correct management compared to progressive multiple sclerosis which can cause a gradual deterioration in health and functioning. Disease trajectories, thus, also affect the adjustment to life that people are trying to make with LTCs, with the disease at times being all-consuming psychologically and physically and existing in the foreground of the person's life (Paterson, 2001). People can, therefore, find themselves fluctuating between 'living a life and living an illness' (Whittemore and Dixon, 2008: 177). The processes of integrating and reconstructing new self-identities with an LTC are important for the health care professional to understand and appreciate when working with people with LTCs. The LTC cannot be separated from the person's life and thus management of their condition must start from this perspective. The impact of the LTC on the person's life will often not be seen in relation to the disease or symptom alone but rather what this disease or symptom means for them in their daily life, for example breathlessness preventing them from not being able to play with their grandchildren or wash independently (Kralik *et al.*, 2004). Working from the impact the condition has on the individual's life encourages integration by allowing 'pieces of life with illness to fit into place' (Kralik *et al.*, 2004: 266).

Self-management approaches

People with an LTC are thought to focus on three main areas in their daily management of their conditions and lives (Corbin and Strauss, 1988; Lorig and Holman, 2003). These areas are:

1. Medical management of the condition: For example taking medication or adhering to special dietary requirements.

2. Role management: This involves maintaining, changing or creating new meaningful behaviours or life roles. For example, someone with arthritis and limited mobility may have to adjust the way they cook and prepare food for their family.
3. Emotional management: This relates to the emotional response to living with an LTC and the emotions that are felt as a result of this, for example frustration, anger or fear.

Self-management approaches need to focus on all three of these areas in order to be effective and to encourage people to keep wellness in the foreground (Paterson *et al.*, 2001). Patient education programmes often focus on the medical and behavioural management of LTCs, but few deal with all three areas systematically (Lorig and Holman, 2003). This can result in the 'self' in self-management being ignored and the individual being seen as a patient rather than a person (Koch *et al.*, 2004). Self-management requires the narrative and the impact of the disease on an individual's life to be heard and understood across these three areas. Such a shift means that the voices of the ill are equal to those of the professionals (Thorne and Paterson, 2000). This ideally allows the health care professional and the individual to develop a shared understanding of the LTC and encourages an alliance to form in managing the individual's life with the LTC.

Self-management approaches can be implemented within a one-to-one relationship with individuals or within a programme set up for a group of individuals. Recently, the government has supported the implementation of the Expert Patients Programme (EPP) (Department of Health, 2001). This self-management programme is based on the work of Kate Lorig and colleagues who have carried out extensive work on self-management with people living with arthritis in America (Lorig *et al.*, 2001; Lorig and Holman, 2003). The EPP consists of a 6-week programme run by a trained lay tutor who is also living with an LTC. The programme content is set out in a self-management guide that all participants receive and aims to develop five key skills which are thought to be necessary in promoting self-management strategies (NHS EPP, 2002) (see Box 8.2). As the programme content is generic and not condition specific, participants living with varying conditions can attend and benefit from the same course.

Box 8.2   Five key self-management skills.

1. Problem-solving
2. Decision-making
3. Utilisation of resources
4. Partnership working with health care professionals
5. Taking action or self-efficacy

Problem solving

Problem solving in self-management does not seek to teach people the solutions to their problems, but aims to teach basic problem-solving skills which can be taken away and applied to current or future problems as they arise (Lorig and Holman, 2003). Problem solving is thus arming people with the skills to self-manage their lives now, but also preparing them for any future changes that may occur with their condition or life. Problem solving focuses on teaching people how to define exactly what the problem is, identify potential solutions to this problem and how to evaluate any solutions tried (see Box 8.3 and Table 8.1).

Box 8.3   Summary of problem-solving steps taught in EPP (NHS EPP 2002).

1. Identify problem: This involves carefully thinking about the issue and getting to the heart of what the problem actually is. For example, a problem may be identified as difficulty in breathing at night. Careful thought about this problem and possibly exploring this with a health care professional may identify that the actual problem is fear of being alone at night which causes anxiety and the consequent difficulties in breathing.

2. List ideas to solve problem: Individuals are encouraged to think widely and consult with others on generating possible solutions to this problem. The generation of ideas can be carried out with a health care professional who can work with the individual in brainstorming possible solutions. It is important that all ideas are accepted as valid and are written down. Once both the individual and health care professional have saturated all ideas then the list can be considered again and ideas that are felt to be unacceptable to either can be ruled out. The resulting solutions can then be considered.

3. Select one method to try: The person chooses one possible solution that they are willing to try. This solution and action must be something that the individuals actually want to do for themselves. It should not be something that they are doing to please their family or health care professional. This solution is then implemented using an action plan. An action plan lists the precise actions that the person is going to undertake, for example, in the next week. The plans need to be achievable, linked to an exact behaviour and should be as detailed as possible, for example listing what, when and how often the action will be carried out. This plan should be written down and used to give feedback and motivation on the person's achievements. For example, ticking when the action has been done, encouraging them to share achievements with family and friends and making sure that health care professionals also give timely feedback on progress and achievements made. The action plan can also include a discussion about what the barriers might be to achieving the goal and what support or resources the person has which will help them to overcome these barriers (Von Korff *et al.*, 2002). The EPP also recommend the person giving themselves a score between 0 and 10 as to how confident they feel in achieving their goal.

4. Think about the results: At the end of the action plan period the individual is encouraged to review their progress. This can be done alone, with family or a friend or with a health care professional.

5. Try another idea if the first didn't work: If little or no progress is being made then the individual is encouraged to try another of their problem solving ideas; writing an action plan and reviewing the progress as before.

6. Use other resources (ask friends, family or professionals for ideas): If there is still no progress and the problem still exists then the individual is encouraged to seek further advice.
7. Accept that the problem may not be solvable for now: It may be that even with professional advice and trialing several possible solutions, the individual's solution still exists. The person will then need support to accept that, for now, the problem is not solvable.

Table 8.1 Example of action plan for someone who identified that they want to be more independent.

No.	Goal (expressed in behaviour)	Barriers to achieving goal	Action plans to address barriers	Comments
1	To cook dinner for myself once a week on a Wednesday with dessert.	Motivation and meaningless cooking just for self.	Invite friend over for dinner with me or tell myself 'I'm worth it'. Buy flowers for the table.	Consider a reciprocal arrangement with friends.
		Tiring standing up in kitchen for long periods.	Contact OT or buy stool for kitchen. Pace the preparation throughout day.	Local chemist has stools available – discuss with son about driving me to collect.
		Not thinking ahead and planning menu and food shopping.	Plan menu on Monday so ready for shopping on Tuesday. Buy flowers whilst shopping.	Go to library and look at cookery books for ideas to motivate me.

Decision-making

Decision-making can be viewed as a part of the process of problem-solving and is a necessary skill in deciding what problem the individual wishes to focus on and which solution they wish to try first. In addition, decision-making is also a daily part of living with an LTC (Lorig and Holman, 2003). Individuals are forced continually to make decisions on the basis of ongoing changes to their condition and the necessary responses to this. This can include knowing when to alter treatment, whether to adapt their activities, and when and who to contact if certain symptoms are present. Effective decision-making needs to be based on appropriate and clear information which is tailored to the individual's condition and circumstances. For example, a health care professional may work with an individual and develop a system which the individual is able to follow when certain known changes occur to their condition. This information needs to be discussed when the person is well and focused on activities which have been helpful in the past (see Table 8.2).

Table 8.2 System to support someone to identify changes in their depression and actions to take.

Risk	Observation	Action
GREEN	Motivated to undertake activities. Interested in others; socialising. Self-caring; eating, washing, allowing treats. Sleeping usual amount. Anxiety levels low; no persistent thoughts.	Congratulate yourself for doing so well. Plan a small celebration for your success each week!
YELLOW	Undertaking activities requiring more effort. Not as interested in socialising; starting to consider cancelling appointments. Self-caring only because you know you must. Not feeling hungry, lacking energy to wash. Sleeping more than usual; feeling fatigued and going to bed early evenings. Beginning to feel that you're not able to work and would rather hide away.	You agreed the following activities: (1) Ring the three identified people and tell them how you feel. Arrange for them to ring and see you every day until you feel better. (2) Start swimming again. You agreed twice a week and have a shower at the pool. (3) Eat out in a café twice a week. (4) Tell your manager at work as agreed and negotiate flexible hours. (5) Remember you've been here before and with the activities above have successfully gone back into the green.
RED	No interest to undertake activities. Feeling like you're 'going through the motions'. No interest in others and not socialising. Interest in self-care minimal. Sleeping excessive amounts and can't wait to get into bed to 'escape'. Persistent thoughts of meaningless and 'what's the point'. Little wish to carry on with work.	You need to visit your GP urgently and arrange for your medication to be reviewed. Communicate your feelings to your three support people and arrange to stay with one of them as agreed. Communicate with work and if necessary take a few days sick to self-care. Continue with swimming and increase this to alternate days. Remember that this will pass.

Utilisation of resources

The self-management approach teaches people not just what resources are available, but how to actually search themselves to locate different resources. This approach equips individuals with the skills to search for different resources in the future, should the need arise. People are taught where they can go to find information, for example internet sources, telephone book, the local library. In addition, people are taught the skill of contacting a wide range of sources at the same time and gathering all this information together, rather than the more time-consuming approach of contacting one source at a time.

Partnership working with health care professionals

This key skill has been included in self-management programmes in acknowledgement of the different management approach that an LTC requires. People with LTCs are taught the importance of working in partnership with health care professionals and how to present information about their condition in a consultation. Although this skill is undoubtedly valuable in assisting health care professionals to assess the benefits of different treatment regimes, it has also been criticised as teaching people how to adhere to the medical model of condition management rather than demanding that health care professionals change their approach (Wilson *et al.*, 2007). Despite this, there is value in teaching people how to use health care professionals, and in particular medical expertise, so that they can seek medical advice on their own terms and remain in control of this.

Taking action or self-efficacy

One of the benefits of the self-management programme reported by participants has been an increased sense of control over their condition (Lorig and Holman, 2003; Creer, 2008). The concept of control has been linked to the self-efficacy theory and has formed the basis for further research on this area (e.g. Wasson *et al.*, 2008; Jerant, 2008). Self-efficacy is based on the work by Bandura (1997) on expectations. Bandura identified two types of expectation: outcome expectation, which relates to our belief about the possible consequences of our actions, and self-efficacy, which is our belief that a particular behaviour will lead to a particular outcome. Self-efficacy therefore relates to the degree of control an individual feels they have over their condition. Self-efficacy is thought to be the most powerful determinant of behaviour change as it determines the following factors:

1. The initial decision to perform the behaviour. A person is more likely to decide to make a behavioural change if they feel that their behaviour directly influences an outcome.
2. How much effort the person is prepared to put into the behavioural change. If the person believes strongly that the behaviour will bring about the desired outcome, for example stopping smoking will improve their breathing, then they will expend more effort in trying to make the change.
3. The extent to which the person is prepared to persevere even when faced with extreme difficulties. For example, continuing not to smoke despite a series of very stressful events happening in the person's life, which would normally increase their cigarette use.

Self-efficacy is therefore a key ingredient in self-management approaches. Self-management strategies need to include opportunities for encouraging people to feel more in control of their condition and their life. Bandura (1997) has identified four key ways to promote self-efficacy:

1. Performance mastery: Individuals are encouraged to become actively involved in the management of aspects of their life with their condition. Within the EPP this includes encouraging participants to make a specific action plan for an activity they want to carry out over the next week. This could also include teaching people how to perform

clinical skills to gain more control over their condition, for example blood glucose monitoring or carrying out and recording peak flow readings, or encouraging them to seek out a new resource or group and report back to the health care professional.

2. Modelling: People gain support and encouragement from seeing positive models of other people managing and living their life successfully with an LTC. This helps people to start to believe that it is possible to have control over their life. With a self-management programme, modelling can occur through interactions with peers or the lay tutor, or by using videos or information about other people living with a similar LTC. This demonstrates the value of support groups where people gain the opportunity to meet with other people in similar situations.

3. Interpretation of symptoms: People may need support to interpret the symptoms they are experiencing and making sense of the causes. Lorig *et al.* (2001) highlight the importance of teaching people that symptoms have multiple causes and thus have multiple self-management solutions. This means that there are more possibilities available to manage the symptoms and thus individuals have the potential for more control over these. This prevents individuals becoming stuck in a belief that they are unable to control the cause and thus the symptom and its effect. For example, the symptom of fatigue can have several causes including disease itself, depression, pain, anxiety, poor nutrition, insomnia, medication or interactions. A belief that fatigue is a symptom of the disease itself can lead to low self-efficacy, whereas exploring the other potential causes offers greater self-efficacy.

4. Social persuasion: People are more likely to undertake a behavioural change if other people around them are also engaged in this activity. For example, someone is more likely to stop smoking if everyone else around them, no longer smokes. People can be encouraged to attend specific support groups or join with friends and families in making behavioural changes and supporting each other though this. For example, if the whole family changes their diet, then this will encourage the person with an LTC to persevere with this change.

Conclusion

People with an LTC have no choice but to manage their condition in a way that is meaningful for them. The nurse's role in self-management is to work in alliance with the person to develop the most effective management strategies that fit with the person's life. Nurses also need to be aware of the impact that living with an LTC can have on one's self-identify and the complex and fluctuating process of adjustment and integration required to the losses and changes in the person's life. Nurses can support and facilitate self-management through accepting and validating the individual's experiences of living with LTCs and starting from this perspective when planning and negotiating care. Nurses also need to develop knowledge of strategies and self-management techniques, beyond medical management, that have been used successfully by people with LTCs. The generic approach to self-management strategies has been discussed in this chapter. Chapter 9 offers more detailed strategies related to generic symptoms that are commonly experienced in people with LTCs.

References

Bandura, A. (1997) *Self Efficacy: The Exercise of Control*. WH Freeman, New York.

Barlow, J., Wright, C., Sheasby, J., Turner, A. & Hainsworth, J. (2002) Self management approaches for people with chronic conditions: a review, *Patient Education and Counselling*, 48(2), pp. 177–187.

Bodenheimer, T., Lorig, K., Holman, H. & Grumbach, K. (2002) Patient self management of chronic disease in primary care, *Journal of the American Medical Association*, 288(19), pp. 2469–2475.

Bury, M. (1982) Chronic illness as biographical disruption, *Sociology, Health and Illness*, 4, pp. 67–82.

Cicutto, L., Brooks, D. & Henderson, K. (2004) Self-care issues from the perspective of individuals with Chronic Obstructive Pulmonary Disease, *Patient Education and Counselling*, 55, pp. 168–176.

Coleman, M. & Newton, K. (2005) Supporting self management in patients with chronic illness, *American Family Physician*, 72(8), pp. 1503–1510.

Corbin, J. & Strauss, A. (1988) *Unending Work and Care: Managing Chronic Illness at Home*. Jossey-Bass, San Francisco.

Coster, S. & Norman, I. (2009) Cochrane reviews of educational and self management interventions to guide nursing practice: a review, *International Journal of Nursing Studies*, 46, pp. 508–528.

Cotterell, P. (2008) Striving for independence: experiences and needs of service users with life limiting conditions, *Journal of Advanced Nursing*, 62(6), pp. 665–673.

Creer, T. & Christian, W. (1976) *Chronically Ill and Handicapped Children: Their Management and Rehabilitation*. Research Press Champaign, Illinois.

Creer, T. (2008) Behavioural and cognitive processes in the self management of Asthma, *Journal of Asthma*, 45, pp. 81–94.

Department of Health (2001) *The Expert Patient: A New Approach to Chronic Disease Manageme*. Department of Health, London.

Department of Health (2005) *Promoting Optimal Self-Care Consultation Techniques that Improve Quality of Life for Patients and Clinicians*. Department of Health, London.

Department of Health (2008) *Your Health, Your Way – a Guide to Long-Term Conditions and Self-Care*. Department of Health, London.

Ek, K. & Ternestedt, B. (2008) Living with chronic obstructive pulmonary disease at the end of life: a phenomenological study, *Journal of Advanced Nursing*, 62(4), pp. 470–478.

Hall, B. (1996) The Pschiatric model: a critical analysis of its undermining effects on nursing in chronic mental illness, *Advances in Nursing Science*, 18(3), pp. 16–26.

Jerant, A. (2008) Depressive symptoms moderated the effect of chronic illness, self management training on self efficacy, *Medical Care*, 46, pp. 523–531.

Kelly, M. (1992) Self-identity and radical surgery, *Sociology of Health and Illness*, 14(3), pp. 390–415.

Kendall, E. & Rogers, A. (2007) Extinguishing the social?: state sponsored self-care policy and the chronic disease self-management programme, *Disability and Society*, 22(2), pp. 129–143.

Kleinman, A. (1988) *The Illness Narratives: Suffering, Healing and the Human Condition*. Basic Books, New York.

Kralik, D., Koch, T. & Webb, C. (2001) The domination of chronic illness research by biomedical interests, *Australian Journal of Holistic Nursing*, 8, pp. 4–12.

Kralik, D. (2002) The quest for ordinariness: transition experienced by midlife women living with chronic illness, *Journal of Advanced Nursing*, 39(2), pp. 146–154.

Kralik, D., Koch, T., Price, K. & Howard, N. (2004) Chronic illness self-management: taking action to create order, *Journal of Clinical Nursing*, 13, pp. 259–267.

Koch, T., Jenkin, P. & Kralik, D. (2004) Chronic illness self management: locating the 'self', *Journal of Advanced Nursing*, 48(5), pp. 484–492.

Lau-Walker, M. (2007) Importance of illness beliefs and self-efficacy for patients with coronary heart disease, *Journal of Advanced Nursing*, 60(2), pp. 187–198.

Leventhal, H., Nernez, D. & Steele, D. (1984) Illness representations and coping with health threats. In: *Handbook of Psychology and Health* (eds A. Baum, S. Taylor & J. Singer). Lawrence Erlbaum Associates, New York, pp. 219–252.

Lorig, K., Sobel, D., Ritter, P., Laurant, D. & Hobbs, M. (2001) Effect of a self-management program on patients with chronic disease, *Effective Clinical Practice*, 4, pp. 256–262.

Lorig, K. & Holman, H. (2003) Self-management education: history, definition, outcomes and mechanisms, *Annals of Behavioural Medicine*, 26(1), pp. 1–7.

Lundman, B. & Jansson, L. (2007) The meaning of living with a long-term condition. To revalue and be revalued, *Journal of Clinical Nursing*, 16(7b), pp. 109–115.

NHS Expert Patients Programme (EPP) (2002) *Self-Management of Long-Term Health Conditions, A Handbook for People with Chronic Disease*. Bull Publishing Company, Colorado.

Paterson, B. (2001) The shifting perspectives model of chronic illness, *Journal of Nursing Scholarship*, 33(1), pp. 21–26.

Paterson, B., Russell, C. & Thorne, S. (2001) Critical analysis of everyday self-care decision making in chronic illness, *Journal of Advanced Nursing*, 35(3), pp. 335–341.

Rogers, C. (1967) *On Becoming a Person*. Constable, London.

Telford, K., Kralik, D. & Koch, T. (2006) Acceptance and denial: implications for people adapting to chronic illness: literature review, *Journal of Advanced Nursing*, 55(4), pp. 457–464.

Thorne, S. & Paterson, B. (2000) Two decades of insider research: what we know and don't know about chronic illness experience, *Annual Review of Nursing Research* 18, pp. 3–25.

Toombs, K. (1992) *The Meaning of Illness: A Phenomenological Account of the Different Perspectives of Physicians and Patients*. Kluwer Academic Publishers, London.

Von Korff, M., Glasgow, R. & Sharpe, M. (2002) Organising care for chronic illness, *British Medical Journal*, 325, pp. 92–94.

Wasson, J., Johnson, B. & Mackenzie, T. (2008) The impact of primary care patients' pain and emotional problems on their confidence with self-management, *Journal of Ambulatory Care Management*, 31(2), pp. 120–127.

Whittemore, R. & Dixon, J. (2008) Chronic illness: the process of integration, *Journal of Nursing and Healthcare of Chronic Illness* in association with, *Journal of Clinical Nursing*, 17(7b), pp. 177–187.

Williams, G. (1984) The genesis of chronic illness: narrative reconstruction, *Sociology of Health and Illness*, 6(2), pp. 175–200.

Wilson, P., Kendall, S. & Brooks, F. (2007) The expert patients programme: a paradox of patient empowerment and medical dominance. *Health and Social Care in the Community*, 15(5), pp. 426–438.

World Health Organisation (1983) *Health Education in Self-Care: Possibilities and Limitations*. World Health Organisation, Geneva.

Chapter 9

Managing common symptoms of long-term conditions

Kerri Wright[1], Pia Sweet[1,2], Natasha Ascott[3], Harry Chummun[1] and Jenny Taylor[4]

[1]School of Health and Social Care, University of Greenwich, Eltham, London, UK; [2]South London Health NHS Trust, UK; [3]Basildon and Thurrock University Hospital, UK; [4]St Christopher's Hospice, South London, UK

Introduction

The chapter explores some of the common generic symptoms which people with long-term conditions (LTCs) experience. The symptoms of fatigue, depression, stress, pain and breathlessness will be considered along with appropriate strategies and ideas that could help people to manage living with these symptoms more effectively. Lastly, the benefits of increasing physical activity are discussed.

Fatigue

Fatigue is a difficult and debilitating symptom of many LTCs. It is experienced by many people who are living with a wide range of different LTCs, such as multiple sclerosis (MS), chronic obstructive pulmonary disease (COPD), rheumatoid arthritis (RhA), cancer, chronic fatigue syndrome and Parkinson's disease (Repping-Wuts *et al.,* 2008). In MS and RhA, studies have highlighted that over half of people with these conditions experience fatigue on a daily basis (Branãs *et al.,* 2000; Bol *et al.,* 2009; Repping-Wuts *et al.,* 2008). Fatigue is also described by many people as one of the most debilitating symptoms and the most difficult to live with. People living with RhA and MS have both reported that after pain, fatigue is the most frequent and difficult to manage symptom of their condition (Repping *et al.,* 2007; Bol *et al.,* 2009; Neill *et al.,* 2006).

Fatigue related to living with an LTC is described as 'physical, exhausting and frustrating having consequences for role, relationships, leisure time, with emotional aspects requiring everyday adaptation' (Repping-Wuts *et al.,* 2008: 1000). It is experienced as unpredictable and fluctuating from day-to-day. This can increase frustration as it cannot be planned for and results in constant changes to the person's routine and plans; leading to cancellations and a feeling of letting people down (Repping-Wuts *et al.,* 2008). Frustration is also felt because there is not always a specific reason for the experience of fatigue which makes it harder for the person and those around to understand and accept:

Long-Term Conditions: Nursing Care and Management, First Edition. Edited by Liz Meerabeau and Kerri Wright.
© 2011 Blackwell Publishing Ltd. Published 2011 by Blackwell Publishing Ltd.

'I think most people, unless they have experienced it themselves, don't understand about fatigue and think it is simply being tired. I know I speak to my partner about being 'wiped' out and at first he just thought this meant I merely needed sit down (I wish)!!! But now he knows I mean utterly exhausted, physically and mentally and emotionally. It is like nothing I have ever had before. . .and I hate it!!!'

(Kralik *et al.*, 2005: 376)

'Frustrating, my mind is full of energy but my body doesn't have that energy, is unwilling to react . . . it is just tired and nothing else, totally worn out.'

(Repping-Wuts *et al.*, 2008: 999)

Fatigue is described as being different from the everyday experience of feeling tired. Normal tiredness is generally related to some identifiable form of exertion and is relieved by resting. In contrast, one of the features of fatigue is that it is not linked to any identifiable exertion and is not always relieved or improved with rest (Neill *et al.*, 2006).

The invisibility of fatigue and the difficulties in articulating how this experience feels can make the problem difficult to accept by the person themselves, by friends and family and health care professionals (Kralik *et al.*, 2005). This can lead to people feeling stigmatised as the experience is believed to be unreal and 'all in their head'. Fatigue is a subjective experience and is, therefore, unquantifiable. This can result in health care professionals dismissing this problem or misunderstanding what this experience means for the individual (Trendall, 2000). In addition, research into fatigue has been criticised as using a biomedical perspective in an attempt to ascertain the cause of fatigue and provide medical treatment (Kralik *et al.*, 2005). This could explain why many studies report that people experiencing fatigue do not discuss this symptom with health care professionals and feel that they have to manage it on their own (Repping-Wuts *et al.*, 2008; Kralik *et al.*, 2005; Hewlett *et al.*, 2005):

'It's funny that you don't get much response from doctors or consultants when you try and explain that, there's a big chunk of what's wrong isn't something they can touch or feel or x-ray or blood tests.'

(Hewlett *et al.*, 2005: 701)

'I don't think I have ever raised it because I honestly think I have been blaming myself for being tired or sick or not able to do things!!! . . . '

(Kralik *et al.*, 2005: 377)

'I just don't mention it anymore to the (general practitioner), as I have so many times and he has just ignored it so I have given up . . . '

(Kralik *et al.*, 2005: 377)

Fatigue is a real experience felt by people living with LTCs which greatly affects their quality of life and ability to manage their life with their condition. The unpredictability, invisibility and debilitating effects of fatigue when experienced can affect individuals' roles from being a family member, such as an active grandparent, to the ability to maintain employment. Relationships can be challenged, with family and friends finding it difficult to understand and accept; frequently being let down or having to take on more respon-sibilities. In addition, there can be frustration from being incapacitated by fatigue for no obvious reason and the inability to fulfil their plans for that day. It is understandable, therefore, that the experience of fatigue is also often associated with psychological distress in people trying to manage this symptom (Kralik *et al.,* 2005).

> '...before the fatigue hits you feel as if you are physically being drained. Like someone has pulled a plug on you somewhere and your entire 'life force' is being drained off. Also often a feeling of utter despair comes at the same time. It is an awful, and often frightening experience.'
>
> (Kralik *et al.,* 2005:376)

Living with fatigue is challenging physically, psychologically, spiritually and socially for people (Kralik *et al.,* 2005). Fatigue, therefore, cannot be viewed in isolation, but must be considered within the context of the person's life experiences (Kralik *et al.,* 2005). As people experiencing fatigue do not often mention this problem to health care professionals, it is important that nurses are aware that this is likely to be a common experience for people living with an LTC and question people about this. Opportunities need to be made to allow people to communicate their experiences of fatigue. These experiences need to be heard and validated by health care professionals and their fears and frustrations acknowledged as real and important. The exploration of fatigue experience with people needs to include the social, emotional and spiritual realms of the person's life as well as the physical symptoms. This involves exploring what the physical symptoms and the effect they have on their life mean to them and their relationships around them. Having one's experiences being validated, legitimised and heard in itself is therapeutic and is felt to be an important role for health care professionals in supporting people who are experiencing fatigue (Kralik *et al.,* 2005).

There are a number of different strategies that people living with fatigue employ to help them manage this symptom of their LTC. These strategies are useful for health care professionals to be aware of when assessing and supporting people living with LTCs. The strategies can be divided into two main areas: problem-based strategies and emotional strategies (Repping-Wuts *et al.,* 2008), although the two areas are also closely related.

Problem-based strategies for the management of fatigue

Problem-based strategies are physical activities that people engage in, or omit, in an attempt to manage and alleviate their fatigue. These strategies are unique to the person and are based on their experience of what helps them. The most commonly cited interventions by people are pacing and rest.

Pacing

Pacing involves the person limiting the number of activities that need to be completed in a day and taking one's time in completing these. People tended to conserve energy for their most valued activities (Kralik *et al.,* 2005; Neill, 2005), for example a visit from a grandchild or a walk in the park. Nurses can support people in prioritising and being creative about the activities that they feel need to be completed in a day and utilising resources which could allow people to conserve vital energy. For example, occupational therapists may be able to suggest aids that allow people to conserve energy such as a chair to allow the person to sit whilst washing and cooking or home carers to take over cleaning and shopping activities to allow energy to be saved for more valued activities. Nurses need to work closely with the individual to problem solve the issue of pacing and energy conservation throughout the day, respecting what is valued and vital for the individual and working with these to find acceptable strategies or solutions.

Rest

Rest involves activities that encourage the person to physically or mentally rest their body. These include planning an afternoon sleep, sitting down after each activity completed or spending time relaxing through having a bath, listening to music or reading a book. Again these activities are unique to the individual and they may require time to experiment with several of these strategies to find the ones that are most effective for them.

Exercise

Exercise has also been identified as effective in managing the symptom of fatigue (Neill *et al.*, 2006; Bol *et al.*, 2009). The exercise programme needs to be tailored to the individual and could be designed by the individual themselves based on their own knowledge of their fatigue patterns. Exercise has been found to be effective in the management of a number of common symptoms found with LTCs such as depression and stress. As physical exercise is such an important strategy for self-management, it will be discussed in more detail later in this chapter.

Emotional strategies for the management of fatigue

Acceptance

One of the difficulties for people living with fatigue is that it is invisible and, therefore, difficult for the person and their friends and family to always understand. This can make accepting the symptom of fatigue difficult for the individual and their family. Engaging in self-care activities, such as pacing or conserving energy, can then become problematic as the person feels compelled to complete activities that they or their family expect of them. One of the most important strategies for managing fatigue, therefore, is gaining the understanding and support of friends and family and of health care professionals to firstly validate what the person is feeling and experiencing (Repping-Wuts *et al.*, 2008; Kralik *et al.*, 2005). This can give the person 'permission' to rest or be exempt from certain activities and can give vital support as friends and families become involved in helping practically and sharing the problem of managing their fatigue together (Hewlett *et al.*, 2005), illustrating the 'sick role' exemption discussed in the Chapter 4. Accepting the symptom of fatigue and adjusting the expectations people have of themselves, therefore, can help the individual to begin to integrate the experience of fatigue into their life (Small and Lamb, 1999).

Self-efficacy

The experience of gaining mastery over the effects of fatigue and the feeling of being able to control and manage this symptom can also have a beneficial effect on the person's emotional well-being (Kralik *et al.,* 2005). Increased self-efficacy has been correlated in studies with a reduction of fatigue (Riemsma *et al.,* 1998) and has been shown to positively affect a person's willingness and ability to engage in self-care activities (Scruggs, 2009; Hoffman *et al.,* 2009). Self-efficacy can be increased by validating the individual's experiences of living with fatigue, involving family and friends in supporting and working with the individual to develop self-management strategies to manage their fatigue (Hewlett *et al.,* 2005).

Cognitive behavioural therapy (CBT)

The debilitating effects, both emotional and physical, of fatigue can mean that some people do not have the motivation or strength to begin to engage in any self-management activities and cannot, therefore, begin to gain control of their symptoms. For these people, CBT could be useful in helping them to challenge the beliefs which are contributing towards their negative thoughts and preventing them from engaging in activities which could help them to manage their fatigue (see Chapter 6 for more information about CBT).

This section has discussed the effect fatigue can have on a person's life and outlined the main strategies that are useful for supporting people to manage these symptoms. The importance of nurses assessing and validating an individual's experience of fatigue has been highlighted and the necessity of planning and supporting individuals to manage their fatigue based on their current value and belief system. Box 9.1 summarises the main roles for a nurse in supporting a person to self-manage fatigue.

Box 9.1 Nurses' responsibilities in supporting people with fatigue.
(Adapted from Neill *et al.* 2006).

1. Ask about and validate the person's experience of fatigue and how it affects their life.
2. Assessing the person individually based on what is important to them.
3. Consider the possibility of other causes for symptom of fatigue and testing for these, for example hypothyroidism, anaemia, depression, but remain accepting of the experience of fatigue regardless of any tangible cause.
4. Encourage a balance between rest and optimal level of exercise for individual.
5. Support the individual in educating family and friends about fatigue and provide health education where appropriate.
6. Consider referrals to other health care professionals to support individual, for example homecare, occupational therapist, physiotherapist.
7. Recommend other community resources available, for example support groups, leisure facilities and clubs.
8. Monitor and continually assess symptoms of fatigue.

Depression

As discussed in Chapter 5, depression is a common co-morbidity of many physical LTCs. There is evidence of high prevalence of depression in particular in people with cardiovascular disease, diabetes, Parkinson's disease and stroke (Ormel and Von Korff, 2000; Anderson *et al.,* 2001; Goldney *et al.,* 2004; National Institute for Health and Clinical Excellence (NICE), 2006a). Depression can be both a consequence of living with an LTC and the associated effects this could have on someone's life and also the cause of a physical condition developing, for example coronary heart disease (Care Services Improvement Partnership (CSIP), 2006; NICE, 2009a). Living with an LTC and managing symptoms and self-care can be impeded by the development of depression and can result in the exacerbation of physical symptoms and emotional distress. Prevention and early detection of depression is thus an important role for nurses in LTC management.

Depression is characterized by a persistent low mood, loss of interest and enjoyment in ordinary things and experiences and a range of other cognitive, behavioural and emotional symptoms that impair the person's ability to function on a day-to-day basis (NICE, 2009a). Some of the common symptoms experienced are fatigue, sleep disturbances, an inability to concentrate, preoccupation with negative thoughts, emotional numbness, feeling guilty or self-blaming and feelings of worthlessness and hopelessness (see Table 9.1 for more symptoms). Depression is usually characterised by the intensity and persistence of the feelings that people experience on a continuum from mild to severe and is diagnosed through assessment questionnaires based on a person's subjective experiences such as the Beck Depression Inventory or Hospital Anxiety and Depression Scale (HADS).

Screening and diagnosing for depression has recently been advised in the NICE guidelines for depression (NICE, 2009b). Depression has recently been included as an additional National Quality Indicator to encourage case finding for depression within the coronary

Table 9.1 Symptoms of depression.

Behavioural and physical	Emotional	Cognitive
Tearfulness	Anxiety	Poor concentration
Irritability	Agitation	Reduced attention
Social withdrawal	Loss of interest or	Pessimism
Reduced sleep	enjoyment in everyday life	Recurrent negative thoughts
Exacerbation of pre-existing	Feelings of guilt,	about oneself, one's past
pains	worthlessness	and the future
Muscular tension and	Deserved punishment	Mental slowing
associated pain	Low self-esteem	Rumination
Loss of appetite	Loss of confidence	
Reduced libido	Feelings of helplessness	
Fatigue	Suicidal ideation	
Reduced physical activity		
Attempts at self-harm or		
suicide		

Source: NICE, 2009a.

Table 9.2   Physical manifestations of psychological distress.

Physical manifestations	Examples
Pain	Pain, migraines, abdominal pains or exacerbation of current pain
Sleep disturbances	Waking early, difficulty getting to sleep, waking unrefreshed
Fatigue	Lethargy, no energy or motivation, exhaustion after minimal activity
Change in bowel habits	Constipation or irregular or loose stools

heart disease and diabetes practice populations where there is significant evidence of prevalence and assessments for severity of depression at the onset of any treatment (British Medical Association (BMA), 2009; NICE, 2009b). The NICE guidelines also recommend screening for all people with a significant physical illness and especially if this illness causes disability (NICE, 2009a). In addition, research has indicated that people are more likely to present for help with a physical complaint than with a psychological complaint. These people may feel that physical complaints are a more valid reason for a health consultation or could be experiencing somatised feelings (where psychological distress is manifested in physical symptoms; see Table 9.2) possibly related to depression. Health professionals need to undertake a full assessment in order to ascertain potential causes and treatment and not be side-tracked into focusing on any pre-existing known chronic disease as the cause, to the exclusion of assessing the person's psychological well-being and overlooking potential depression (NICE, 2009a).

Depression can be a difficult illness for people to understand and accept. Like fatigue, it is invisible and it can, therefore, be difficult for friends and family to understand or for the individual themselves to accept. There is still a stigma regarding depression and a view that it is not a real illness and that people need to just 'snap out of it'. Such views can prevent people from acknowledging that they have a problem and from seeking help and can lead to an exacerbation of some of the symptoms of low self-worth and self-blame. Depression can sometimes be viewed as understandable and 'to be expected' considering the circumstances that someone has experienced. This is especially apparent in the older population who may be more reluctant to waste the time of their GP or nurse for something that they do not consider to be a 'real illness'. It is important to challenge these thoughts and validate the feelings that the person is experiencing, reassuring them that it is a genuine illness which can be treated and managed.

Depression is a debilitating and isolating illness that can have a devastating impact on all aspects of a person's life. It affects cognitive, physical, emotional and spiritual realms of the person as can be seen by the list of symptoms in Table 9.1. At its worst, depression can lead to feelings of utter despair, hopelessness and a preoccupation with suicidal thoughts. The person may be emotionally withdrawn and it may be difficult to make emotional contact with them. The symptoms of depression also interrelate and create a negative cycle of despair. For example, sleeplessness can lead to tiredness and low-energy levels which can prevent someone from being physically active. This can contribute to the person feeling and thinking that they are useless because they cannot undertake an activity and lead to more feelings of despair and anxiety, which could cause further sleeplessness. In severe depression, this cycle is incredibly difficult to break as the person may be too low and withdrawn to make any emotional contact.

> 'People rarely discuss the absolute humiliation of severe depression, the punishing helplessness, the distressing, child-like impotence. When well –intentioned friends and family say to the depressive, 'pull yourself together', they may as well be saying it to a baby crying in its cot. We cannot. It is not that we don't want to. We simply can't. But, unlike the baby in the cot, our adult brain is sufficiently engaged to know that we should, to believe that if we tried hard enough, we could. Then every attempt and every failure brings with it its own additional depression, its own profound and hopeless despair. And every contemptuous glance, every irritated sigh from family and friends drives us still further into the cold, black night.'
>
> (Brampton, 2008: 43)

The feelings of depression can fluctuate. There can be times when someone may feel their mood lift slightly and then other times when they can feel it sinking lower. One of the strategies of managing depression is to help people to use the 'windows' created by their mood lift to undertake an activity which could further lift their mood (Samaritans, 1996). This can create a positive cycle. For example, if someone felt their mood lift slightly they may be able to go for a short walk to the corner shop. The effect of the physical activity, the sense of achievement and the social interaction in the shop can further improve the person's mood as well as reducing sleeplessness and contribute to further 'windows'. Creating 'windows' and challenging the symptoms of depression to break the negative cycle are the basis for many of the strategies to treat and manage depression that will be discussed in the next section.

Strategies for managing depression

Validation and education

One of the most important strategies for managing depression is validating the person's experience and feelings. The stigma of depression and the invisibility of the illness can lead to feelings of self-blame and frustration in family and friends that can further exacerbate the person's feelings of worthlessness. Validating and educating everyone involved in supporting the individual with depression can help the individual to accept their depression and access appropriate support and help. There are a number of free leaflets about depression available on mental health websites, such as Depression Alliance and MIND, which can be downloaded and given to family and friends and the individual to help them accept their illness and consider different ways of treating and managing this.

Talking therapies

The recommended treatment for severe depression is anti-depressants or talking therapies (NICE, 2009b). There are a large number of anti-depressants available (see British National Formulary (BNF) for details). Often, several types may need to be trialled before the right one is found for the individual, so it is important that people are encouraged to try a different type of anti-depressant rather than stop taking medication if they do not get on with a particular type. Anti-depressant medication can lift a person's mood and create 'windows' so that other treatments such as talking therapy or exercise can be used. Anti-depressant medication alone is unlikely to treat depression, and other treatments and strategies are needed alongside this.

There are several different types of talking therapies available that people with depression could try. The most common therapy, which can be accessed through the GP, is CBT. This therapy aims to challenge an individual's negative thoughts which could be contributing to their behaviour in order to break the negative cycle of depression. CBT has been shown to be effective in the treatment of depression and is discussed in more detail in Chapter 6. Other talking therapies involve counselling with various different approaches from exploring the individual's present feelings (humanistic) to analysing past experiences to make sense of the individual's depression (psychodynamic) (see Chapter 6 for more details on talking therapies). Not all of these therapies are available through the NHS and they may require accessing privately. Therapists registered with the British Association of Counselling and Psychotherapy (BACP) and available in local areas are listed on the BACP website.

Exercise

Exercise has been increasingly shown to lift a person's mood and is, therefore, seen as a useful strategy for treating and managing depression (NICE, 2009b; Mead *et al.,* 2009). As discussed below, physical activity does not have to be vigorous or involve taking part in a formal sport, but can be any physical activity adapted for the individual according to their limitations. Sitting in a chair and doing arm lifts with tin cans or standing three times every hour could all contribute. The activity needs to be achievable with a measurable outcome to increase motivation and a sense of achievement when completed. Motivation can also be increased by linking the activity with a social occasion or group activity, such as a walking group or chair aerobics classes.

Social interaction

Social isolation is another common symptom of depression that can again exacerbate some of the other symptoms and lead to individuals having a preoccupation with their thoughts and feelings which can become negative. Encouraging social interaction can alleviate some of the isolation and loneliness that exacerbate depressive symptoms and can encourage people to develop an interest outside of themselves. Initially, people may not wish to socialise due to feelings of low self-esteem and feeling that they will make other people miserable and bored. Educating the person as well as friends and family as to the importance of socialising could give an added incentive for the person to try to meet other people, for example attending a day centre or luncheon club or arranging for family or friends to visit once a week.

The treatment for depression requires that the individual try to help themselves to create windows of opportunity, through talking therapies or medication for example, and then use these windows to undertake an activity which can further help their depression, for example exercise or socialising. Unfortunately, people with depression can find it difficult to generate the energy or feel so despairing that they cannot help themselves. It is important that nurses work with people who are experiencing depression so that they can begin to reflect on what is causing it, understanding the negative cycle and how it applies to them and can work out what helps *them* to break this cycle and lift their mood and feelings (see Table 9.3 which can be photocopied and given out, or worked through with people). Nurses may need to work with other health care professionals such as counsellors or GPs to access treatment that helps to lift a person's mood so that they can work with the 'windows' of opportunity this treatment may create.

Stress

The stress reaction is elicited by a wide variety of biopsychosocial events that are perceived as physiologically or emotionally threatening. People's responses to events and whether they are perceived to be threatening are unique to each individual. Perceived threats are dependent on, for example, an individual's past experiences, their social and cultural values and beliefs as well as genetic factors. It is vital, therefore, to listen to the person and their perceptions of the event or situation to understand how they maybe feeling and how their body may be responding to the stress. It is also possible that a person may feel stressed, but not know the reason. Unknown stress reactions can occur if the threat experienced is not in the person's conscious awareness, but is being experienced unconsciously by the body. The body's response to these threats will be the same and we need to respect the feelings and experiences of the individual and try to understand the situation from their perspective in order to support them.

Stress is experienced when the body perceives itself to be under threat, and responds by making psychological and biologically adjustments. These adjustments are important to enhance performance and protect the body from harm; in the short term, therefore, stress is a useful response to threatening situations. However, in the long term, if the body is continually or regularly perceived to be under threat, the prolonged biological and psychological adjustments required can result in physical and psychological disorders (Epel *et al.,* 1998). This section discusses the biological and psychological adjustments to perceived threats and strategies to manage and reduce the effects of chronic stress.

The general adaptive syndrome

The stress response is an innate response to protect the body from threats which were likely to be life-threatening, for example when humans were hunters and at risk from physical attacks. Even though the situations that are perceived as threats are not often life-threatening today, for example an appointment with a consultant, the physiological and psychological adjustment the body makes in response to this threat is the same.

Table 9.3 Challenging depressive symptoms.

Symptom	Action
Loss of feeling, lack of reaction, numbness	Try to give yourself possibilities to feel some emotion. You may need to actively seek these experiences to allow space for these feelings to emerge: Get angry, e.g. shout loudly, try shouting what you are angry about, e.g. 'I'm sick of this pain' or 'I hate being stuck inside' (play music loudly if you are worried that the neighbours may hear!); throw or punch cushions. Cry, watch or read a sad story, play music that moves you or look at old photographs – give yourself the opportunity and space to feel and cry. Laugh, watch funny films, smile at yourself in the mirror, make yourself laugh; after a while the sheer absurdity of what you are doing may bring a genuine laugh!
Loss of sensation	Creating strong sensory stimulation can help you to begin to feel again: Play some music loudly and feel the beat of the music within you. Do some exercise; the pain of this will take your mind off your depression! Take a hot or cold shower. Wear some aftershave or perfume you used to like. Eat spicy or tasty food or have a drink you are not used to, to challenge your taste buds. If you are able to, have a massage or have your hair cut and ask for a head massage too.
Loss of self- expression or creativity	Give yourself the opportunity to be creative. If it does not feel right on your own then find some children you can 'play' with to give you the perfect excuse: Paint or draw; you are not looking to create art but to use the colours and physical act of drawing to express how you feel, use brushes or dip your fingers in the paint. Pottery or play dough can be another way of expressing yourself, make models, squeeze the material or make models and squash them violently to express your feelings. Dance to music. This can be in your chair or even while lying in bed.
Distance from other people	These are ideas that can help you to reduce the distance that your depression may have brought between you and family and/or friends: Be honest and say what you think and feel. Put judgement and blame of others aside. Put judgement and blame of yourself aside and say what you need to say.
Difficulty in sleeping	Change your sleeping habits: Try a different room, go to bed or get up earlier or later, devise a different bedtime routine, use new bedding, buy a new pillow. Get so tired physically that you need more sleep; this will also help you to relax as well as give you a sense of achievement.

(Continued)

Table 9.3   Challenging depressive symptoms. (*Continued*)

Symptom	Action
Difficulty in getting up in the morning	Set your alarm: Put it on a plate on the other side of the room or even downstairs where you cannot ignore it and have to get up! Try to find an incentive to get up: Make sure that food and drink is in another room, so you have to get up for it. Set up something that you are responsible for, e.g. walking a dog, collecting the neighbour's paper, doing voluntary work.
Feeling worse in the morning	Get your body moving: Do some stretches, walk to the corner shop, visit your local cafe, try not to think about the activity, but have something that you do without thinking, so before you know it you are active. Create a timetable of morning activities that you follow each week. Postpone any activity requiring concentration or initiative to later in the morning.
Difficult in getting moving, tiredness, feeling there is little energy in your body	Do some cleaning: Sort out a bookshelf, tidy a cupboard, open a window and air the room. However small, the sense of achievement and the act of 'sorting' and 'cleaning' can lift your mood. Take some form of physical activity; it does not matter how small as long as you start to move those muscles! Do some aggressive physical activity: Punch or kick a pillow, throw balled socks across the room, do cooking that involves crushing ingredients, e.g. biscuits or nuts and go to town with the rolling pin. The combination of the physical exercise and the aggressiveness can act as a powerful natural antidepressant.
Slumped body, bent back	Try to stand more upright. Do some stretching exercises. Consider getting a different mattress for your bed, so that you lie flatter or get someone to put some boards under your mattress.
Slowness of movement	Try to speed up your movement if you can. If you are able to, gradually increase your speed of walking and maybe even start to run (check with your GP first). If you are unable to walk, try to increase the speed of your thought; try a crossword or word search and challenge yourself to do these more quickly.
Miserable expression	Try to smile. Every morning look in the mirror and smile at yourself. The act of changing a bodily gesture or expression can have a feedback effect on the feeling.
Constipation	Make sure your diet includes plenty of fresh fruit, vegetables and fibre. Try to do more physical exercise; this stimulates the gut to work faster. Make sure you drink plenty of fluids, not just tea or coffee. Talk to a health care professional if the constipation causes pain or does not improve.

Table 9.3   Challenging depressive symptoms. (*Continued*)

Symptom	Action
Loss of initiative and difficulty in getting started at anything	Get someone else to give you orders and organise you. Make a list of everything you need to do. From this list take two things, one that you will like and one that you will hate. Both must be things that are realistic and can be done in a short time – a few hours at the most. The goals must be realistic and achievable. Arrange to do things with other people. Make an appointment with somebody, so there is a little pressure to be somewhere by a certain time. Do the shopping or the crossword with a friend or family.
Indecisiveness	Consider the fact that not making a decision is more likely to cause failure than the actual decision you make. Therefore, decide one way or another and tackle that course of action without further thought. If you really cannot decide, flip a coin or use dice and obey the result. This advice obviously does not apply to major life decisions!
Loss of concentration and short-term memory	Write things down. If you find you are continuously forgetting things keep a pen and note pad close at hand to remind you and help you concentrate. Use a separate page for written questions or concerns to discuss with forthcoming health care professionals appointments.
Loss of care about your appearance	How you look can be an expression of yourself and can have a strong effect on how you feel. Buy some new clothes or ask family members to do this for you. Consider doing exercise to try to change your body shape, if you are not happy with this. Get your hair done; maybe try a new look. Have a manicure or a pedicure or get a wet shave.
Loss of care about your environment	Changing how the physical environment looks can change how you feel. Consider cleaning and decorating or arranging to have this done. Put up some different photographs, take down the net curtains, move a lamp; little changes can make a difference.
Giving up responsibility of action, blaming yourself	Ask yourself if your depression gives you a way out of responsibility and, therefore, whether it is a genuine temptation to stay depressed. Do not be afraid to admit this if it is true. Accepting it is the first step to changing it. Make yourself responsible for something or somebody. Get some plants to look after, look after somebody's dog or get a cat. Concern yourself with somebody else's needs. You can be helped by others, but there is no doubt that you have the final say. The powers of self-healing are already within you.

(*Continued*)

Table 9.3   Challenging depressive symptoms. (*Continued*)

Symptom	Action
Hating yourself, hating the world, losing self-respect, believing the world is bad, believing you are bad	Forgiving yourself and forgiving others are both healing processes. The more you can forgive yourself, the more you can forgive others and vice versa; the two are intimately connected. Find ways to self-care and treat yourself; make a list of things you enjoy or used to enjoy doing and then choose an activity in the list and do it just for fun and no other reason, e.g. bake a cake or buy a treat from the shops, plant some seeds, do some painting, buy a new DVD, go for a ride on a bus around town, go to the park and feed the ducks and sit and have an ice cream. If you find yourself reading the newspapers and using them to support your view of the world, stop reading them for a while or write to the newspaper with a positive opinion. Put love into the things you do. Whether you are caring for someone or talking to the home carer; do it out of love rather than duty. The love you put out with trust and no expectation will come back to you somehow.
Negative thinking	Remember that positive thought is as powerful as negative thoughts. Just a few seconds of positive thinking maybe long enough to initiate a positive activity. Positive thinking requires an activity to affirm it; be patient with the activity and don't expect miracles! Write down a list of your assets; get family and friends to help if you wish. Read the list of assets every day. Pin it to your wall in the bathroom or bedroom.
Believing there is nothing inside of you	Give. If necessary make yourself give something. Give of yourself, your memories, your thoughts, and your dreams. There is no greater proof that there is something inside of you.
Negative colouration of the past; on looking back everything seems awful	Make a list of all the positive things you have done in your life and of all the people you have helped even in the smallest way. If you are too depressed to do this on your own get someone who knows you to help you remember. Stick the list next to your list of assets and read this every day too. Make another list of all the moments of pleasure you have had. You may have negative thoughts about these moments thinking 'oh yes but these will never happen again' Put these thoughts aside for a moment and try to read and enjoy your list.
The future seems blank and everything is getting worse; negative colouration of the future; loss of purpose; loss of hope	It may not be your privilege to know what your purpose is. When you feel a slight upswing in mood write down some achievable and realistic goals for the future and plan how you are going to work towards these. If you cannot feel hope, remember there is always the hope of hope. Know that depression, even when untreated, gets better.

Source: Adapted from Gillet, 1987 (137–141).

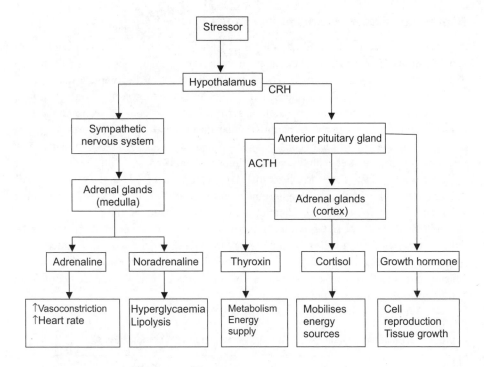

CRH – Corticotropin-releasing hormone

ACTH - Adrenocorticotropic hormone

Figure 9.1   The stress hormones and their functions.

There are three stages to the adaptive response to stress often referred to as the General Adaptation Syndrome or GAS. The hormones and neural responses and the effect they have on the body can be seen in Figure 9.1.

1. *'Fight or flight' response/phase:* When first exposed to a stressor, the adrenal medulla and the sympathetic nerves from the autonomic nervous system respond by releasing the hormones adrenaline and noradrenaline to help the body overcome the stressor. These hormones activate a series of physiological responses to prepare to fight or run away from the stressor.
2. *The resistance phase:* During exposure to a sustained stress period, the adrenal cortex produces cortisol to continue supporting various organs in their struggle to overcome the stressor with the support of thyroxin and growth hormone.
3. *The exhaustion phase:* If the resistance phase is inadequate, pathological changes occur in the anatomical structures with severe reduction in physiological functioning, resulting in chronic disorders and, ultimately, organ failure. Recovery from this is almost impossible.

Biopsychosocial effects of chronic stress

The long-term effects of raised adrenaline and noradrenaline decrease the immune response, alter protein and fat metabolism, impair tissue repair, increase blood pressure and decrease digestion and libido (Everly and Lating, 2002). If complete relaxation is not achieved, cortisol will be released in larger amounts to continue the adjustment. Prolonged hypercortisolaemia causes long-term muscle and connective tissue wastage, hyperglycemia, increased risk of cardiovascular disease and chronic suppression of the immune response and of the healing process (Gianaros *et al.*, 2007). A summary of the responses to chronic stress can be seen in Tables 9.4 and 9.5.

Chronic stress can, therefore, lead to the development of LTCs such as heart failure, diabetes and irritable bowel syndrome, and psychological disorders such as depression and anxiety. In addition, chronic stress can also exacerbate the physiological and psychological effects of LTCs and make the management of some conditions more difficult, for example hyperglycaemia in people with diabetes, increased risk of infection in respiratory conditions and increased pain in neurological or musculoskeletal conditions. Chronic stress can also cause anxiety and low mood, contributing to reduced confidence and motivation to self-manage LTCs.

Table 9.4 The common signs and symptoms associated with chronic stress.

Physical	Psycho-emotional	Behavioural
Headache and backache	Loss of concentration	Overeating
Fatigue	Confusion	Nervous habits, e.g. nail
Insomnia, sleep disturbance	Inability to complete	biting
Dry mouth	allocated tasks	Procrastination, indecision
Nausea	Inability to undertake	Withdrawal
Abdominal pain	cognitive exercises	Alcohol abuse
Indigestion	Irritability/short temper/	Increased smoking
Diarrhoea/constipation	impatience/argumentative	Substance abuse
Loss of appetite	Problems with personal	Suicidal thoughts
Chest pain	relationships	
Palpitations	Anxiety, constant worrying	
Sweaty hands	Depression, apathy	
Hypertension	Intense mood swings	
Hyperglycaemia	Feeling of helplessness	
Loss of libido	Feeling of worthlessness	
Low thyroxin hormone	Feeling of doom	
Decrease in muscle mass	Seeing only the negative	
Increased abdominal fat	Hypersensitivity	
Development of metabolic		
syndrome		
Decreased bone density		
Lowered immunity and		
inflammatory responses		
Reduced wound healing		
Higher levels of low-density		
lipoprotein and lower levels		
of high-density lipoprotein		

Table 9.5 The main physiological effects of chronic stress.

Cardiovascular system	Musculoskeletal system
Increased strength and rate of heartbeat Hypertension Thickening and narrowing of arteries Ventricular hypertrophy Increased cardiac effort Reduced blood flow and fatigue Hyperglycaemia Hypercholesterolaemia	Chronic muscular tension and pain Migraine and tension headaches Exaggeration of reflexive postural patterns Bone demineralisation Loss of bone mass Reduced bone healing
Digestive tract	**Reproductive system**
Increased hydrochloric acid production Gastritis Stomach and duodenal ulcers Gastric distension Obesity or weight loss Irritable bowel syndrome Diarrhoea	Infertility Menstrual disorders Impotence or premature ejaculation Loss of libido
Urinary system	**Immune system**
Bladder urgency Incontinence	Allergies Increased susceptibility to illness such as common cold Autoimmune conditions
Metabolism	**Respiratory system**
Reduced metabolic rate Diabetes mellitus	Asthma symptoms often worsen under mental or emotional stress Frequent chest infections

Strategies for reducing stress

To normalise cortisol levels, the body's relaxation response must be activated after the fight or flight response. During the relaxation response, the mind is trained not to perceive the stressor as a threat, but as a challenge. Therefore, as the mind does not perceive a threat, it may not lead to an acute physiological response and thus cortisol synthesis will remain within or very close to therapeutic ranges. During the relaxation process, the body moves from a state of heightened physiological arousal, such as increased heart rate and blood pressure, slowed digestive functioning, decreased blood flow to the extremities and increased release of hormones like adrenaline and cortisol, to a state of physiological relaxation, where blood pressure, heart rate, digestive functioning and hormonal levels return to normal.

A relaxation response can best be achieved when the stressed person simultaneously adopts a change in lifestyle and participates fully in programmes of external support from suitably trained therapists. Changing lifestyle may include learning to care for one's self better – getting plenty of sleep and exercise, eating more healthily, setting realistic goals, prioritising tasks and learning to say 'no' to give the body the best chance of fending off the stressor. Changing a lifetime of maladjusted behaviour, which initially leads to the chronicity of the stress, may not be easy and it is more helpful to discuss problems with professionals, such as a counsellor or a therapist. Some external support such as visual imagery, relaxed breathing, progressive muscle relaxation, meditation or yoga may be adopted by stressed individuals to complement lifestyle changes. However, for more persistent stress, more intensive therapy such as a mindfulness-based stress reduction (MBSR) programme should be considered.

Guided visual imagery

Visualization, or *guided visual imagery*, is a relaxation technique in which the person is encouraged to imagine a peaceful and tranquil scene. This helps to reduce the perception of the threat and induce a state of relaxation, by reducing sympathetic neural responses to dampen stress emotions. The unconscious mind cannot differentiate between images from experience and something imagined, so it can be fooled into producing a sense of relaxation.

Deep breathing

This quick relaxation technique focuses attention on inhaling deeply, holding the breath for a few seconds and then exhaling. This technique improves cardiovascular efficiency by increasing venous return and strengthening ventricular output which effectively increases oxygenation of the tissues under stress. More oxygen facilitates a cellular response and improves tissue adaptation to the stressor through improved internal respiration and metabolism. Deep breathing triggers the relaxation response in the body, thus helping to stop the release of cortisol (Brown *et al.*, 2005).

Deep muscle relaxation

Deep, or progressive, muscle relaxation aims to reduce overall tension in the muscles by tensing and releasing specific muscle groups. This can be achieved through massage to muscles or by exercises, where muscles are tensed and relaxed in turn. When muscles are tense there is a reduction in blood flow, nerve communication is inhibited and nutrient assimilation is decreased. Deep muscle relaxation improves blood and energy supply to every area of the body to improve local tissues' ability to overcome adverse conditions such as lactic acid, carbon dioxide and free radical accumulation.

Yoga

Yoga offers a means to connect, join or gain a balance between body and mind. Practicing regular yoga, sometimes in conjunction with meditation, enhances the relaxation response, trains the body to alter its responses to stressors and promotes a state of insight and tranquillity by reducing the influence of the pre-frontal cerebrum over the autonomic nervous system. Yoga allows the parasympathetic system to function fully to bring about the relaxation response. The hormones activated by the sympathetic nervous system are deactivated by the parasympathetic system, and so the system slows down body processes (except those that are suppressed by the sympathetic, i.e. the digestive system and the skin functions). Yoga decreases blood supply to the heart and skeletal muscles by redistributing it to inactive organs such as the gut and skin; metabolism slows down, respiration rate is reduced, digestion speeds up, the inflammation response is restored and the central nervous system is taken out of the arousal state. Yoga also significantly decreases self-reported depression, anxiety and low mood, as well as fatigue associated with cerebral neurotransmitters such as serotonin and cortisol (Malathi *et al.*, 2004).

Mindfulness-based stress reduction programmes

MBSR programmes were proposed by Jon Kabat-Zinn (1992) as a source of support to promote coping strategies and help stressed individuals to understand the theory related to stress management and the mind–body connection. Mindfulness-based stress reduction brings together mindfulness, meditation and yoga. Although MBSR has potential benefits to improve daily stress, historically, it is most effective for a wide range of chronic disorders and diseases. Mindfulness approaches are not relaxation or mood management techniques, but a form of mental training to reduce cognitive vulnerability to reactive modes of mind that may heighten stress and emotional distress, or that may otherwise perpetuate psychopathology (Kabat-Zinn, 1990). Mindfulness practice is ideal for cultivating greater awareness of the unity of mind and body, as well as of the ways the unconscious thoughts, feelings and behaviours can undermine emotional, physical and spiritual health. The mind is known to be a factor in stress and stress-related disorders, and meditation has been shown to positively affect a range of autonomic physiological processes, such as lowering blood pressure and reducing overall arousal and emotional reactivity. It strengthens coping skills relating to chronic medical conditions, such as irritable bowel syndrome, depression and chronic fatigue (Baer, 2003). This approach has been shown to reduce neural activity associated with reduced cortisol synthesis (Grossman *et al.*, 2004) and is now also used to reduce psychological morbidity from chronic illness (Kabat-Zinn, 1998).

During stress, the body responds psychologically and biologically to adjust and manage the perceived threat. In the short term, the responses provide the initial energy necessary to cope with increased physiological demand placed on the organs by the stressors. Long-term exposure to the hormones involved in the stress response can lead to physiological disorders which can cause exacerbation of LTCs, such as diabetes, or over a prolonged period can cause LTCs to develop. Recognising the signs and symptoms of progressive stress, adopting lifestyle changes and implementing stress strategies, such as relaxation through yoga, meditation, visual imagery and deep breathing exercises, can improve the quality of life for people with LTCs and potentially reduce the incidence of LTCs.

Pain

Pain is an unpleasant sensation with both physical and emotional components. The International Association for the Study of Pain (1994: 209) defines pain as 'an unpleasant sensory and emotional experience associated with actual or potential tissue damage or described in terms of such damage'. This definition is widely accepted throughout the world as it encompasses both the physical and the emotional effects of living with pain. Pain affects millions of people nationally and has far-reaching consequences on the national economy through loss of work and expenditure on NHS treatments; within the NHS half a billion pounds are spent annually on pain medication alone (Chief Medical Officer, 2009). Long-term pain can have devastating effects on a person's life, and combined with other LTCs and associated symptoms can seriously impact on a person's ability to manage their life.

The impact of living with pain can have wide-reaching implications for a person's life. Pain can impact on a person's psychological well-being and can cause, for example, stress, anxiety and depression. The psychological impact of living with pain can also exacerbate the sensation of pain and the ability to manage other self-care activities. Pain also causes physical sensations related to the cause of pain or how this pain is experienced, for example increased temperature, nausea or muscle spasms. This can impact on other areas of the person's life, for example mobility, sleep and appetite. Finally, pain can also impact on a person's social world – their ability to interact with others and the effect of social isolation, ability to work and fulfil other important social roles, such as being a caregiver, and the resultant impact on friends and family. Understanding and helping someone to manage their pain, therefore, requires a biopsychosocial approach to pain management.

Pain is commonly classified into nocioceptive and neuropathic pain. Nocioceptive pain is experienced as a result of an injury to a part of the body. Nocioceptors close to the injured site become stimulated and transmit information about the injury to the brain. This could be pain due to inflammation in a muscle, pain within the joints or pain in a person's foot. Neuropathic pain, however, is a sensation of pain that results from a problem in the nerves themselves. This can be caused by neurological conditions where the nerves are affected, for example MS, or long-term damage to the nerves, for example in diabetic neuropathy. In LTCs pain experienced by individuals can be a combination of both nocioceptive and neuropathic pain depending on the LTC they are living with as well as their own unique experiences.

Persistent pain is pain that continues beyond the time of tissue healing. As yet, the reasons for the continued sensation of pain being experienced are not fully understood. The nervous system undergoes artificial changes both peripherally and centrally which seem to contribute to the persistent sensations felt. The exact changes are unique to each individual and are thus experienced uniquely.

Persistent pain is a feature of many LTCs. In people with musculoskeletal conditions such as arthritis, joint pain is a common symptom and is estimated to be experienced by over 8.5 million people (Arthritis Care, 2004). People with neurological conditions such as MS also report pain as a symptom and experience both neurogenic and musculoskeletal pain (NICE, 2003). Other conditions such as diabetes also cause pain through neuropathy which can be problematic to manage (NICE, 2004b). The experience of persistent pain can be exacerbated by other symptoms such as depression or anxiety, but can also cause exacerbation of other LTCs through the impact of trying to manage the pain. Pain can prevent mobility, contribute towards fatigue, lower mood and reduce the feeling of control the person feels about their life. This can exacerbate feelings of depression and consequently the sensation of pain. In addition, pain and the sensations experienced by the individual with LTCs are often familiar and can have specific meanings for the person which can affect how they perceive this pain. Supporting a person to manage their pain, therefore, involves an approach that encompasses the intertwined aspects of pain within the unique experience of the person.

Pain assessment is, therefore, unique to the individual. The assessment of someone presenting with pain requires gaining information about the meaning the pain has for the person and the impact it is having on their life. This requires sound communication skills (described in Chapter 6) in order to promote an accepting and genuine interest in the person and their pain experiences. For example, pain may be an indication for the person that their condition is about to flare up again and the fear and frustration this can cause or result in more time off work and feeling that they are not in control of their condition. Assessment also involves gathering information about the type, duration, intensity and evaluation of management strategies the person is currently using or has used in the past and the success of these strategies. There are a number of pain assessment tools available for health care professionals to use to help gather information about a person's pain, for example the Magill Questionnaire and the Brief Pain Inventory which use descriptive words and numerical rating scales (Melzack, 1975; Cleeland, 1989). Successful management of persistent pain requires repeated evaluation of the patient's pain and its response to treatment or intervention.

Assessment leads to an agreed treatment plan to manage the person's pain. Complete pain relief in the treatment of pain is rarely achieved; more often a balance must be made between the effect of the treatment in managing the person's pain and the impact that this has on their life, for example side effects of pharmacological pain relief such as constipation or inability to drive, or the financial cost of treatments such as massage or psychotherapy. There are many common misconceptions about the treatment plan, and it is vital that time is made to explore the treatment agreed and the expectations and beliefs of the individual. Some of the common misconceptions are listed in Table 9.6. There are three main types of treatments/interventions for persistent pain: pharmacological, non-pharmacological and interventional treatments. Each of these will be briefly discussed.

Pharmacological treatment of pain

The drug treatment of persistent pain in LTCs can be approached in a stepwise ladder, similar to the WHO ladder for the treatment of cancer pain. It is important to titrate doses against side effects and constantly evaluate the response to any changes in treatment. The ladder in Figure 9.2 summarises some of the commonly used drugs in the management of persistent pain.

Table 9.6   Common misconceptions about pain treatment.

Misconceptions	Reality
Pain can always be controlled/improved	Often it cannot. A 50% reduction in pain is a good result in persistent pain.
Doctors can always find a cause for pain	Often they cannot, but this will usually mean that there is no sinister underlying pathology.
It is unsafe to use analgesia to maintain activity for fear of masking damage	This is untrue. Within chronic pain, the cause is often unknown and continues after any injury has healed. Analgesia is useful, therefore, in allowing activities to be continued which have many other benefits, and will not cause further damage.
Rest is good and allows healing	There may be a role for rest in acute pain but remaining active and exercise are positively beneficial in persistent pain.

Non-pharmacological treatments for pain

Transcutaneous electrical nerve stimulation (TENS)

TENS is a simple, cheap, portable self-administered device that some patients may find beneficial, which uses a low dose of electricity to stimulate the nerves. The TENS device usually has two electrodes that are placed on the area affected and apply a variable

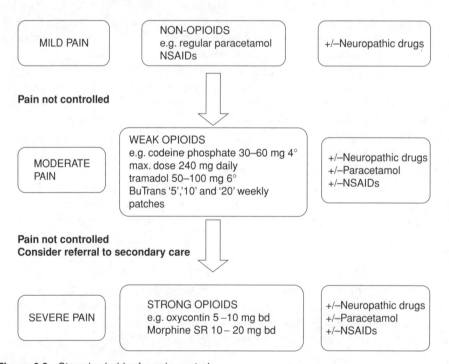

Figure 9.2   Stepwise ladder for pain control.

small electrical current which has been found to be effective in managing pain in chronic musculoskeletal pain (Johnson and Martinson, 2006) but could be beneficial for any persistent pain. There are few contraindications to TENS and minimal side effects and it is therefore a useful treatment or adjunct to treatment for pain.

Acupuncture

Acupuncture is based on the principle that illness and pain occur when the body's energy is not allowed to flow freely due to blockages that can be the result of injury, infection or emotional stresses. Treatment consists of fine needles being inserted into specific acupuncture points to re-establish the free flow of energy and stimulate healing. Acupuncture is gaining popularity and becoming more widely available on the NHS with recent NICE guidance endorsing acupuncture for low back pain (NICE, 2009d). As an effective treatment for some individuals with persistent pain, it has few adverse effects. A course of treatments with top-up is usually required for the management of LTCs.

Physical therapy

Physiotherapy, chiropractors or osteopaths can be accessed for hands-on manipulative treatment which can be useful in the early stages of pain management. This can help, for example, with realigning joints, releasing muscle tension and increasing joint mobility that could be causing or exacerbating pain. However, in persistent pain in LTCs, staying active and exercising regularly is more appropriate. The beneficial effects of physical exercise will be discussed in the section on 'physical activity' and are a useful treatment for persistent pain. Exercise strengthens joints, bones and muscles and encourages greater flexibility and suppleness in joints and is a recommended treatment for chronic back pain. Exercise also has psychological benefits that indirectly improve the person's experience of pain, such as improving depression and reducing fatigue. Massage is also an additional therapy that some people find beneficial in managing their pain, helping to relax muscles and reduce stress.

Psychological therapy

The role of psychological therapies in the treatment of persistent pain has been increasingly recognized and is recommended for the treatment of low back pain (NICE, 2009d). Early identification of psychological factors in the causation of pain will help the introduction of this therapy to an individual's treatment plan. Often, access to psychological treatment is limited by resources and it may then be possible to offer treatment in a multidisciplinary pain management programme, where patients are seen in a group setting.

Interventional treatments

Some individuals may benefit from interventional treatments, such as epidural steroids, hip blocks and facet joint injections and denervations. These treatments are available through pain clinics in secondary care. Other more specialized techniques include peripheral nerve stimulation and spinal cord stimulators.

Pain management programmes (PMP)

A PMP is a psychologically based rehabilitative pain management programme for people who have chronic pain that has not been resolved through other treatments. The programme is delivered in a group setting where people with similar pain are taught and supported to manage their life with pain and to remain as active as possible. Programmes are delivered by an interdisciplinary team and can include education and psychotherapy as well as complementary therapies. Programmes can be delivered in pain clinics where groups of people with similar pain are brought together, in residential settings, or can be encompassed in other programmes such as the Expert Patients programme (Department of Health, 2001).

Pain is an emotional and physical sensation that is experienced uniquely by individuals. Assessment and management of persistent pain requires firstly understanding the meaning that pain has for the person and how this is impacting on their life. As complete pain relief in people with persistent pain is rarely achieved, assessment and treatment involves close working with the person to help them achieve optimal quality of life with their pain.

Breathlessness (Dyspnoea)

Breathlessness is a frequent and distressing symptom of COPD, heart failure and advanced cancer. It is described as a 'subjective experience of difficult, laboured or uncomfortable breathing' (Zhao and Yates, 2008: 693) which can have a debilitating impact on a person's life. The symptom of breathlessness is multidimensional and involves a complex interplay between the biopsychosocial effects of experiencing and living with this symptom (Corner, 1999). For example, the distressing experience of not being able to breathe, a fundamental process to preserving life, can lead to avoidance of situations that could exacerbate the feelings of breathlessness (Ek and Ternestedt, 2008). Such avoidance can contribute towards social isolation, decreased physical endurance through muscle weakness and anxiety which can further exacerbate the experience of breathlessness. As a result of the multidimensional and subjective experience of breathlessness the exact cause is not always obvious; this can make planning and evaluating interventions for breathlessness problematic.

There are a range of different interventions for breathlessness. Most have been developed through the end of life care interventions used for people with advanced cancer. Both the COPD strategy and NICE guidelines for heart failure mention breathlessness as a symptom of the conditions, but offer few strategies for the management of these apart from pharmaceutical interventions at the end of life stage in COPD (NICE, 2004) and exercise and the possible benefit of breathing exercises in heart failure (NICE, 2003). Considering that breathlessness is such a distressing symptom and requires complex management by the individual experiencing this in an attempt to maintain the quality of their life (Bausewein *et al.,* 2008), the scarcity of treatment approaches is surprising.

The evidence for effective interventions to manage breathlessness is limited with many reviews highlighting the need for further research into these areas (for example Polosa *et al.*, 2002; Cranston *et al.*, 2008; Bausewein *et al.*, 2008). However, as the experience of breathlessness is subjective, the effectiveness of interventions is likely to be subjective also. In this case, a scientific evidence base is perhaps not as important as the individual's experience of relief through the use of a specific intervention. For this reason, the main interventions used in breathlessness will be discussed, regardless of the evidence base.

The first intervention for managing breathlessness is to ensure that the treatment for the underlying condition is optimised. Breathlessness should not be assumed to be an accepted symptom of an LTC, but attempts should be made to assess this symptom and ascertain if there is an underlying cause which could be reversible (NHS Lothian, 2009). This could be due to an exacerbation or advancement of the condition, the development of a complication or a symptom of another LTC. For example, increased breathlessness could be a result of an infection, pleural effusion or pulmonary embolism, cardiac arrhythmia (such as atrial fibrillation) or anaemia. Assessment and diagnosis of specific causes such as these can result in successful treatment. For people with LTCs experiencing breathlessness as a regular symptom of their conditions, it is useful to develop strategies to assess exacerbations of this symptom, both for the nurse and the person with the condition, so that changes can be assessed. This could be the use of a Visual Analogue Score (VAS) where people are asked to rate their breathlessness on a scale of 0 (no breathlessness) to 10 (extreme breathlessness); regular dyspnoea assessment using a tool such as the Medical Research Council (MRC) breathlessness tool (see Table 12.2 in Chapter 12); or facilitating the person through discussion to have more awareness of their subjective experiences of breathlessness and any changing signs. Breathlessness requires regular and thorough assessments to ensure that treatable causes are identified and managed effectively first before palliative intervention is considered. Palliative interventions aim to manage the experience of breathlessness rather than treat the cause. They can be divided into non-pharmacological and pharmacological interventions.

Non-pharmacological interventions for breathlessness

Breathing exercises

Breathing is an autonomic response regulated through a biofeedback mechanism that is driven by carbon dioxide levels. When carbon dioxide levels rise this stimulates the body to draw air into the lungs (inspiration). The sensation of breathlessness can mean that people feel they are fighting to draw enough air into their lungs and never feel satiated. The anxiety and overwhelming survival instinct to acquire sufficient air can result in an over-focus on the drawing in of breath (inspiration) at the expense of exhaling (expiration). People may begin to take short breaths in at speed as they focus on drawing air into their lungs and may recruit their accessory muscles of respiration to lift the rib cage in an attempt to increase their lung capacity. This has several effects. Firstly, rapid and shallow inspiration prevents the lungs from exhaling effectively and leads to an increase in carbon dioxide levels. The increase in carbon dioxide stimulates the body to increase the respiratory rate and exacerbates the feeling of breathlessness already felt. Secondly, the rapid inspiration rate means that full lung capacity isn't being utilised and each inspiration is unsatisfying. Using accessory muscles combined with persistently fighting for breath is both physically exhausting and uses a large amount of energy. Ensuring that each inspiratory breath is as effective as possible is a useful intervention for breathlessness.

Exercises can be taught to reduce the sensation of breathlessness by a nurse or a physiotherapist (Bott *et al.,* 2009). These exercises are aimed at improving tone and resilience of often de-conditioned respiratory muscles, achieving enhanced control of their breathing or the removal of secretions that may impede breathing. People who are managing breathlessness have also found benefit when taught the anatomy and physiology of normal respiration and the causes of their breathlessness, as an adjunct to learning breathing control technique and exercises, because enhanced understanding helps mastery of this debilitating symptom (Taylor, 2007).

Teaching someone with breathlessness to regain some control over their breathing can have both physical and psychological benefits. The hyperventilation pattern can be broken by encouraging the person to focus on their exhalations. Exhalations need to be prolonged to expel the carbon dioxide that has built up from excessive inspirations and can be achieved by instructing the person to sigh out and then out further or by concentrating on counting up to five for the exhalation. The reflex breath in that follows this is consequently deeper and uses the lung capacity more effectively. Initially, the controlled breathing technique can feel counter-intuitive for the person, but once practised with encouragement can dramatically improve their breathlessness:

'I've struggled for so long to get more air in, not understanding how breathing works. Using this way [controlled breathing technique], I feel air coming in right down deep in my chest. I feel I can fly!'

(Taylor 2007:25)

Pursed-lip breathing

This is often used by people with COPD and entails air being exhaled slowly through pursed lips. Although acknowledged by the Lung Function Association as a method of allowing each breath to feel more effective by enhancing control, it actually increases the work of breathing. Pursed-lip breathing acts by keeping the airways open for longer which can ease the sensation of breathlessness. As this pattern can rapidly become habitual, it can be very difficult to modify, but it can sometimes be helpful to encourage a more relaxed style, and thus reduce anxiety.

Removing secretions

Other breathing exercises involve the person being encouraged to inhale deeply, using the diaphragm to increase lung capacity, holding the inhalation for a count of three to five (depending on capability) and exhaling forcefully again and contracting the diaphragm to force the air out. This is known as 'huffing' and can easily be taught by a physiotherapist. This breathing exercise is a useful method for clearing secretions from the lungs and airways and can increase the person's lung capacity (see also Section 'Chest physiotherapy').

Positioning

The way a person sits or lies can affect their experience of breathlessness. The ideal position is for the thorax to be as straight and upright as possible to allow the air to be easily drawn into the lungs and for the lungs to inflate fully. When sitting in bed the person can be supported in an upright position by using pillows or making use of the bed's multi-positional features. A small pillow can be used to support the natural hollow of the lower spine and help to open up the rib cage. Arms can be supported with pillows so that the shoulders and accessory respiratory muscles are relaxed.

For some people this position is not comfortable and does not relieve breathlessness. An alternative position is for the person to use a forward leaning position to maximise their chest capacity. This can be achieved by sitting in a chair and leaning forward onto a table positioned at a comfortable height in front of the chair, using pillows for comfort. This position fixes the rib cage in an open position and reduces the work of the accessory respiratory muscles to open the rib cage, thereby reducing the work of breathing. A similar position can be used in bed, but can be uncomfortable for long periods due to the strain on the lower spine and hamstring muscles, so frequent repositioning may be required to find a tolerable position for the person.

Environment

A well-ventilated room can reduce the sensation of 'airlessness' that can exacerbate feelings of breathlessness. Ensuring that windows and doors are open when possible or positioning a chair by a window can counteract an illusion of breathlessness. A fan can also be used to provide the sensation of air availability and should be directed to pass air across the person's face. The effect of the fan can be enhanced by applying a cool damp cloth to the face or using a fine cool mist spray.

Oxygen

Oxygen is used as a treatment for hypoxia and is, therefore, useful for people who are experiencing breathlessness as a result of hypoxia, broadly with an oxygen saturation of less than 90% (NHS Lothian, 2009). However, for some people with breathlessness who are not hypoxic, oxygen therapy has been found to be useful and is worth consideration (Cranston *et al.*, 2008). However, people can become psychologically dependent on oxygen therapy – sometimes viewing it as 'life support' (Taylor, 2007: 20). This can be restrictive and distressing for the individual. Oxygen therapy can also restrict the activity of people causing further social isolation and difficulties in meeting basic care requirements. In addition, there are other considerations, such as cost, fire hazard and the community provision of oxygen. Therefore, oxygen therapy should only be used following a thorough assessment to rule out other interventions, and should be used on a trial basis only, evaluating and stopping it if it is not effective. Although oxygen is a non-pharmacological intervention, oxygen therapy does need to be prescribed and is therefore subject to pharmacological guidelines.

Saline nebulisers

Saline nebulisers have been found in some cases to be as effective in reducing the experience of breathlessness as oxygen therapy. Saline nebulisation moistens the air breathed into the lungs and is primarily used to loosen secretions and facilitate expectoration. Usually, 5% 5 mL sodium chloride is used in a nebuliser and as often as the person finds beneficial. Like oxygen therapy, saline nebulisers are a non-pharmacological intervention, but need to be prescribed and pharmacological guidelines applied.

Physical exercise

There are many physiological as well as psychological benefits to being physically active which can also benefit people experiencing breathlessness. In relation to breathlessness, physical exercise increases muscle efficiency and enables people to gradually improve their exercise tolerance which can contribute to reducing their associated breathlessness. Exercise can also improve lung function which can again reduce breathlessness and has been found to improve quality of life. It can, for example, improve breathlessness and reduce hospital admission in people with heart failure (Davies *et al.*, 2010). Both of these effects can increase a person's feeling of psychological well-being – through decreased anxiety linked to physical exertion and positive feelings of achievement and control. A physical exercise programme should be planned in conjunction with a thorough health assessment and should ideally incorporate a physiotherapist or exercise trainer where possible. A range of gentle thoracic and shoulder girdle exercises will include rotation, side flexion and general stretching within comfort zones to improve intercostal and postural muscle functions. Possible progression to appropriately modified pulmonary rehabilitation exercises which incorporate carefully supervised pacing should be considered, preferably in a group context, as this can greatly increase coping capacity and well-being.

Pacing and planning

One of the most effective interventions for managing breathlessness is planning and pacing activities to conserve energy and reduce breathlessness (Christenbery, 2005). People living with this symptom are required to plan their day according to their breathlessness and prioritise and pace their activities (Ek and Ternestedt, 2008). Some functional activities may have to be forgone or planned extensively in order for the person to manage simple activities of daily living, for example a trip to the shops may need to be planned with frequent stops for rest or through booking a wheelchair or mobility aid such as a rollator to assist in pacing their breathing (Bausewein *et al.*, 2008). Pacing and planning requires experience and awareness of the individual's body, its strengths and limitations, alongside problem solving approaches in order to prioritise and plan activities appropriately. A nurse can support and facilitate a person in this process. Suggestions to minimise the impact of breathlessness in everyday activities are given in Table 9.7.

Table 9.7 Suggestions for pacing in everyday activities.

Activity	Strategy	Rationale
Dressing	Dress and undress as much as possible sitting down	Reduces exertion for standing
	Place all clothes on bottom half of body whilst sitting as far as possible and then stand to pull up in one go	Maximises effort used in standing
	Put footwear on by crossing leg at the knee and not bending	Bending compresses the chest and increasing breathlessness
	Wear clothes that have front openings	This reduces need to twist which increases exertion
	Wear slip-on shoes	Prevent need to bend down for laces/straps, etc.
Personal hygiene	Use a stool or chair in the shower	Reduces exertion of standing
	Ensure bathroom is well ventilated	Prevents build up of steam which exacerbates sensation of breathlessness
	Avoid very hot water	Increases the sensation of breathlessness
	Wear a towelling robe after bathing or showering	This reduces the need to towel the body dry and reduces exertion
	Dry shave rather than wet	This reduces prolonged arm movements required
	Use an electric toothbrush	Reduces arm movements
	Avoid strong mint toothpaste	Reduces risk of involuntary inhalation which can provoke respiratory distress
Mobility	Consider using a walking aid such as a walking stick or rollator	Reduces exertion in walking, and provides stable support to enable pauses for pacing and breathing control
	Consider using a wheelchair for longer distances	Reduces exertion in walking
Miscellaneous	Inhale to reach and exhale to bend down	Helps to avoid breath-holding. The rib cage movement also complements the mechanical impact of changing lung capacity through bending
	Pace and pause during eating and drinking activities	Both activities prevent intake of air and require careful breathing control
	Limit time spent talking on the telephone	During face-to-face conversations we unconsciously 'mirror' breathing patterns. Using a telephone, in the absence of visual cues, we may be subject to an imposed breathing pattern as well as a pressure to maintain constant audibility

(Continued)

Table 9.7   Challenging depressive symptoms. (*Continued*)

Activity	Strategy	Rationale
	Consider other adaptations that could reduce exertion in the home through own research for adaptations or in consultation with an occupational therapist	Reduces exertion

Source: Modified from Taylor, 2007.

Psychological management

There is a complex relationship between breathlessness and the psychological effects it has on a person (Duranti, 2006). Breathlessness and the limitations that it places on a person can challenge the concept of self and meanings that life has for that person (Ek and Ternestedt, 2008). In addition, the experience of not feeling able to breathe and consequent lack of control felt over one's body can also give rise to psychological distress and anxiety not only in the person affected, but also in loved ones witnessing this. Interventions aimed at increasing control, as well as reducing anxiety and stress and promoting relaxation, can therefore have a beneficial effect on the experience of breathlessness. Strategies of distraction, for example listening to music, or playing a board game, and complementary therapies to reduce stress such as massage, aromatherapy or acupuncture can all help; and talking therapies such as CBT or humanistic approaches are useful tools to explore the experiences and thought processes relating to breathlessness. Encouraging the person with breathlessness to understand how this affects them and assisting and supporting them to find interventions to help them manage can, in itself, increase the confidence and control the person feels over both their breathlessness and life.

Chest physiotherapy

Chest physiotherapy can be helpful for those people whose breathlessness experience is attributable (either wholly or in part) to increased lung secretions and accumulation of sputum. The most common techniques aimed to loosen secretions and thereby improve lung aeration are chest wall vibrations (CWV) and percussion. CWVs are applied during expiration and after a deep inspiration. The physiotherapist's hands are placed flat over the rib area and a fine vibration applied, aimed at increasing turbulence in the airways. This encourages secretions to move upwards. CWVs have been shown to be effective in improving breathlessness in people with a range of conditions (Bausewein *et al.,* 2008). In contrast, percussion, also performed by a physiotherapist, does not rely on a controlled breathing pattern so is often more easily tolerated by the breathless person. Rhythmic energy is transmitted through cupped hands and relaxed wrists, with the aim of loosening secretions from the lung passages. Care must be taken with regard to any rib pathology or osteoporosis.

Neuro–electrical muscle stimulation (NEMS)

The electrical stimulation of leg muscles in people experiencing breathlessness has been shown to have some benefits (Bausewein *et al.,* 2008). NEMS uses an electrical impulse applied to the leg muscle which mimics the electrical impulse from the central nervous system and causes the muscle to contract. Used repeatedly this intervention increases muscle tone and strength and is of benefit in reducing the effects of breathlessness linked to physical exertion.

Pharmacological Interventions for Breathlessness

Bronchodilators

Bronchodilators are used to open up the airways and are usually used in respiratory conditions where there is inflammation or narrowing of these airways, contributing to the experience of breathlessness (NICE, 2004). However, bronchodilators may also be beneficial to other people without respiratory disease but with breathlessness and can be trialled to see if an effect is noted (NHS Lothian, 2009). Bronchodilators can be taken with an inhaler or spacer. Nebulisers, which allow a larger dose of the bronchodilator to be administered, may also be beneficial for some people. The benefit of the bronchodilator needs to be assessed and it should be discontinued if no effect is noted.

Steroids

Steroids such as dexamethasone can be useful in reducing inflammation which could be exacerbating the experience of breathlessness (NICE, 2004). This is especially useful if someone's breathlessness has responded well to steroids before. Steroids can be taken orally or in an inhaled form. They should be used for a week and then reduced slowly to the smallest effective dose; they should be stopped if not effective.

Opioids

Opioids can be useful in reducing breathlessness experienced whilst at rest and in the terminal phases of a condition (NICE, 2004a). The choice of opioid and dosage needs to be tailored to the individual and their previous medical history, for example whether they already take an opioid for pain relief or the breathlessness is continuous or on exertion. Opioids have a number of side effects, notably respiratory depression, hallucinations and opioid-induced constipation and will have addictive properties if used inappropriately. Therefore, the person's response to the opioids needs to be assessed and monitored carefully. More information about the recommended dosages for opioids for specific clinical situations can be found in the palliative care guidelines for breathlessness (NHS Lothian, 2009).

Anxiolytics

These medications are useful in helping the person manage feelings of anxiety which can exacerbate breathlessness. In some cases, anxiety can be extreme and experienced as a 'panic attack' where the feelings of anxiety are overwhelming and affect the person's breathing leading to hyperventilation and extreme distress. Panic attacks or episodes of anxiety can also be caused by the fear of not being able to breathe and can be extremely distressing for the person and observing family members. Anxiolytics such as lorazepam or diazepam can be helpful in alleviating and helping to manage some of this anxiety.

There are many interventions available for managing breathlessness. Not all the interventions have been proven to be clinically effective and research is still ongoing to evaluate the benefit of many of these interventions. However, breathlessness is a subjective experience and thus the interventions and the benefits of these will be experienced individually regardless of the clinical evidence for the intervention. Therefore, the management of breathlessness requires comprehensive knowledge of the range of interventions available and entails working closely with the person experiencing breathlessness to find the most beneficial intervention for them.

Physical activity

Physical activity is defined as 'any force exerted by skeletal muscle that results in energy expenditure above resting level' (Caspersen *et al.,* 1985). Physical activity is classified according to the intensity, time, mode and volume of activity carried out:

- *Intensity* refers to the exertion that is expended doing the activity, for example a gentle walk or a vigorous run, and is usually calculated according to the kilocalories that are expended per kilogram weight of the individual or the metabolic activity. The intensity of the activity varies according to the health, weight and fitness of the individual. For someone who is very inactive and overweight a gentle slow walk may be a moderate intensity exercise. The intensity of this activity will reduce as the individual's fitness increases.
- *Time* refers to the length of time the activity is continued for.
- *Mode* is the type of exercise.
- *Volume* is the total amount of exercise completed in a set period, for example per week.

The national recommended amount of physical activity for an adult in England to improve general health is to build up to 30 minutes of moderate exercise at least five times per week. The recommendation is the same for older adults (Department of Health, 2009b). The activity is effective whether undertaken in smaller amounts such as 10–15 minute activities or for the whole 30 minutes. The British Heart Foundation (BHF) has further recommended that 30–60 minutes should be spent on strength and endurance exercises for each major muscle group two to three times a week and flexibility exercises should be undertaken on a daily basis (BHF, 2003).

The benefits of physical activity on general health have been widely accepted and incorporated into national health policy (Department of Health, 2004; Department of Health and Physical Activity, Health Improvement and Prevention, 2004). Research has indicated strong links between reduced physical activity in people and the increased incidence of a number of LTCs and risk indicators such as depression, hypertension and obesity (Department of Health, 2004a; Thomas *et al.,* 2006; Rietberg *et al.,* 2005; Mead *et al.,* 2009). This has led to recent campaigns to increase physical activity across the population and the publication of guidance stipulating recommendations for physical activity for different age groups (Department of Health and Physical Activity, Health Improvement and Prevention 2004; Department of Health 2009; NICE 2009c). Primary care professionals have also been tasked with identifying and supporting people to meet the recommendations for physical activity and need to have strategies that can be used to promote people meeting these targets (NICE, 2006b).

Physical activity is also beneficial in moderating a number of symptoms that are common within people living with LTCs. For example, physical activity can increase joint mobility, muscle strength and balance in people living with musculoskeletal conditions (NICE, 2008), reduce hypertension in cardiovascular disease (NICE, 2006c) and reduce feelings of breathlessness in people living with COPD (Chavannes *et al.,* 2002). Physical activity has also been found to decrease feelings of fatigue, reduce stress and increase the depth and length of sleep in people with a number of LTCs (Rietberg *et al.,* 2005; Department of Health and Physical Activity, Health Improvement and Prevention, 2004).

There have also been psychosocial benefits identified in research through undertaking increased physical activity. People have reported an increase in their mood levels, in particular studies focusing on mild to moderate depression (Mead *et al.,* 2009), reduced anxiety levels (Taylor, 2000) and also feeling generally better about themselves (Taylor and Fox, 2005). Physical exercise is thought to impact on a person's body image and their self- worth and allow them to develop more confidence in themselves and their capabilities, creating greater self-efficacy (Bol *et al.,* 2009).

The psychosocial benefits of physical activity are acknowledged as being complex and having multiple effects, and are thus difficult to research and find causal links. However, it is thought that the benefits of physical activity come from the activity itself rather than the accompanying fitness level obtained, although this does contribute towards a sense of achievement and confidence. There are three main areas that have been identified as contributing towards psychosocial wellness (Department of Health, 2004b):

1. *Biochemical:* Exercise promotes the release of the chemicals endorphins and noradrenaline which promote feelings of wellness; and serotonin which affects sleep, depression and memory.
2. *Physiological:* Exercise increases the body's core temperature and cerebral blood flow promoting vascular perfusion. Musculoskeletal tension is decreased and neurotransmitters increase in efficiency.
3. *Psychosocial:* Exercise increases the individual's perception of competence and confidence about their body and what they are capable of. It can improve body image, lead to a sense of achievement and promote feelings of mastery.

Strategies to increase physical activity

The recommended amount of physical activity a week is a target for generally healthy adults to work towards and to maintain. People who are living with an LTC may find this target unrealistic, and indeed unhelpful, if it feels unachievable and beyond their capabilities. The physical activity needs to be planned and tailored to the individual according to their knowledge of their capabilities and condition. The activity needs to be easily achievable initially and gradually increased once confidence and endurance improve.

The actual activity does not have to be a recognised sport or activity. Bearing in mind the definition of physical activity, anything that promotes skeletal muscle movement above rest is a physical activity. This can involve walking to the toilet or up the stairs, leg and arm exercises in a chair or bed, housework such as washing up or dusting or light gardening. There are also now recognised chair exercises that are being incorporated into LTC management systems which have been shown to be effective (Witham *et al.,* 2005; McMurdo *et al.,* 2000). These various activities can open up a whole range of different ways that someone could incorporate physical activity into their daily life at a manageable level for them.

Motivation

Motivation to continue with a physical activity can be difficult and people can struggle to continue with an activity they once started with enthusiasm. Firstly, it is important to check that the activity was an appropriate one to start with and to consider reducing or changing the activity so that it is more manageable to maintain. Secondly, it is worth considering whether there is someone or a group that the individual could join to help keep the motivation strong. For example, someone who is housebound could perhaps do their exercises with the home carer when they visit, or with a supportive family member.

Sometimes having a target or goal can provide additional motivation for someone to continue with an activity, especially if they are finding it difficult initially. This goal or target needs to be meaningful for the individual and something that they want to achieve for themselves. For example, a patient may wish to take her grandchild to the playground opposite her flat when she visits in the summer which is considered an achievable aim. The patient can gradually build up her physical activity endurance through increasing her walking and stair exercises, for example, so that she can eventually walk to the playground and back with ease.

Nurses have an important role in promoting the benefits of physical activity in people living with LTCs. Physical activity can improve a number of symptoms that commonly occur and can also enhance feelings of self-efficacy and well-being which can further feed into people's ability to self-manage other aspects of their conditions. Physical activity needs to be tailored to the individual's life style and based on their knowledge and experience of living with their LTC.

References

Anderson, R., Freedland, K., Clouse, R. & Lustman, P. (2001) The prevalence of comorbid depression in adults with diabetes: a meta-analysis, *Diabetes Care*, 24, pp. 1069–1078.

Arthritis Care (2004) *OA Nation*. Arthritis Care, London.

Baer, R. A. (2003) Mindfulness training as a clinical intervention: a conceptual and empirical review, *Clinical Psychology: Science and Practice*, 10, pp. 125–143.

Bausewein, C., Booth, S., Gysels, M., *et al.* (2008) Non-pharmacological interventions for breathlessness in advanced stages of malignant and non-malignant diseases, *Cochrane Database of Systematic Reviews*, (2), p. CD005623.

BMA (2009) *Quality and Outcomes Framework Guidance for GMS Contract 2009–10*. The NHS Confederation (Employers) Company Ltd, London.

Bol, Y., Duits, A., Hupperts, R., Vlaeyen, J. & Verhey, F. (2009) The psychology of fatigue in patients with multiple sclerosis: a review, *Journal of psychosomatic Research*, 66, pp. 3–11.

Bott, J., Blumenthal, S., Buxton, M., *et al.* (2009) Guidelines for the physiotherapy management of the adult, medical, spontaneously breathing patient, Joint BTS/ACPRC Guideline, *Thorax*, 64(Suppl.1), pp. i1–i52.

Brampton, S. (2008) *Shoot the Damn Dog: A Memoir of Depression*. Bloomsbury, London.

Branãs, P, Jordan, R., Fry-Smith, A., Burls, A. & Hyde, C. (2000) Treatments for fatigue in multiple sclerosis: a rapid and systematic review, *Health Technology Assessment*, 4, 27, pp. 1–61.

British Heart Foundation (2003) *Active for Later Life: Promoting Physical Activity with Older People*. British Heart Foundation, London.

Brown, R. P., Gerbarg, P. L. & Sudarshan, K. (2005) Yogic breathing in the treatment of stress, anxiety, and depression: part II: clinical applications and guidelines, *Journal of Alternative and Complementary Medicine*, 11(4), pp. 711–717.

Caspersen, C., Powell, K. & Christensen, G. (1985) Physical activity, exercise and physical fitness: definitions and distinctions of health-related research, *Public Health Reports 1985*, 100, pp. 126-131.

Chavannes, N., Vollenberg, J., Van Schayck, C. & Wouters, E. (2002) Effects of physical activity in mild to moderate COPD: a systematic review. *British Journal of General Practice*, 52, pp. 574–578.

Chief Medical Officer (2009) *150 years of the Annual Report of the Chief Medical Officer: on the State of Public Health 2008*. Department of Health, London.

Christenbery, T. (2005) Dyspnea self-management strategies: use and effectiveness as reported by patients with COPD, *Heart Lung*, 34(6), pp. 406–414.

Cleeland, C. (1989) Measurement of pain by subjective report. In: *Advances in Pain Research and Therapy, Volume 12: Issues in Pain Measurement* (eds C. R. Chapman, & J. D. Loeser). Raven Press, New York, pp. 391–403.

Corner, J. (1999) Development of a breathlessness assessment guide for use in palliative care, *Palliative Medicine*, 13, pp. 375–384.

Cranston, J., Crockett, A. & Currow, D. (2008) Oxygen therapy for dyspnoea in adults, *Cochrane Database of Systematic Reviews*, (3), CD004769.

CSIP (2006) *Long-term Conditions and Depression: Considerations for Best practice in Practice Based Commissioning*. Department of Health, London.

Davies, E., Moxham, T., Rees, K., *et al.* (2010) Exercise based rehabilitation for heart failure, *Cochrane Database of Systematic Reviews*, (4), CD003331.

Department of Health (2004) *Choosing Health, Making Healthier Choices Easier*. Department of Health, London.

Department of Health and Physical Activity, Health Improvement and Prevention (2004) *At Least Five a Week*. Department of Health, London.

Department of Health (2009a) *Change4Life – Eat Well, Move More, Live Longer*. Available at: http//:www.dh.gov.uk/changeforlife (accessed 20 May 2010).

Department of Health (2009b) *Annual Report of the Chief Medical Officer*. Department of Health, London.

Duranti, R. (2006) Dyspnea: the importance of a psychological approach, *Respiration*, 73, pp. 739–740.

Ek, K. & Ternestedt, B. (2008) Living with chronic obstructive pulmonary disease at the end of life: a phenomenological study, *Journal of Advanced Nursing*, 62(4), pp. 470–478.

Epel, E. S., McEwen, B. S. & Ickovics, J. R. (1998) Embodying psychological thriving: physical thriving in response to stress. *Journal of Social Issues*, 54(2), pp. 301–322.

Everly, G. S. & Lating, J. M. (2002) *A Clinical Guide to the Treatment of the Human Stress Response*. Kluwer Academic, New York.

Fox, K. R. (1999) The influence of physical activity on mental well-being, *Public Health Nutrition*, 2, pp. 411–418.

Gianaros, P. J., Jennings, J. R., Sheu, L. K., Greer, P. J., Kuller, L. H. & Karen, A. (2007) Prospective reports of chronic life stress predict decreased grey matter volume in the hippocampus, *NeuroImage*, 35(2), pp. 795–803.

Gillet, R. (1987) *Overcoming Depression: a practical self help guide to prevention and treatment*. Dorling Kindersley, London.

Goldney R, Phillips P, Fisher L and Wilson (2004) Diabetes, depression, and quality of life: a population study. *Diabetes Care*. 27(5):1066–7

Grossman, P., Niemann, L., Schmidt, S. & Walach, H. (2004) Mindfullnes-based stress reduction and health benefits- a meta-analysis, *Journal of Psychosomatic Research*, 57, pp. 35–43.

Hewlett, S., Cockshott, Z., Byron, M., Kitchen, K., Tipler, S., Pope, D. & Hehir, M. (2005) Patient's perceptions of fatigue in rheumatoid arthritis: overwhelming, uncontrollable, ignored, *Arthritis and Rheumatism*, 33(5), pp. 697–702.

Hoffman, A., Von Eye, A., Gift, A., Given, B., Given, C. and Rothert, M. (2009) Testing a theoretical model of perceived self efficacy for cancer-related fatigue self management and optimal physical functional status, *Nursing Research*, 58(1), pp. 32–41.

International Association for the Study of Pain (1994) Part III: pain terms, a current list with definitions and notes on usage. In: *Classification of Chronic Pain* (2nd edn, pp. 209–214) (eds H. Merskey, & N. Bogduk). IASP Task Force on Taxonomy, IASP Press, Seattle. Available at: http://www.iasppain.org/AM/Template.cfm?Section=Pain_Defi...isplay.cfm&ContentID=1728 (accessed 16 June 2010)

Johnson, M. & Martinson, M. (2006) Efficacy of electrical nerve stimulation for chronic musculoskeletal pain: a meta-analysis of randomized controlled trials, *Pain*, 130(1), pp. 157–165.

Kabat-Zinn, J. Massion, A. O. Kristeller, J., *et al.* (1992) Effectiveness of a meditation-based stress reduction program in the treatment of anxiety disorders, *American Journal of Psychiatry*, 49, pp. 936–943.

Kabat-Zinn, J. (1990). *Full Catastrophe Living: Using the Wisdom of your Body and Mind to Face Stress, Pain and Illness*. Random House Publishing Group, New York.

Kabat-Zinn, J. (1998). Meditation. In: *Psycho-oncology* (ed J.C. Holland). Oxford University Press, New York.

Kralik, D., Telford, K., Price, K. & Koch, T. (2005) Women's experiences of fatigue in chronic illness, *Journal of Advanced Nursing*, 52(4), pp. 372–380.

Malathi, A., Damodaran, A., Saha, N., Patil, N. & Maratha, S. (2004). Effects of yogic practices on subjective well being, *Indian Journal of Physiology and Pharmacology*, 44, pp. 202–206.

McMurdo, M., Millar, A. & Daly, F. (2000) A randomized controlled trial of fall prevention strategies in old peoples' homes. *Gerontology*, 46(2), pp. 83–87.

Mead, G., Morley, W., Campbell, P., Greig, C., McMurdo, M. and Lawlor, D. (2009) Exercise for depression, *Cochrane Database of Systematic Reviews*, (3), CD004366.

Melzack, R. (1975) The McGill Pain Questionnaire: major properties and scoring methods, *Pain*, 1, pp. 277–299.

National Institute for Health and Clinical Excellence (NICE) (2003) *Management of Multiple Sclerosis in Primary and Secondary Care*. National Institute for Health and Clinical Excellence, London.

National Institute for Health and Clinical Excellence (NICE) (2004a) *Chronic Obstructive Pulmonary Disease - Management of Chronic Obstructive Pulmonary Disease in Adults in Primary and Secondary Care*. National Institute for Health and Clinical Excellence, London.

National Institute for Health and Clinical Excellence (NICE) (2004b) *Diagnosis and Management of Type 1 Diabetes in Children, Young People and Adults*. National Institute for Health and Clinical Excellence, London.

National Institute for Health and Clinical Excellence (NICE) (2006a) *Parkinson's Disease: Diagnosis and Management in Primary and Secondary Care*. Royal College of Physicians, London.

National Institute for Health and Clinical Excellence (NICE) (2006b) *Promoting Physical Activity, Active Play and Sport for Pre-School and School-Age Children and Young People in Family, Pre-School, School and Community Settings*. National Institute for Health and Clinical Excellence, London.

National Institute for Health and Clinical Excellence (NICE) (2006c) *Hypertension: Management of Hypertension in Adults in Primary Care*. National Institute for Health and Clinical Excellence, London.

National Institute for Health and Clinical Excellence (NICE) (2008) *The Care and Management of Osteoarthritis in Adults*. National Institute for Health and Clinical Excellence, London.

National Institute for Health and Clinical Excellence (NICE) (2009a) *Depression With a Chronic Physical Health Problem*. National Institute for Health and Clinical Excellence, London.

National Institute for Health and Clinical Excellence (NICE) (2009b) *Depression The Treatment and Management of Depression in Adults (update)*. National Institute for Health and Clinical Excellence, London.

National Institute for Health and Clinical Excellence (NICE) (2009c) *Promoting Physical Activity, Active Play and Sport for Pre-School and School-Age Children and Young People in Family, Pre-School, School and Community Settings*. National Institute for Health and Clinical Excellence, London.

National Institute for Health and Clinical Excellence (NICE) (2009d) *Low Back Pain: Early Management of Persistent Non-Specific Low Back Pain*. National Institute for Health and Clinical Excellence, London.

Neill, J. (2005) Exploring underlying life patterns of women with multiple sclerosis or rheumatoid arthritis: comparison with NANDA dimensions, *Nurse Science Quarterly*, 18(4), pp. 344–352.

Neill, J., Belan, I. & Reid, K. (2006) Effectiveness of non-pharmacological interventions in adults with multiple sclerosis, rheumatoid arthritis or systemic lupus erythematosus: a systematic review, *Journal of Advanced Nursing*, 56(6), pp. 617–635.

NHS Lothian (2009) *Palliative Care Guidelines: Breathlessness*. NHS Lothian. Available at: www.palliativecareguidelines.scot.nhs.uk/documents/breathlessnessfinal.pdf (accessed 3 June 2010).

Ormel, J. and Von Korff, M. (2000) Synchrony of change in depression and disability, *Archives of General Psychiatry*, 57, pp. 381–382.

Polosa, R., Simidchiev, A. & Walters, E. (2002) Nebulised morphine for severe interstitial lung disease, *Cochrane Database of Systematic Reviews*, (3), CD002872.

Riemsma, R., Rasker, J., Taal, E., Wouters, E. and Weigman, O. (1998) Fatigue in rheumatoid arthitis: the role of self efficacy and problematic social support, *British Journal of Rheumatology*, 37(10), pp. 1042–1046.

Repping-Wuts, H., Uitterhoeve, R. and Van Riel, P. (2008) Fatigue as experiences by patients with rheumatoid arthritis (RA): a qualitative study, *International Journal of Nursing Studies*, 45(7), pp. 995–1002.

Rietberg, M. B., Brooks, D., Uitdehaag, B. M. J. and Kwakkel, G. (2005) Exercise therapy for multiple sclerosis. *Cochrane Database of Systematic Reviews 2005*, Issue 1. Art. No.: CD003980. DOI: 10.1002/14651858.CD003980.pub2.

Samaritans (1996) *Dealing with Depression*. Vermilion, London.

Schwartzstein, R., Lahive, K., Pope, A., Weinberger, S. and Woodrow Weiss, J. (1987) Cold facial stimulation reduces breathlessness induced in normal subjects, American Review, *Respiratory Disease*, 136(1), pp. 58–61.

Small, S. and Lamb, M. (1999) Fatigue in chronic illness: the experience of individuals with chronic obstructive pulmonary disease and asthma, *Journal of Advanced Nursing*, 30(2), pp. 469–478.

Scruggs, B. (2009) Fatigue: assessment and management, *Home Healthcare Management and Practice*, 22(1), pp. 16–25.

Taylor, A. (2000). Physical activity, anxiety, and stress: a review. In: *Physical Activity and Psychological Well-Being* (eds S. Biddle, K. Fox & S. Boutcher), Routledge, London, pp 10–45.

Taylor, A. and Fox, K. (2005). Changes in physical self-perceptions: findings from a randomised controlled study of a GP exercise referral scheme, *Health Psychology*, 24, pp. 11–21.

Taylor, J. (2007) The non pharmacological management of breathlessness, *End of Life Care*, 1(1), pp. 20–27.

Thomas, D., Elliott, E. J. and Naughton, G. A. (2006) Exercise for type 2 diabetes mellitus. *Cochrane Database of Systematic Reviews 2006*, Issue 3. Art. No.: CD002968. DOI: 10.1002/14651858.CD002968.pub2.

Trendall, J. (2000) Concept analysis: chronic fatigue, *Journal of Advanced Nursing*, 32(5), pp. 1126–1131.

Witham, M., Gray, J., Argo, I., Johnston, D., Struthers, A. and McMurdo, M. (2005) Effect of a seated exercise program to improve physical function and health status in frail patients > or = 70 years of age with heart failure, *American Journal Cardiology*, 95(9), pp. 1120–1124.

Zhao, I. and Yates, P. (2008) Non-pharmacological interventions for breathlessness management in patients with lung cancer: a systematic review, *Palliative Medicine*, 22, pp. 683–701.

Chapter 10

Medicines management

Shivaun Gammie
Medway School of Pharmacy, Kent, UK

Introduction

Taking a prescribed medicine is the commonest health intervention within the NHS. During 2009, community pharmacists in England dispensed 886 million prescription items at a net ingredient cost of £8,539.4 million (Health and Social Care Information Centre, Prescribing Support Unit, 2010). This equates to an average of 17.1 prescription items dispensed per year per head of population, excluding medicines supplied within hospitals.

People with long-term conditions (LTCs) are much more likely to be prescribed numerous medicines; it is not unusual for patients to be taking more than six different medicines at different times during the day and many people take considerably more than this. As a result, medicines management (see definition Box 10.1) is an important component of health care for patients with LTCs.

The examples below (Tables 10.1–10.3) show typical, standard medications for patients with chronic heart failure, type 2 diabetes and chronic obstructive pulmonary disease. It is important to remember that patients with later stages of these conditions often require more intensive therapy, for example a patient with type 2 diabetes may well be taking two or more antihypertensive medications. In addition, it is unusual for patients to just have one clinical condition and it is common for people with LTCs to additionally take, for example, analgesics, medication for dyspepsia or medication for skin conditions.

Therefore, for a person with an LTC – many of whom will be elderly – the array of medicines that they take can be a confusing minefield with uncertainty around what medicine does what, and what benefits and harms can be expected from the different medicines. Similarly, health care professionals caring for people with LTCs may feel confused about the best way to optimise a patient's medication to ensure that they receive maximum benefit and minimum harm.

The Medicines and Older People section of the National Services Framework for Older People (Department of Health, 2001: 3) recommended:

'Appropriate medicines management systems should be in place so that the medication needs of older people are regularly reviewed, discussed with older people and

Long-Term Conditions: Nursing Care and Management, First Edition. Edited by Liz Meerabeau and Kerri Wright.
© 2011 Blackwell Publishing Ltd. Published 2011 by Blackwell Publishing Ltd.

Table 10.1   Typical medication taken by a patient with chronic heart failure secondary to ischaemic heart disease.

Medication	Dosing instructions	Indication
Furosemide 40 mg tablets	One tablet each morning	Diuretic for heart failure
Lisinopril 10 mg tablets	One tablet each morning	Heart failure (target
Lisinopril 20 mg tablets	One tablet each morning	dose 30 mg daily)
Bisoprolol 10 mg tablets	One tablet each morning	Heart failure/symptom control in angina
Spironolactone 25 mg tablets	One tablet in the morning	Heart failure
Aspirin 75 mg tablets	One tablet each morning with food	Cardiovascular disease prevention
Simvastatin 40 mg tablets	One tablet to be taken at night	Cardiovascular disease prevention (lipid lowering)
Glyceryl trinitrate 400 μg spray	1–2 sprays sub-lingually when required for chest pain	Chest pain
Isosorbide mononitrate tablets 20 mg	One tablet to be taken twice a day at 8 am and 2 pm	Prevention of chest pain
This equates to nine doses (plus when required glyceryl trinitrate spray) of eight different medications that need to be taken at three different times during the day (plus when required glyceryl trinitrate spray).		

Source: NICE (2003, 2006, 2008b).

their carers, and information and other support provided to ensure older people get the most from their medicines and that avoidable adverse events are prevented.'

This chapter explores the issues regarding medicines management and provides guidance on how to help people with LTCs manage their medicines effectively.

Table 10.2   Typical medication taken by a patient with type 2 diabetes who also has hypertension.

Medication	Dosing instructions	Indication
Metformin 850 mg tablets	One tablet twice a day	Type 2 diabetes
Gliclazide 80 mg tablets	Two tablets each morning	Type 2 diabetes
Aspirin 75 mg tablets	One tablet each morning with food	Cardiovascular disease prevention (antiplatelet)
Simvastatin 40 mg tablets	One tablet to be taken at night	Cardiovascular disease prevention (lipid lowering)
Lisinopril 20 mg tablets	One tablet in the morning	Hypertension
This equates to seven doses of five different medications that need to be taken at three different times during the day.		

Source: NICE, 2008b.

Table 10.3   Typical medication taken by a patient with chronic obstructive pulmonary disease with an FEV_1 less than 50% experiencing more than two exacerbations per year.

Medication	Dosing instructions	Indication
Salbutamol 100 μg/ metered dose inhaler	Two puffs four times a day and when required	Treatment of breathlessness
Tiotropium bromide inhalation capsules 18 μg	One capsule inhaled once a day	Treatment of breathlessness
Beclomethasone 200 μg/ metered dose	Two puffs twice a day	Prevention of exacerbations
This equates to at least 13 inhalations of five different inhalers that need to be taken at least four different times during the day.		

Source: NICE, 2004.

What do patients want to know about their medicines?

Medicines Management (Box 10.1) will be important for a person with an LTC because, as introduced above, they are likely to be prescribed a number of medicines. Box 10.2 identifies some of the questions that a person with an LTC may have for the health professionals caring for them. A priority for health care professionals caring for people with LTCs should be to help patients answer the questions that they have regarding their medicines and so assist them in medicines taking.

Box 10.1   Definition of medicines management.
(National Prescribing Centre, 2002).

Medicines management has been defined as a system of processes and behaviours that determines how medicines are used by patients and by the NHS. Effective medicines management places the patient as the primary focus, thus delivering better targeted care and better informed individuals.

Box 10.2   Questions patients may ask about medicines.
(National Prescribing Centre, 2002).

- Do I need a medicine?
- How do I find out about different treatments?
- Who decides which medicines I get?
- How am I involved?
- How do I find out about my medicines?
- How do I get my medicines?
- How can I make sure my medicines suit me?
- Do I keep taking my medicines or when can I stop?

Source: National Prescribing Centre, 2002.

The National Prescribing Centre (2002) has identified a number of tools and resources that are available to patients and health care professionals to help address patients' concerns about their medicines.

Do I need a medicine?

It can be very difficult for people with LTCs to understand why they need to take the medicines that they are prescribed. Whilst the prescriber will spend time explaining the importance of the medicines that they are prescribing patients may find it difficult to recall and understand this information, especially if the consultation has introduced a diagnosis or worsening of a medical condition that the patient was not expecting. Therefore, people with LTCs may need to increase their awareness of the reasons for the medicines that they have been prescribed.

In addition to the prescriber, health care professionals, especially pharmacists when dispensing prescriptions and nurses when reviewing patients, will be a valuable source of information on the reasons for medication. Patients can also be encouraged to contact advice services such as NHS Direct and may benefit from participation in programmes such as the Expert Patients Programme.

How do I find out about different treatments?

People with LTCs may require more detailed information on the treatment options available to them. Again patients should be encouraged to discuss their specific questions with their prescriber as well as other health care professionals providing them with care. Patients may require support to work out exactly what their question is. For example, a patient asking about different treatments may have specific concerns about one or two of their medications. Perhaps they believe that a new symptom that they are experiencing has occurred as a result of one of their medications.

Who decides which medicines I get?

Patients and their relatives may seek reassurance that they are being asked to take medicines that are 'right' for their condition. In the current age of information technology it is not unusual for patients or their relatives to seek information on what the recommended treatment is for their condition.

Patients may need assurance that decisions about the medicines that they have been prescribed are based on the best evidence and are in line with appropriate national and local guidance, for example the National Institute for Health and Clinical Excellence (NICE) produces a range of guidance which is supported by information designed for people who use NHS services.

How am I involved?

Many, but not all, patients will want to be involved in decisions regarding their medication. The challenge for health care professionals is to provide information in a way that patients can understand to ensure that they can become true partners in their treatment. The Medicines Partnership programme (see Section 'Medicines Information Resources') provides a variety of support around medicine taking for health care professionals working with patients. Medication reviews, which are discussed later in this chapter, should involve patients to the extent that they want to be involved.

How do I find out about my medicines?

Patients will have a number of questions regarding their medicines. A number of patient information sources are available to both patients and those caring for them. For example, NHS Direct, Medicines Information Services, the Expert Patients Programme, pharmaceutical companies, the media and the Internet. Further information is given in the section on 'Medicines Information Resources' at the end of this chapter.

How do I get my medicines?

The majority of people with LTCs will need to obtain regular supplies of their medication through repeat prescription services run by their GP and community pharmacist. The traditional system for supplying repeat medication can be summarised as follows:

- Generally, patients will be supplied with a fixed quantity of medicine, for example 1 month's supply.
- When the supply is running low, the patient will be asked to complete a slip of paper provided with the original prescription to specify that they require a further supply of medication.
- They will take or send this slip to the GP surgery where a new prescription will be generated for collection some time later, for example within 48 hours of receipt.
- The patient will collect the prescription (which will also include the ordering slip for next time) and take it to their community pharmacy for dispensing.

A number of variations have developed to help with this process. For example, many community pharmacies provide a 'collection and delivery' service whereby the patient can nominate a pharmacy to collect their prescription so that the patient avoids a trip to the GP surgery. In some cases the community pharmacist will deliver the dispensed medicines to housebound patients.

Repeat dispensing (Department of Health, 2007) also offers a valuable service to patients on long-term medication that is unlikely to change. The prescriber produces a prescription covering a set period of time and a number of 'batch issues' which allow the community pharmacist to dispense the required items without the need for the patient to return to the prescriber each time they require a further supply of their medication. Some medicines, for example schedule 2 and 3 controlled drugs, cannot be prescribed on repeatable prescriptions. The Department of Health (2007) has also signalled its intention to introduce electronic repeatable prescribing through the Electronic Prescription Service (EPS).

The system of obtaining repeat prescriptions can seem daunting and confusing to people with LTCs and can be extremely difficult for those living alone with limited mobility. Health care professionals have an important role to play in supporting people with LTCs to obtain their supplies of medicines in the easiest, appropriate way.

How can I make sure my medicines suit me?

People with LTCs want to know that their medicines are helping them by having the desired outcome with minimal adverse effects. As discussed above, people with LTCs may have asked about why they need a medicine and the different treatment options available to them but a frequent concern is that of adverse effects.

No medicine is completely safe and patients reading the patient information leaflets enclosed in dispensed medicines will receive information on reported adverse effects. This does not mean that they will experience the adverse effects listed but people can be put off by the information presented. Others will trust their prescriber and take the medication preferring not to read about possible adverse effects.

People with LTCs may experience adverse effects from their medicines and it is a challenge for health care professionals to firstly ask the right questions of patients to determine whether an adverse effect could be occurring and secondly to work with the patient to weigh up the risks from the adverse effects against the benefit that the patient is obtaining from the medicine. Thus, it is important that the patient is encouraged to talk about symptoms that have occurred or worsened since a change in their medications and for health care professionals to have access to good information on potential adverse effects of medication. The information in the section on 'Medicines Information Resources' at the end of this chapter directs readers to sources of information on adverse effects of medicines. The section on 'Medication Review' discusses adverse effects further.

Do I keep taking my medicines or when can I stop?

People with LTCs are often concerned that they will have to take medicines for the rest of their lives. Opportunities to reinforce the need for regular medication taking should be taken at every opportunity. They should be encouraged to attend Medication Review Clinics (see the section on 'Medication Review') and review appointments (often referred to as Disease Management Clinics) with their primary or secondary care teams.

Thus, medicines (often a large number) are commonly prescribed for people with LTCs and patients will have questions and concerns about their medicines. The section above has illustrated some of the questions that patients will ask and provided guidance on how health care professionals can support patients to get the answers that they need.

What can go wrong with medicines used?

A variety of problems can occur when medicines are not used effectively. Patients may experience adverse effects from their medicines and in some cases these can be serious enough to necessitate an admission to hospital or cause the patient to experience an effect that causes them harm and impairs their quality of life. For example, adverse effects of medicines are a potential cause of falls in elderly patients taking medication such as blood pressure lowering medication. People who take a number of medicines are at greater risk of experiencing adverse effects of medicines. As discussed previously people with LTCs are often prescribed a number of medicines and so it is important to be aware of what can go wrong with medicine use.

It is also important to consider what happens when a patient doesn't take the medication prescribed for them. This can lead to wastage and unnecessary expense to the NHS but also patients may be experiencing unnecessary symptoms from their LTC because they are not taking a medication that would help alleviate their symptoms.

The National Service Framework for Older People (Department of Health, 2001) included a section on medicines and older people and, whilst not all people with LTCs will be older people, the problems identified with medicines (Box 10.3) appear applicable.

Box 10.3   Problems with medications identified in the NSF for older people.

Many adverse reactions to medicines could be prevented: They are implicated in 5–17% of hospital admissions, while in hospital 6–17% of older inpatients experience adverse drug reactions.

Some medicines are under-used in older people (as well as in others). For example, anti-thrombotic treatments to prevent stroke, preventive treatment for asthma, and antidepressants are not always prescribed for patients that would benefit.

Medicines not taken: As many as 50% of older people may not be taking their medicines as intended. Older people and their carers need to be more involved in decisions about treatment and to receive more information than they currently do about the benefits and risks of treatment.

Inequivalence in repeat prescription quantities causes wastage: Campaigns for people to return unwanted medicines confirm that large amounts of medicines, probably worth in excess of £100m, are never taken. Inequivalence in quantities on repeat prescriptions means that patients have to order different items at separate times, and may unintentionally receive the same medicine on separate prescriptions. The wastage that results from this inequivalence has been estimated to account for 6–10% of total prescribing costs.

Changes in medication after discharge from hospital: Following discharge, changes to medication are frequently made by patients and GPs. These changes may be intentional, but nonetheless unintentional changes are too frequent.

Poor two-way communication between hospitals and primary care: In secondary care, communication needs to be improved to reduce the delay in transfer of medication recommendations to primary care; to ensure treatment that was only intended short term, while the patient was in hospital, is discontinued on discharge; and to improve explanation for medication changes. In primary care, interpretation and implementation of discharge medication is not always optimal and full medication histories are not always provided to hospitals at admission.

Repeat prescribing systems need improvement: Most of the medicines taken by older people are obtained on repeat prescription. Careful consideration needs to be given to the processes for ordering, synchronising quantities, ensuring regular review of the need for each medicine, and monitoring that the medicine is being taken and the patient is benefiting from it. General Practice computer systems that target patients at higher risk of medication problems, and that link medicines added to prescription records at different times and identify duplication of medication would enable more effective reviews to be undertaken.

Dosage instructions on the medicine label are sometimes inadequate, such that neither the patient nor carer has access to the correct dosage information, for example 'Take as directed' or 'Take as required'. The Royal College of Physicians (RCP) Sentinel Audit of Evidence Based Prescribing for Older People showed that up to 25% of medicines were prescribed 'as required'.

Access to the surgery or pharmacy can be a problem: Some older people may have difficulty getting to the doctor's surgery to collect their prescription, or to the pharmacy to have it dispensed. People who are housebound or who have limited mobility have particular difficulties in accessing advice and help with their medicines.

Carers' potential contribution and needs not addressed: Carers are in a position to support older people in medicine taking but their potential contribution is under used. Local operating procedures often prevent social services staff from providing support. Formal carers (e.g. home care workers) need training in medicines and their use. Home care workers regularly assist people with medicine taking, even though their job description discourages them from doing so. Informal carers (e.g. family members), together with those they care for, could be more involved in, and consulted about, treatment decisions. Their wealth of knowledge about the patient's health and any adverse changes is too often untapped. Carers want to know more about possible side effects of treatment, about which combinations of medicines should be avoided, and about the reasons for changes in medication.

Detailed medication review minimises unnecessary costs: Medication review for older people usually results in a reduction in the number of prescribed medicines. Studies in general practices and nursing homes have shown that every £1 spent on employing pharmacists to review patients' medication resulted in a £2 cost savings.

Some long-term treatments can be successfully withdrawn: Diuretic treatment, for example, often needs to be continued for a long term but can be stopped in about half of patients provided progress is monitored.

Source: Department of Health, 2001.

What does medicines management involve?

The National Prescribing Centre (2002) has described four stages in achieving optimal medicines management for patients. These aim to address patients' needs for information as well as addressing issues of best practice:

1. Selection of correct and appropriate drug
2. Ensuring and enabling medicines partnerships
3. Getting the right drug to the right patient at the right time
4. Outcome monitoring

1. Selection of correct and appropriate drug

It is the responsibility of the prescriber to make appropriate prescribing decisions which are based on the best available evidence. The National Institute for Health and Clinical Excellence (NICE) has produced clinical guidelines covering the main LTCs, for example chronic heart failure (NICE, 2003), type 2 diabetes (NICE, 2008a) and COPD (NICE, 2004) which are easily accessible and supported by patient information. Similarly, the Department of Health has produced a number of National Service Frameworks which are freely available to the public (Department of Health, 2010).

In addition, local decisions will play a part in treatment choices. Primary Care Trusts and local acute trusts will have groups that make recommendations on the choice of medicines, and in many areas a prescribing formulary will be in place. These have many advantages, for example ensuring consistent prescribing across primary and secondary care, reducing the number of medicines that prescribers need to be familiar with and promoting cost effective use of medicines.

2. Ensuring and enabling medicines partnerships

Between a third and a half of medicines prescribed for LTCs are thought not to be taken as recommended (NICE, 2009). The National Institute for Health and Clinical Excellence (2009) produced a clinical guideline on Medicines Adherence which discusses how to involve patients in decisions about prescribed medicines and supporting adherence. NICE (2009: 1) defines adherence to medicines 'as the extent to which the patient's action matches the agreed recommendations'. It is important to recognise that non-adherence is not the patient's problem; rather it represents a problem with the delivery of health care. Thus, it is a key responsibility of health care professionals to identify and address issues of non-adherence.

Two overlapping categories of medicines non-adherence have been identified (NICE, 2009): intentional or non-intentional. In intentional non-adherence, the patient makes a decision not to follow the treatment recommendations, whereas in non-intentional non-adherence the patient wants to take their medication as intended but is unable to do so as a result of factors outside of their control, for example forgetting to take medication, being unable to pay for it, or being unable to use medicines, for example lacking the manual dexterity to remove medication from a blister pack.

The key principles of the NICE Medicines Adherence Clinical Guideline (2009) are shown in Box 10.4. However, readers are referred to the full guidance for a full description of medicines adherence and strategies to support it. At the heart of maximising adherence is exploring patients' perspectives of medicines and the reasons why they may not take their medicines as intended by the health care professional. It is important to recognise that patients may have beliefs about their medicines that differ from those of health care professionals. Adopting an open dialogue with patients to explore their beliefs and concerns will identify potential problems which once identified can lead to a joint approach to finding solutions.

Box 10.4   Key principles of the NICE Medicines Adherence Clinical Guideline.

- Health care professionals should adapt their consultation style to the needs of individual patients so that all patients have the opportunity to be involved in decisions about their medicines at the level they wish.
- Establish the most effective way of communicating with each patient and, if necessary, consider ways of making information accessible and understandable (e.g. using pictures, symbols, large print, different languages, an interpreter or a patient advocate).
- Offer all patients the opportunity to be involved in making decisions about prescribed medicines. Establish what level of involvement in decision-making the patient would like.
- Be aware that increasing patient involvement may mean that the patient decides not to take or to stop taking a medicine. If in the health care professional's view this could have an adverse effect, then the information provided to the patient on risks and benefits and the patient's decision should be recorded.
- Accept that the patient has the right to decide not to take a medicine, even if you do not agree with the decision, as long as the patient has the capacity to make an informed decision and has been provided with the information needed to make such a decision.
- Be aware that patients' concerns about medicines, and whether they believe they need them, affect how and whether they take their prescribed medicines.
- Offer patients information that is relevant to their condition, possible treatments and personal circumstances, and that is easy to understand and free from jargon.
- Recognise that non-adherence is common and that most patients are non-adherent sometimes. Routinely assess adherence in a non-judgemental way whenever you prescribe, dispense and review medicines.
- Be aware that although adherence can be improved, no specific intervention can be recommended for all patients. Tailor any intervention to increase adherence to the specific difficulties with adherence the patient is experiencing.
- Review patient knowledge, understanding and concerns about medicines, and a patient's view of their need for medicine at intervals agreed with the patient, because these may change over time. Offer repeat information and review to patients, especially when treating long-term conditions with multiple medicines.

Source: NICE, 2009.

A range of 'compliance devices' are available to support patients who have difficulty taking their medication and are unintentionally non-adherent. Examples of devices that are available for patients who have specific physical difficulties using their medicines include the following:

- Use of alternative inhaler devices for patients unable to coordinate actuation of a metered dose inhaler with inhalation.

- Use of a device that actuates a metered dose inhaler by squeezing rather than pressing for patients who have insufficient strength to actuate the inhaler.
- Use of specific devices to help patients with poor manual dexterity to remove tablets from 'blister' strips of medicines.
- Use of specific devices to help patients use eye drops.
- Use of large print or talking labels for patients with poor eyesight who are unable to read standard labels.

The use of multi-compartment compliance devices for patients who forget to take their medicines is not a universal solution for patients with poor memory. They may be difficult to manipulate and the patient has to have sufficient memory to remember to open the device, remove and take the medication at the correct time. An important factor when considering whether to use a multi-compartment compliance device is whether the prescribed medications can be dispensed in the device. The following medicines are examples of medicines that cannot be dispensed in a multi-compartment compliance device:

- Liquid medication.
- Dispersible tablets, for example aspirin dispersible tablets 75 mg and other formulations that are known to be pharmaceutically unstable.
- Medicines taken 'when required'.
- Medicines which are subject to frequent dose changes, for example warfarin.
- Medicines prescribed after the compliance device has been dispensed without the issue of a new prescription covering all the required medication.

3. Getting the right drug to the right patient at the right time

As mentioned previously, patients can find the system for obtaining supplies of their medicines challenging. It is important that health care professionals ensure that patients are given information about how to obtain their medicines. The NSF for Older People (Department of Health, 2001) promoted the following good practice in repeat prescribing systems:

- Written explanation of the repeat prescribing process for the patient and carers.
- Practice personnel with dedicated responsibility for ensuring that patient recall and regular medication review takes place.
- Agreed written practice policy on the length of medication supply on repeat prescriptions.
- Authorisation check made each time a repeat prescription is signed.
- Training of practice staff on the elements of good practice and how to spot poor patient compliance.
- Compliance check made on every repeat prescription.
- Regular housekeeping changes made to keep records up to date.

4. Outcome monitoring

It is important that patients with LTCs are regularly assessed to ensure that the aims of treatment are being achieved. This could include assessing patients' symptoms or undertaking investigations to determine whether the condition is improving or could involve assessing whether the patient is adhering to the medication regime that has been prescribed.

Medication review

A key component of medicines management, which runs alongside the four stages discussed above, is medication review. Responsibility for undertaking medication review has traditionally been assigned to the prescriber. However, the emergence of health care professionals with responsibility for supporting patients with LTCs, for example, community matrons, has increased the number of people undertaking medication reviews.

A medication review has been defined as a structured, critical examination of a patient's medicines with the objective of:

- reaching an agreement with the patient about treatment;
- optimising the impact of medicines;
- minimising the number of medication-related problems; and
- reducing waste.

(Task Force on Medicines Partnership and the National Collaborative Medicines Management Services Programme, 2002).

More recently three types of medication review have been adopted for use in the National Health Service (Clyne *et al.*, 2008):

- *Type 1 (prescription) reviews* are reviews of patients' prescription items. The patient does not need to be present and their purpose is to address technical issues relating to the prescription.
- *Type 2 (concordance and compliance) reviews* take place in partnership with the patient and explore the patient's medicines-taking behaviour.
- *Type 3 (clinical medication) reviews* are holistic reviews that involve the patient, their medical notes and any relevant laboratory results.

An example of a type 1 (prescription) medication review is medicines reconciliation which may occur when a patient is admitted to hospital. A health care professional will ensure that an accurate list of the medicines that the patient takes is available. For example, the medicines prescribed on admission to hospital could be compared to the General Practitioner's repeat prescription record to identify any anomalies, for example a medicine unintentionally omitted from the hospital prescription.

An example of a type 2 (concordance and compliance) medication review is Medicines Use Review (MUR) which is an advanced service within the community pharmacy contract. MURs are designed to help patients get the most out of their medicines and involve patients having an appointment with their pharmacist to discuss the medicines being taken.

Type 3 (clinical and medication) reviews are undertaken holistically with the patient when all their clinical information is available. This type of medication review will be especially important for patients with LTCs who are taking multiple medicines. The Medicines and Older People section of the National Service Framework for Older People (Department of Health, 2001) recommended that medication reviews should be targeted at those known to be at higher risk of medicines-related problems, namely:

• Those prescribed four or more medicines (polypharmacy)
• Post-discharge from hospital
• In care homes
• Where medicines-related problems have been identified
• Patients aged over 75
• Following an adverse change in health

More recently, the National Prescribing Centre (NPC Medical Review, 2008) has provided more detailed guidance for targeting medication reviews (Table 10.4).

There are many schemes and checklists available to support health care professionals undertake clinical medication reviews. The author has found an approach which considers the following seven questions adapted from Gammie and Luscombe (1995) helpful:

• What is the INDICATION for therapy?
• Is the DOSE suitable?

Table 10.4 Targeting medication reviews.

Target group	Specific issues
Patient-related triggers	
Older people (>75 years)	• Complex medication regimen • Multiple drugs (polypharmacy) • Multiple diseases (co-morbidity) • Compliance issues • Physical problems (swallowing, arthritis) • Resident in care home • Mental state (confusion, anxiety, depression, forgetfulness) • Living alone or poor carer support • Frequent hospital admissions
Condition-related triggers	
Long-term or complex conditions	• Newly diagnosed long-term condition • Polypharmacy • Co-morbidity • Drugs that need special monitoring • Adverse effects and/or drug interactions • Care plan is not up-to-date
Complex conditions	• Coexisting physical and mental health problems • Care plan not up-to-date

Table 10.4   Targeting medication reviews.(*Continued*)

Target group	Specific issues
Medication-related triggers	
Medication regimens	• Four or more medicines • More than 12 doses in a day • More than four changes in medication in past 12 months • Recent changes to medication regimen • Medicines from more than one prescriber
'Specialist' drugs	• Narrow therapeutic index, for example warfarin, amiodarone, lithium • Drugs not commonly used in primary care • Drugs that need special monitoring
Medication-related event	• Recent falls • Adverse drug reaction • Unexpected or exaggerated reaction to one or more medicines • High incidence of self-medication with non-prescription medicines or alternative remedies
Environmental triggers	
Change in care provider	• Newly registered patient • Recent discharge from hospital • Transfer to a care home
Care homes	• Polypharmacy • Enteral feeding • Inappropriate use of home remedies • Long-standing prescription of psychotropic medication, for example antipsychotics/hypnotics

Source: Clyne *et al.*, 2008.

- Is the drug WORKING?
- Is the drug causing any SIDE EFFECTS?
- Is the drug INTERACTING with another drug or medical condition?
- Is the patient TAKING the medication?
- What's MISSING?

What is the INDICATION for therapy?

Medicines should be prescribed for specific indications but sometimes it is not clear why a medicine is being prescribed or the medicine may be prescribed for an indication that is no longer present or has exceeded its recommended duration. Examples of situations where there may not be a valid indication include the following:

- Warfarin prescribed as a 6-month treatment for a deep vein thrombosis when 6 months of treatment has been completed and the patient has experienced no recurrence of the deep vein thrombosis.
- A proton pump inhibitor initiated for a patient presenting with pain where the differential diagnosis was dyspepsia and chest pain. A myocardial infarction was subsequently confirmed and treated.

Is the DOSE suitable?

Medicines should be prescribed at the correct dose for the individual patient. Patients with, for example, renal impairment require reduced doses of renally excreted medicines, for example digoxin. Doses of medicines can also be too low. For example, patients with heart failure may not be receiving the recommended dose of ACE inhibitors.

Is the drug WORKING?

When medicines are initiated there should be a clear idea of the purpose of the medication and, therefore, how the patient and health care professional will know whether the medication is working. For example, a patient treated with medicines for their heart failure would be expected to be less short of breath and able to walk further if the medication is working. When patients are on a number of medications it is important to regularly review the medication to ensure that the desired effects are occurring. Where a benefit is not clear, stopping the medication should be considered.

Is the drug causing any SIDE EFFECTS?

Medicines cause side effects and patients who are taking a large number of medications are more prone to the adverse effects of medicines. It is important to consider whether a medicine could be causing the patient's new symptom rather than assuming that it is a new medical condition. For example, a patient who experiences swollen ankles when taking a calcium-channel blocker may be experiencing a side effect rather than developing heart failure.

Is the drug INTERACTING with another drug or medical condition?

Drug interactions are common and all patients should have their list of medication reviewed to ensure that there are no unintended drug interactions. It is also important to ensure that drugs are not interacting with a patient's medical condition. For example, non-steroidal anti-inflammatory drugs (NSAIDs) are contraindicated in all patients with severe heart failure as they cause fluid retention which worsens heart failure.

Is the patient TAKING the medication?

As explained previously, any review of a patient's medication needs to consider whether the medication is being used as intended.

What's MISSING?

As discussed previously, national and local guidelines specify evidence-based treatments for LTCs. A medication review should ensure that all the recommended treatments have been considered and prescribed, if appropriate for the individual patient. For example, all patients with heart failure should be considered for ACE inhibitors.

The following case studies are example of patients who present for a medication review. Suggested answers are included at the end.

Case Study 10.1

Mrs A is an 86-year-old lady with hypertension, and congestive cardiac failure following a myocardial infarction some years ago, who presents for a medication review and is found to be taking the following medicines:

- Aspirin 75 mg in the morning
- Simvastatin 40 mg at night
- Amlodipine 5 mg in the morning
- Furosemide 40 mg in the morning
- Lisinopril 10 mg in the morning
- Paracetamol 500 mg to 1 g four times a day when required

From her medical notes you find that her most recent blood pressure was 120/65; when measuring her lying and standing blood pressure you record a 15 mm Hg postural drop. Her chest appears clear and she says that she rarely has difficulty breathing.

Mrs A tells you that she has had a number of falls in recent months and is extremely worried about her swollen ankles which she describes as painful and have 'stopped her getting around'.

Mrs A appears to know exactly when she should take her medicines and links this to her regular activities. However, she does not know why she takes the various medicines and what benefits she can expect from them.

What issues could be addressed during a medication review?

Case Study 10.2

Mr B is a 75-year-old gentleman with COPD with worsening symptoms who presents for a medication review and is found to be taking the following medicines:

- Salbutamol 100 μg inhaler two puffs four times a day, and when required
- Tiotropium bromide 18 μg inhalation capsules twice a day

You notice in his medical notes that he has called out the emergency doctor on two occasions recently. On both occasions, he was very short of breath but recovered quickly after receiving nebulised salbutamol.

What issues could be addressed during a medication review?

Case Study 10.3

Mrs C is an 84-year-old lady who has had a number of admissions to hospital for heart failure who presents for a medication review and is found to be taking the following medicines:

- Lisinopril 5 mg each morning
- Furosemide 40 mg each morning
- Aspirin 75 mg each morning
- Diclofenac 50 mg three times a day with food
- Simvastatin 40 mg at night

Her medical notes indicate that she also suffers from osteoarthritis. When you talk to Mrs C about her medicines she has a good understanding of them, is able to describe why she takes each medication and she appears extremely motivated to take her medicines to best effect as she wants to control her heart failure symptoms as best she can.

What issues could be addressed during a medication review?

Suggested answers to the case studies

Case Study 10.1

Issues that could be addressed during the medication review:

Drug-related falls: Mrs A has experienced a number of falls recently and on examination her blood pressure is low and there is evidence of a postural drop. Her past medical history includes hypertension which is presumably why she is taking amlodipine and possibly lisinopril (although the primary indication may be heart failure). Furosemide may also decrease blood pressure. Stopping the amlodipine may reduce the postural hypotension and number of falls and any increase in blood pressure is likely to still keep her within the NICE target of less than 140/90.

Swollen ankles: It would be easy to attribute Mrs A's swollen ankles to her heart failure but calcium-channel blockers such as amlodopine are also associated with peripheral oedema. This provides another reason to consider stopping the amlodipine.

Understanding of medicines: Mrs A appears to have a good system for taking her medicines. However, she does not appear to understand why she is taking the various medications. It would be useful to have a discussion with Mrs A to explore what information she would like about her medicines.

Case Study 10.2

Issues that could be addressed during the medication review:

Adherence with inhaled therapy: The story presented is very suggestive of poor adherence to medication. Mr B appears to recover well when nebulised salbutamol is administered. He is receiving two different types of inhaler devices (a metered dose inhaler and inhalation capsules) and he may have difficulty using the devices. It will be important to explore Mr B's beliefs about his medication with him as well as asking him to demonstrate how he uses both inhalers.

Optimal management of COPD: Little information is given in this scenario about Mr B's COPD. It will be important to ensure that appropriate spirometry has been undertaken and once the results are known compare his treatment with that recommended by NICE. For example, an inhaled steroid should be considered if Mr B's FEV$_1 \leq$ 50% and he has had two or more exacerbations in 12 months.

Case Study 10.3

Issues that could be addressed during the medication review:

Suffering an adverse drug reaction: Mrs C is prescribed the maximum daily dose of diclofenac, a NSAID, presumably for osteoarthritis. NSAIDs cause fluid retention and should be used with caution in heart failure (and are contraindicated in severe heart failure). A priority should be to review Mrs C's analgesic requirements. She is not prescribed paracetamol. It may be that she takes this as required but many patients can get satisfactory pain relief from regular paracetamol. Since the restrictions on the quantity of paracetamol that can be sold over the counter many patients have reduced the amount of paracetamol that they take. In Mrs C's case, regular paracetamol should be considered as it is much less likely than diclofenac to cause harm.

Optimal management of heart failure: When Mrs C's medication is compared to the NICE clinical guideline for heart failure she is receiving less than the target dose of lisinopril (NICE recommends a daily dose of 30–35 mg) and she is not prescribed a beta-blocker such as bisoprolol or carvediol. He blood pressure is 140/90 with no postural drop so it should be possible to maximise her heart failure treatment in accordance with NICE.

Developing a shared treatment plan: Mrs C appears to have a good understanding of her medication and it will be important to discuss your suggested management plan with her to gain a shared decision about her future treatment. She may express concerns about stopping diclofenac and you may need to discuss the benefits and risks carefully and come to a compromise perhaps involving Mrs C undertaking a trial of regular paracetamol to see if it helps her before abandoning all NSAIDs.

Medicines management services

This chapter has identified that patients with LTCs are frequently prescribed complex medication regimes. It is, therefore, important both that patients have access to the information that they require and that health care professionals ensure that everything is done in order to maximise the benefits (and minimise the harms) from medicines. Medicines management services should be an integral part of the services available for people with LTCs. Of particular importance are the need to work with patients to maximise adherence and regular medication review to ensure that the patients receive appropriate treatment at all times.

Pharmacists are important sources of information regarding medicines management but it is the responsibility of all health care professionals to identify and address patients' medicines management needs.

Medicines information resources

It is not possible in a chapter of this length to give comprehensive information on all aspects of medicines management and readers are referred to the list of medicines information resources and list of references for further information. The following is a list of medicines information resources that may be helpful for patients and health care professionals.

NHS Direct

NHS Direct provides health advice and information to the general public 24 hours a day, 365 days a year through its telephone advice line, Internet site, self-help guides, digital TV and a variety of other services.

Full information available at: http://www.nhsdirect.nhs.uk/.

British National Formulary (BNF)

The BNF is compiled with the advice of clinical experts; this essential reference provides up-to-date guidance on prescribing, dispensing and administering medicines. It aims to provide prescribers, pharmacists and other health care professionals with sound up-to-date information about the use of medicines. An updated book is produced twice a year in addition to an online version (fees may be charged).

Full information available at: http://www.bnf.org/bnf/.

National Institute for Health and Clinical Excellence (NICE)

NICE is an independent organisation responsible for providing national guidance on the promotion of good health and the prevention and treatment of ill health. Guidance is produced in three areas of health: public health, health technologies and clinical practice.

Full information available at: http://www.nice.org.uk/.

Medicines Information Services

The Medicines Information (MI) Service in the United Kingdom is provided on a national basis by specialist pharmacists, the majority of whom are based within hospital trusts located across the United Kingdom. Their work is supported by regional MI centres which provide additional resources and support to local centres. Information on any aspect of drug therapy can be obtained from Regional and District Medicines Services.

Full information (including the facility to search for your local Medicines Information Service) available at: http://www.ukmi.nhs.uk/.

Medicines Partnership Programme

The Medicines Partnership Programme was established by the Department of Health in 2002 and has promoted the concept of concordance – or shared decision-making – as an approach to help patients get the most from their medicines.

Full information available at: http://www.keele.ac.uk/pharmacy/npcplus/workstreams/medicinespartnershipprogramme/.

Expert Patients Programme

The Expert Patients Programme is a lay-led self-management programme specifically for people living with LTCs. The aim of the programme is to support people in increasing their confidence, improving their quality of life and better managing their condition. Having been successfully piloted, the Expert Patients Programme offered around 12,000 course places a year in 2008.

Full information available at: http://www.dh.gov.uk/en/Aboutus/Ministersand DepartmentLeaders/ChiefMedicalOfficer/ProgressOnPolicy/ProgressBrowsable Document/DH_4102757.

Medicines use reviews

The Pharmaceutical Services Negotiating Committee provides a range of resources to support Medicines Use Reviews.

Full information available at: http://www.psnc.org.uk/pages/advanced_services.html.

References

Clyne, W., Blenkinsopp, A. & Seal, R. (2008) *A Guide to Medication Review 2008*. National Prescribing Centre. Available at: http://www.npci.org.uk/medicines_management/review/ medireview/resources/agtmr_web1.pdf (accessed 28 February 2010).

Department of Health (2001) *Medicines and Older People: Implementing Medicines-Related Aspects of the NSF for Older People*. Available at: http://www.dh.gov.uk/en/Publications andstatistics/Publications/PublicationsPolicyAndGuidance/DH_4008020 (accessed 28 February 2010).

Department of Health (2007) *Repeat Dispensing Schemes in England*. Available at: http://www. dh.gov.uk/en/Healthcare/Medicinespharmacyandindustry/Prescriptions/DH_4000157 (accessed 28 February 2010).

Department of Health (2010) *National Service Frameworks*. Available at: http://www.dh.gov. uk/en/Healthcare/NationalServiceFrameworks/index.htm (accessed 28 February 2010).

Gammie, S. M. & Luscombe, D. K. (1995) Pharmaceutical care of the elderly, *The Pharmaceutical Journal*, 254, pp. 578–582.

Health and Social Care Information Centre, Prescribing Support Unit (2010) *Prescriptions Dispensed in the Community: England, Statistics for 1999 to 2009*. Available at: http:// www.ic.nhs.uk/webfiles/publications/prescriptionsdispensed/Prescriptions_Dispensed_1999_ 2009%20.pdf (accessed 28 February 2010).

National Institute for Health and Clinical Excellence (NICE) (2003) *Clinical Guideline 5. Chronic Heart Failure. Management of Chronic Heart Failure in Adults in Primary and Secondary Care*. Available at: http://www.nice.org.uk/Guidance/CG5 (accessed 28 February 2010).

National Institute for Health and Clinical Excellence (NICE) (2004) *Clinical Guideline 12. Chronic Obstructive Pulmonary Disease. Management of Chronic Obstructive Pulmonary Disease in Adults in Primary and Secondary Care*. Available at: http://www.nice.org.uk/Guidance/CG12 (accessed 28 February 2010).

National Institute for Health and Clinical Excellence (NICE) (2006) *Clinical Guideline 34. Hypertension: Management of Hypertension in Adults in Primary Care*. Available at: http://www.nice. org.uk/Guidance/CG34 (accessed 28 February 2010).

National Institute for Health and Clinical Excellence (NICE) (2008a) *Clinical Guideline 66. Type 2 Diabetes. The Management of Type 2 Diabetes.* Available at: http://www.nice.org.uk/Guidance/CG66 (accessed 28 February 2010).

National Institute for Health and Clinical Excellence (NICE) (2008b). *Clinical Guideline 67. Cardiovascular Risk Assessment and the Modification of Blood Lipids for the Primary and Secondary Prevention of Cardiovascular Disease.* Available at: http://www.nice.org.uk/Guidance/CG67 (accessed 28 February 2010).

National Institute for Health and Clinical Excellence (NICE) (2009). *Clinical Guideline 76. Medicines Adherence. Involving Patients about Prescribed Medicines and Supporting Adherence.* Available at: http://www.nice.org.uk/Guidance/CG76 (accessed 28 February 2010).

National Prescribing Centre (2002) *Modernising Medicines Management Guide.* Available at: http://www.npci.org.uk/medicines_management/medicines/medicinesintro/library/library_good_practice_guide1.php (accessed 28 February 2010).

National Prescribing Centre (2008) *Moving towards Personalising Medicines Management: Improving Outcomes for People through the Safe and Effective Use of Medicines.* Available at: http://www.npci.org.uk/medicines_management/medicines/medicinesintro/resources/personalising_medicines_management_web.pdf (accessed 28 February 2010).

Task Force on Medicines Partnership and The National Collaborative Medicines Management Services Programme (2002). *Room for Review. A Guide to Medication Review: the Agenda for Patients, Practitioners and Managers.* Available at: http://www.npci.org.uk/medicines_management/review/medireview/resources/room_for_review.pdf (accessed 28 February 2010).

Chapter 11

Management of heart failure

Susan Simpson
South London Healthcare Trust, UK

Introduction

'Heart Failure is a syndrome in which the patient has the following features: symptoms of heart failure, typically shortness of breath at rest or during exertion, and/or fatigue; signs of fluid retention such as pulmonary congestion or ankle swelling; and objective evidence of an abnormality of the structure or function of the heart at rest.'

(European Society of Cardiology (ESC) 2008: 935)

This new definition clearly explains the syndrome of heart failure, and patients faced with the debilitating symptoms associated with this chronic illness rely upon experienced health care professionals to give them care, management and advice to improve the quality, and in some instances, the length of their life.

Heart failure is a common term which is often applied inappropriately. Patients themselves may believe that heart failure means a heart attack or cardiac arrest. In fact, it mainly means weak heart muscle, which leads to the heart (predominantly the left ventricle) being unable to pump an adequate amount of blood to meet the body's metabolic needs leading to the above symptoms. It is a syndrome of symptoms, not a single disease process, and has a number of causes which are discussed below (see Table 11.1). In some patients (particularly in the younger age group), it is referred to as a dilated cardiomyopathy, which indicates the symptoms of heart failure *not* due to coronary artery, valvular or congenital heart disease (ESC, 2008).

This chapter discusses the key issues including ensuring that these vulnerable patients receive a proper diagnosis of heart failure, and then receive evidence-based medication and regular reviews of their condition. Also, emphasis is placed upon the nursing interventions that should be implemented to provide a high-quality heart failure service for patients and their families; *Winning the War on Heart Disease* (Department of Health, 2004) states that research has shown that specialist heart failure nurses improve both quality of life and long-term survival as well as help to decrease readmission to hospital.

Long-Term Conditions: Nursing Care and Management, First Edition. Edited by Liz Meerabeau and Kerri Wright.
© 2011 Blackwell Publishing Ltd. Published 2011 by Blackwell Publishing Ltd.

Table 11.1 Causes of heart failure.

• Coronary artery disease	• Hypertension
• Previous myocardial infarction	• Excessive alcohol intake
• Heart valve disease	• Drugs, for example chemotherapy, Herceptin
• Pregnancy	• Neuromuscular disease
• Inherited condition	

Epidemiology

In the United Kingdom, in excess of 900,000 people are living with heart failure, with 63,000 new cases being diagnosed each year (British Heart Foundation (BHF), 2008). The prognosis of heart failure is worse than that of breast or prostate cancer, and annual mortality varies between 10% and 50% depending upon severity (National Institute for Health and Clinical Excellence (NICE), 2008). In 2007, the overall prevalence rate of heart failure in the population of England was 0.89% (University of Nottingham, 2007). However, the prevalence increases rapidly with age, affecting up to 1 in 10 people over 85 years of age (NICE, 2008).

Heart failure causes a significant economic burden on the NHS. The annual cost of treatment is estimated at £625 million. Of this cost, 60% is attributable to hospitalisation, with heart failure taking up to 1 million bed days per year, and it has the highest readmission rates of any disease category (Department of Health, 2002). Therefore, any interventions which reduce rates of admission to hospital of people with heart failure save NHS resources.

Aetiology

The commonest cause of heart failure is pre-existing coronary heart disease, including previous myocardial infarction (MI). In frail elderly patients with a new diagnosis of heart failure (who tend to be less intensively investigated), it may not always be possible to isolate one clear cause, but long-standing hypertension remains an important factor (ESC, 2008). Heart valve disease, particularly mitral or aortic regurgitation (leaking valve) or stenosis (narrowed valve) can also lead to heart failure. The heart has to work harder in these circumstances, leading to the heart muscle thickening or dilating and eventually becoming weaker.

Viral myocarditis can affect any age group, and in the United States and Europe it is most commonly caused by the Coxsackie B virus, which is associated with inflammation and injury to the myocardium. The patient often gives a history of a 'flu-like' illness and over weeks or months develops symptoms of heart failure, known as viral cardiomyopathy.

Peripartum cardiomyopathy is a rare complication of pregnancy in previously healthy women. The mechanism of the development of this syndrome is uncertain, but it has recently been associated with abnormal prolactin levels which lead to cardiovascular damage (Jahns *et al.*, 2008). Significant heart failure occurs at, or within a few weeks of delivery. Up to 50% recover, but impaired cardiac function persisting beyond 6 months, indicates a poor outcome (Abboud *et al.*, 2007).

Alcoholic cardiomyopathy occurs in a small number of people who habitually drink excessive amounts of alcohol. A study in North London indicated a prevalence of 12% in people with symptoms of heart failure found to have left ventricular systolic dysfunction on echocardiogram (Galasko *et al.*, 2005). If the sufferer completely abstains from alcohol, significant improvement in cardiac function can occur.

Heart muscle function can be impaired by exposure to various drugs, notably some chemotherapy agents such as Epirubicin. Women taking Herceptin for breast cancer must have serial echocardiograms to assess for heart function due to the known cardiotoxic effect of this drug (NICE, 2009).

There are other rarer causes of heart failure and these include thyrotoxicosis and progressive muscle diseases such as muscular dystrophy.

Dilated cardiomyopathy can also be an inherited condition. Although the knowledge of the genetics of this condition is still in its infancy, for anyone with a family history of dilated cardiomyopathy, or those in whom no clear cause of the condition can be found, screening of close family members is advised (Burkett and Hershberger, 2006). In a few people with dilated cardiomyopathy the cause remains uncertain.

Symptoms and classification of heart failure

The major symptom of heart failure is shortness of breath (SOB). In either the acute phase of heart failure or in decompensation (acute worsening of chronic heart failure), this is due to pulmonary oedema. High pulmonary venous pressure due to poor blood flow through the lungs causes fluid to leak out of the pulmonary capillaries and pool in the lung tissue. The patient will be breathless, have a cough and may expectorate pink frothy sputum. In people with chronic heart failure who have no pulmonary oedema, SOB is generally due to poor cardiac output, as on exercise the heart cannot provide enough cardiac output for the body's needs. In severe heart failure even minimal exertion, such as just taking a few steps across a room, leads to significant breathlessness.

An important aspect of assessing patients with known or suspected heart failure is to ascertain their exercise tolerance. Some patients will have suffered from slowly reducing exercise tolerance and may deny significant breathlessness, as they associate their symptoms with getting old. Others will have developed compensating behavioural mechanisms, such as avoiding stairs or situations where they will be expected to walk any distance. Therefore, it is essential to carefully question the patient to accurately assess their functional capacity.

The other classic symptom of heart failure is recurring peripheral oedema. Patients may complain of weight gain, and they should be assessed for fluid retention. Classically, this occurs as swollen ankles which leave a 'pit' when squeezed. However, in a patient who spends a lot of time in bed, or with legs elevated, the pitting oedema can be observed mainly on the sacrum, genitalia and trunk. Patients may also have liver congestion which

Table 11.2   Symptoms of heart failure.

Breathlessness	Fatigue
Orthopnoea	Abdominal distension
Paroxysmal nocturnal	Loss of appetite
dyspnoea	Nausea
Peripheral oedema	Depression
Dizziness	
Palpitations	

leads to ascites, and they will complain of abdominal distension, poor appetite and nausea (see Table 11.2).

Other symptoms the patient may describe include cough, inability to lie flat (orthopnoea) or waking at night with breathlessness (paroxysmal nocturnal dyspnoea (PND)). The inadequate cardiac output of heart failure leads to postural dizziness and fatigue. Patients often learn to pace themselves so they are able to cope with breathlessness and to stand up slowly to minimise the effects of postural dizziness, but fatigue is a symptom that is hard to deal with and leads to many problems in daily life. Defined by Falk *et al.* (2007: 1020) as 'lacking strength and energy and feeling sleepy', in heart failure fatigue is a circular process. This means that the less the person does as a result of feelings of fatigue the worse the fatigue becomes (see Chapter 9 for more information on fatigue).

In advanced heart failure, the patient can experience significant weight loss known as cardiac cachexia. As with patients suffering from malignant disease, this is associated with poor nutrition, malabsorption and a generalised catabolic state, which is associated with a poor prognosis (ESC, 2008).

It has been noted that some patients' cardiac function defined by echocardiography does not necessarily match their level of functioning. Patients with very poor left ventricular function are able to walk miles, whilst others with borderline function are severely de-bilitated. Although co-morbidities play a part in this discrepancy, anxiety and depression serve to amplify symptoms, so this should always be assessed, formally or informally (Skotzko, 2007). The prevalence of significant depression is up to 20% in patients with heart failure (Rutledge *et al.*, 2006), as their symptoms prevent them engaging in their usual activities, and they develop social isolation. Fear of the future can also cause significant psychological morbidity, so it is essential that health care professionals have honest discussions with the patient about prognosis and quality of life (ESC, 2008). Fear of under-taking activities which may lead to breathlessness can also limit patients more than their actual symptoms.

In spite of the developments in quantifying heart failure by echocardiography, the qualitative classification of heart failure, according to the New York Heart Association (NYHA), first developed in 1964 (DOH, 2001a) is still used in clinical practice and research (see Table 11.3). It stratifies patients symptomatically, according to the health care professional's and patient's perception of their functional capacity, NYHA Class I being mainly asymptomatic, and class IV being breathless at rest.

Table 11.3   New York Heart Association (NYHA) classification of heart failure.

NYHA 1: Ordinary physical activity does not cause undue dyspnoea or fatigue.
NYHA 2: Slight limitation of physical activity, comfortable at rest, but ordinary activity results in fatigue or dyspnoea.
NYHA 3: Marked limitation of physical activity, comfortable at rest, but less than ordinary activity results in symptoms.
NYHA 4: Unable to carry out any physical activity without discomfort, symptoms present even at rest.

Diagnosis

Not everyone with swollen ankles and breathlessness on exertion has heart failure (see Table 11.4). It is not a simple diagnosis to make in primary care without access to echocardiography, and there are indications of many people in the community with undiagnosed heart failure; however, there are others who have been given a diagnosis of heart failure who do *not* have it. For this reason, Standard 11 of the National Service Framework for CHD states:

'Doctors should arrange for people with suspected heart failure to be offered appropriate investigations that will confirm or refute the diagnosis.' (Department of Health, 2001a: 4).

Therefore, nurses should ensure that a definite diagnosis of heart failure has been made in the patients for whom they have responsibility. Symptoms of heart failure associated with a history of a previous MI, coronary artery disease, long-standing hypertension or high alcohol intake should be taken seriously and further tests organised.

In a patient suspected of having heart failure due to history, signs and symptoms, the NICE (2010) guidelines for diagnosis of heart failure should be followed (see Figure 11.1). This involves the patient having an echocardiogram – if it is normal, heart failure is unlikely.

Blood samples should be taken to exclude renal, liver and thyroid dysfunction, and anaemia. In addition, a blood test should be taken for B-type natriuretic peptide (BNP). This is secreted predominantly from the ventricles of the heart in response to wall stress. These levels vary according to age and gender, with women having higher levels than men at any age (Hall, 2004). If results show a high BNP level this does *not* indicate the patient has heart failure; instead, it suggests further testing by echocardiography is indicated. However, low levels of BNP can *exclude* heart failure amongst patients in the community

Table 11.4   Other conditions which may present with symptoms similar to heart failure.

• Obesity	• Hypoalbuminaemia
• Chest disease	• Intrinsic renal or hepatic
• Venous insufficiency in lower limbs	impairment
	• Pulmonary embolic disease
• Drug-induced ankle swelling, for example calcium channel blockers	• Depression and/or anxiety disorders
	• Severe anaemia or thyroid disease
• Drug-induced fluid retention, for example NSAIDs	• Bilateral renal artery stenosis

Diagnosing heart failure

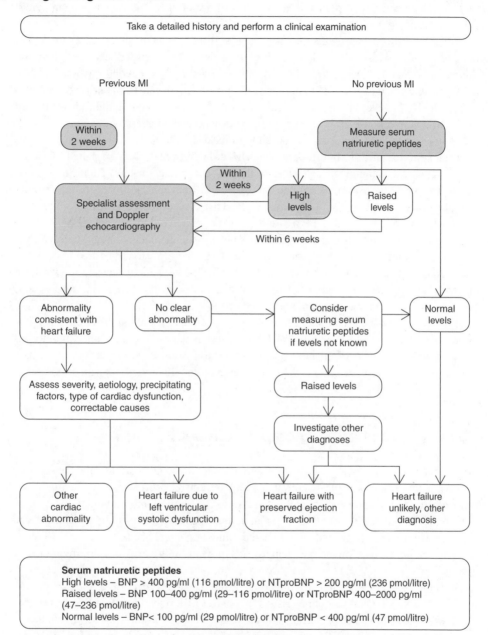

Figure 11.1 Algorithm summarising recommendations for the diagnosis of heart failure (NICE, 2010).

with a confidence value of 95%. Therefore, this test should only be used as a *rule out* test for patients with symptoms of heart failure and should *not* be used as screening tool (Vuolteenaho *et al.*, 2005).

An echocardiogram remains the 'gold standard' for the diagnosis of heart failure, but results should always be correlated with clinical signs. The scan will show valvular and myocardial function. The latter can be quantified by systolic function 'ejection fraction' (EF), i.e. the percentage of blood pumped out of the left ventricle (LV) with each contraction. The LV is never empty, so a normal EF is 60–70%. A rough guide to heart failure is an EF $\leq$ 40%; however, it should not be concluded that a patient with a normal LVEF does not have heart failure, as it is possible to have symptoms of heart failure and have normal systolic function. In this case, the echocardiogram may show so-called 'diastolic dysfunction', which indicates a failure of the LV to relax adequately. This is associated with long-standing hypertension, causing the myocardial muscle fibres to hypertrophy (thicken) and consequently to become 'stiff'. This is also known as heart failure with preserved systolic function (HFPSF), and is most common in older people (ESC, 2008).

When a new diagnosis of heart failure has been made the patient should be seen by a cardiologist for a decision to be made as to whether further investigations are indicated. In the frail older person this may not be feasible, but in all other patients the aetiology should be sought by further investigations, such as coronary angiography, stress echocardiogram, thallium scan or cardiac magnetic resonance imaging (MRI).

If the patient has coronary artery disease, revascularisation could improve cardiac function, thereby alleviating symptoms. Additional tests such as 24 hour Holter monitoring of the patient's heart rhythm should be undertaken to exclude serious arrhythmias, particularly ventricular tachycardia (VT) which are commonly associated with severe heart failure (ESC, 2008).

Overview of pharmacological treatment

In the management of heart failure, the major aims are to reduce mortality and the severity of symptoms. This is achieved through reducing episodes of worsening heart failure (decompensation), and hence hospital admissions, and improving or maintaining quality of life. Evidence-based drug therapy is an essential component of patient management and needs frequent review and alteration according to clinical needs.

This section focuses on the practical aspects of heart failure drug prescribing focusing on ACE inhibitors (ACE I) or angiotensin receptor blockers (ARBs) and beta-blockers. It will include guidelines on up-titrating dosages and the appropriate use of diuretics.

The pharmacological guidelines issued by NICE (2010) (see Figure 11.2) are straightforward in principle, but prescribing in patients with co-morbidities, such as diabetes, COPD or chronic kidney disease, requires a high level of knowledge and skill. Many complex patients are managed by health care professionals not specialising in heart failure care, so they may not receive evidence-based dosages of drugs and hence may suffer preventable morbidity and mortality. A European Survey showed that in accordance with the NICE guidelines, the majority of heart failure patients received an ACE I, but beta-blockers were prescribed in only half of these patients, and the recommended dose was prescribed in only a small minority (ECS, 2001).

Treating heart failure

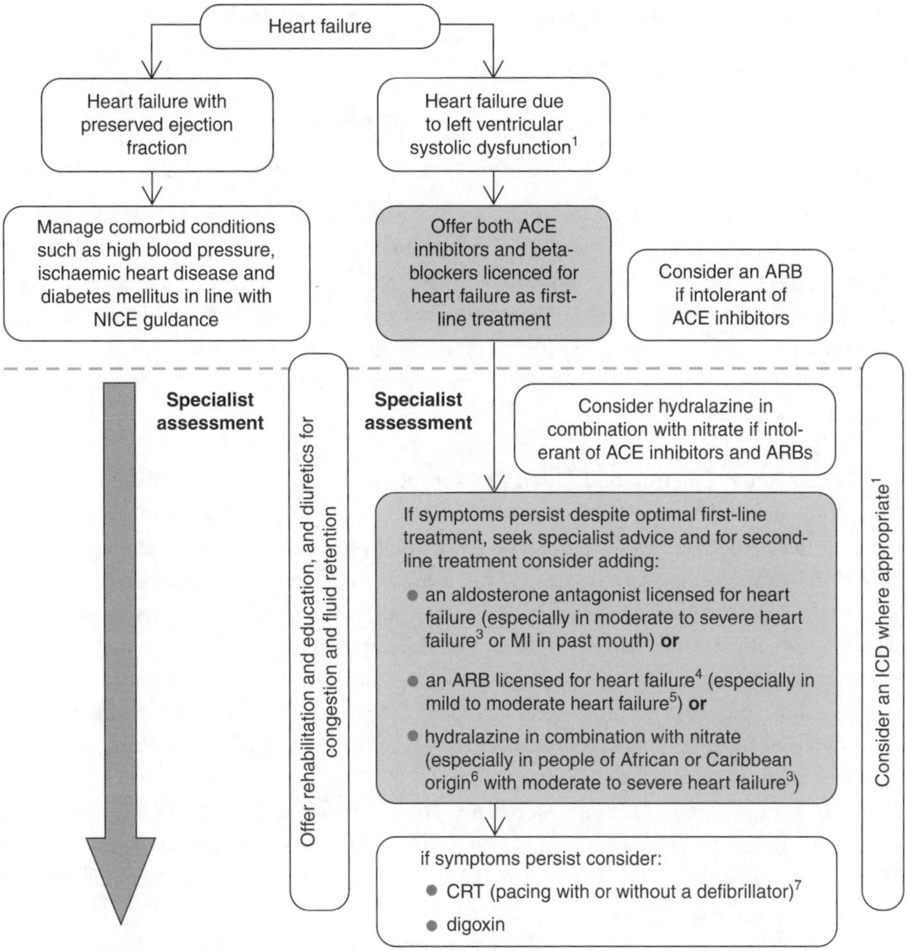
Heart failure
Heart failure with preserved ejection fraction
Heart failure due to left ventricular systolic dysfunction[1]
Manage comorbid conditions such as high blood pressure, ischaemic heart disease and diabetes mellitus in line with NICE guidance
Offer both ACE inhibitors and beta-blockers licenced for heart failure as first-line treatment
Consider an ARB if intolerant of ACE inhibitors
Specialist assessment
Offer rehabilitation and education, and diuretics for congestion and fluid retention
Specialist assessment
Consider hydralazine in combination with nitrate if intolerant of ACE inhibitors and ARBs
If symptoms persist despite optimal first-line treatment, seek specialist advice and for second-line treatment consider adding:
an aldosterone antagonist licensed for heart failure (especially in moderate to severe heart failure[3] or MI in past mouth) or
an ARB licensed for heart failure[4] (especially in mild to moderate heart failure[5]) or
hydralazine in combination with nitrate (especially in people of African or Caribbean origin[6] with moderate to severe heart failure[3])
if symptoms persist consider:
CRT (pacing with or without a defibrillator)[7]
digoxin
Consider an ICD where appropriate[1]

[1] For more information on drug treatment see appendix J and 'Chronic kidney disease' (NICE clinical guideline 73).
[2] Consider an ICD in line with 'Implantable cardiovascular defibrillators for arrhythmias' (NICE technology appraisal guidance 95).
[3] NYHA class III–IV.
[4] Not all ARBs are licensed for use in heart failure in combination with ACE inhibitors.
[5] NYHA class II–III.
[6] This does not include mixed race. For more information see the full guideline at www.nice.org.uk/guidance/CG108
[7] Consider CRT in line with 'Cardiac resynchronisation therapy for the treatment of heart failure' (NICE technology appraisal guidance 120).

Figure 11.2 Algorithm for the treatment of symptomatic heart failure (NICE, 2010).

ACE inhibitors and angiotensin receptor blockers

The poor cardiac output associated with heart failure leads to activation of the renin–angiotensin cascade causing the kidneys to reabsorb salt and water, and the arterioles to vasoconstrict. This leads to the failing heart having to pump an increased blood volume against increased vascular resistance which worsens the vicious cycle of heart

Table 11.5　ACE-inhibitor doses in heart failure.

Drug	Initiating dose	Maintenance dose
Enalapril	2.5 mg BD	10 mg BD
Lisinopril	2.5 mg OD	20 mg OD
Perindopril	2 mg OD	4 mg OD
Ramipril	1.25 mg BD	5 mg BD

failure. ACE I and ARB block the renin–angiotensin cascade at different levels, but have the same effect of reducing salt and water retention, and causing vasodilatation. Treatment has been shown to improve symptoms within days or weeks, and to increase survival. ACE I or ARB should be used in all patients with symptomatic heart failure unless they have specific contraindications, i.e. bilateral renal artery stenosis, previously documented allergy, serum potassium >5.0 mmol/L, serum creatinine >220 μmol/L or severe aortic stenosis (ESC, 2008).

ACE I should be started at a low dose (see Table 11.5), and within 2 weeks of starting therapy, renal function and blood pressure must be checked. A small rise in serum potassium, urea and creatinine should be expected, but ACE I therapy should not be stopped unless the rise is substantial (ESC, 2008). Some patients will complain of dizziness as these drugs cause vasodilatation, but if blood pressure is satisfactory (systolic >90 mm Hg) they can be reassured as this symptom often resolves. If renal function and blood pressure are satisfactory, the ACE I dose should be up-titrated until the maintenance dose is achieved. The dose can be increased every 2–4 weeks, but blood pressure and renal function must be checked after each increase. Once the target dose has been reached, renal function must be checked at least every 6 months, and more often in patients with chronic kidney disease (ESC, 2008).

Some patients develop a troublesome dry cough due to ACE I therapy. It is essential that other causes of a cough are excluded before the ACE I is stopped, but if necessary an ARB can be substituted (see Table 11.6). Currently in the United Kingdom, Candesartan is the only ARB licensed for use in heart failure. This should be prescribed at a roughly equivalent dosage to the ACE I, as if the patient is taking the maintenance dose of ACE I and is changed to the initiation dose of ARB, the sudden loss of ACE inhibition could theoretically cause decompensation. For ARBs, the same precautions and up-titration process should be used as for ACE I.

Beta-blockers

In heart failure the sympathetic nervous system is activated, initiating an increased heart rate and vasoconstriction. This worsens the cycle of heart failure, as the failing heart pumps

Table 11.6　ARB doses in heart failure.

Drug	Initiating dose	Maintenance dose
Candesartan	2 mg OD	32 mg OD
Losartan	25 mg OD	100 mg OD
Irbesartan	75 mg OD	300 mg OD

Table 11.7 Beta blockade dosage in heart failure.

Drug	First dose	Target dose
Bisoprolol	1.25 mg OD	10 mg OD
Carvedilol	3.125 mg BD	25 mg BD
Nebivolol	1.25 mg OD	10 mg OD

faster and less efficiently against an increased vascular resistance. Until relatively recently, it was believed that giving beta-blockers to patients with heart failure would literally kill them, but as has been shown in a number of large research studies over the last 10 years, the opposite is the case. Beta-blockers prevent worsening of heart failure, although patients do not notice symptomatic relief for 3–6 months. Most importantly, beta-blocker therapy improves mortality and reduces hospital admissions. Therefore, beta-blockers should be used in all patients with heart failure unless they have a normal resting heart rate < 50 bpm or 2nd or 3rd degree heart block or sick sinus syndrome (unless the patient has a permanent pacemaker). Other than under specialist care, a systolic BP <100 mm Hg should also preclude the initiation or up-titration of beta blockade. COPD is *not* a contraindication to beta blockade and most patients tolerate this therapy; however, a firm diagnosis of asthma *should* exclude the use of beta blockade (ESC, 2008).

Atenolol and normal preparation Metoprolol are not licensed for use in heart failure and should not be used. Patients already taking these drugs should be switched to either Bisoprolol, Carvedilol, or if they are elderly Nebivolol. Beta-blocker therapy should be initiated at the starting dose (see Table 11.7) when the patient is clinically stable. Now many patients are commenced on beta blockade before discharge from hospital after a new diagnosis of heart failure, but the majority of patients have these drugs started as outpatients.

When starting a beta-blocker, the patient should be warned that an increase in fatigue is common, but passes within a few weeks. However, patients should be encouraged to seek medical attention if they experience new or worsening dizzy spells, or an increase in breathlessness, and/or ankle swelling. The patient should be reviewed within 2 weeks of commencing a beta-blocker and an ECG recorded to exclude any bradyarrhythmia (unless they have a permanent pacemaker). If the patient is suffering from dizzy spells, but heart rate and blood pressure are satisfactory, they should be reassured. Worsening heart failure should initially be treated by temporarily increasing diuretics; it is rare that beta blockade needs to be discontinued.

Assuming the heart rate and BP are satisfactory, beta blockade dose can be up-titrated every 2–4 weeks, but it is essential that the patient is thoroughly assessed before each increase in dose, by recording of ECG and blood pressure, and a physical examination for signs of congestion.

Aldosterone antagonists

Patients with severe symptomatic heart failure (NYHA, Class III–IV), and/or poor LV systolic function (EF <30%) should be considered for treatment with an aldosterone antagonist, i.e. Spironolactone or Eplerenone. At low dose these drugs augment the renin–angiotensin blockade of ACE I or ARBs, thereby improving symptoms and reducing hospitalisations. As these drugs work by promoting the conservation of potassium and the excretion of sodium, they should not be started in patients with serum potassium >5.0 mmol/L or serum creatinine >220 μmol/L. Increasing numbers of patients with heart failure are being treated with an ACE I *and* an ARB. In this case, an aldosterone antagonist *must not* be used due to the risks of hyperkalaemia (ESC, 2008).

The initiation dose of both Spironolactone and Eplerenone is 25 mg OD, and renal function must be checked at 1 and 4 weeks after commencing therapy. If serum potassium rises above 5.5 mmol/L or creatinine >220 μmol/L, the dosage should be reduced to 25 mg on alternate days (it is difficult to break these tablets in half as they crumble), and renal function monitored carefully. If serum potassium rises above 6.0 mmol/L or serum creatinine >310 μmol/L, the drug should be stopped and renal function monitored carefully. In rare cases where severe hyperkalaemia is present, specific treatment in hospital will be required (ESC, 2008).

If the patient tolerates the initiation dose of aldosterone antagonist, it can be increased to 50 mg OD, but again renal function must be checked at 1 and 4 weeks after the increase. Thereafter renal function must be checked at 1, 2, 3 and 6 months, and thereafter at least 6 monthly (ESC, 2008).

Some male patients taking Spironolactone notice breast tenderness and/or gynaeco-mastia (breast enlargement). The patient should be reassured that although this side effect is uncomfortable, it is harmless, and they should be switched to Eplerenone, which has fewer oestrogenic side effects (ESC, 2008).

Diuretics

Most patients with heart failure require a maintenance dose of a loop diuretic (Furosemide or Bumetanide), and at times of decompensation will need an increase in dose. In a patient who has not taken a diuretic previously, low doses should initially be prescribed, and increased if symptoms do not resolve (see Table 11.8). However, it is important that this diuretic dose is reduced when there are no longer any signs of congestion or the patient may become dehydrated. Some well-informed, motivated patients can be taught to manage their diuretic dosage within defined parameters, according to their weight and/or signs of ankle swelling when they wake in the morning (see section 'Monitoring signs and symptoms').

There is evidence that Bumetanide is better absorbed than Furosemide (ESC, 2008), so in patients whose congestion is not responding to high-dose Furosemide, it is worthwhile switching to an equivalent dose of Bumetanide before escalating treatment further.

Table 11.8 Loop diuretic dosages.

Drug	Initial dose	Maximum daily dose
Furosemide	20–40 mg OD	120 mg BD
Bumetanide	0.5–1 mg OD	3 mg am/2 mg pm

In patients with resistant oedema on high doses of loop diuretics, an alternative to admission to hospital for intravenous therapy is to add a thiazide diuretic to the patient's diuretic regime. Caution is needed to avoid dehydration, hypotension and electrolyte imbalances (ESC, 2008). The advised dosage of Metolazone is 2.5 to 10 mg daily (British National Formulary (BNF), 2010), but I have found in clinical practice most patients better tolerate an alternate day regime of Metolazone 2.5 mg, which minimises the debilitating effects of very high-dose diuretic therapy. The patient should be seen *at least* weekly during this time, renal function checked, and the thiazide diuretic stopped as soon as the congestion improves.

Patients find taking diuretics very inconvenient and strategies for promoting concordance are discussed below.

Digoxin

For centuries digoxin was the standard treatment for heart failure, but is now only an adjunct to ACE I/ARB and beta blockade therapy in certain situations. It works by slowing conduction through the atrioventricular (AV) node, thereby reducing heart rate in atrial fibrillation (AF). It has minimal effects in sinus rhythm. Many patients achieve adequate heart rate control on beta blockade and do not require digoxin, but in those patients with AF and a resting heart rate >80 bpm digoxin may be beneficial (ESC, 2008). Some patients with advanced heart failure (NYHA, Class IV) may find some symptomatic relief when commenced on digoxin even if they are in sinus rhythm, but it does not affect mortality or morbidity.

Anticoagulants

Many patients with heart failure have permanent or paroxysmal (intermittent episodes) AF. Poor cardiac output coupled with atria that have uncoordinated contraction means they are at high risk of developing an intra-atrial thrombus which could lead to an embolic stroke. So unless there are strong contraindications these patients should receive warfarin therapy, as this reduces the risk of clot formation and hence reduces the risk of stroke by 60–70% (ESC, 2008). Patients must have their International Normalised Ratio (INR) checked regularly to monitor their level of anticoagulation. In elderly, housebound patients, it is essential that robust systems are put in place to ensure these patients have bloods taken as often as required, to prevent the risks associated with under- or overdosage (notably bleeding). If a decision is taken that the risks of anticoagulation outweigh the benefits this should be recorded clearly in the patients' records.

Promoting concordance in patients with heart failure

All patients with heart failure have to take a substantial number of different drugs, and promoting concordance is vital if the patient is to reap the benefits of the medication. This section examines strategies which can be used to encourage patients to take their medication correctly (see also Chapter 10). The key factor is enabling the patient to understand the reasons why they need to take so many drugs.

In order to thoroughly assess the patient's current medication, they should be asked to show all the medication they are taking including any over-the-counter medication or herbal remedies. It should never be assumed that the GP drug prescription matches what the patient is actually taking! It is also important to ensure that new medication prescribed during a hospital admission has not just been added to the existing prescription. Also, patients become understandably muddled when the same drug is dispensed in boxes from different manufacturers, and it is not unusual to find patients taking two doses of the same drug as the boxes look different. By going through all the patient's medication boxes, it is possible to quickly identify the above problems.

It is important to ensure the patient is not taking any medication that is not indicated, for example the effect of statins to reduce serum cholesterol in patients with non-ischaemic heart failure is unknown. Calcium channel blockers, for example Diltiazem or Amlodipine, are best avoided in heart failure due to their negative inotropic effects, i.e. effects on the force of heart muscle contraction. If the patient does not suffer from angina, nitrates could be stopped (ESC, 2008). This should be discussed with the patient's GP or cardiologist.

It has been shown by Rogers *et al.* (2002) that heart failure patients have little understanding of the purpose of their medication and are concerned about the quantity and the combination of drugs prescribed. Patients have difficulties differentiating between the side effects of drugs and the symptoms of heart failure, and do not possess the knowledge to interpret changing symptoms.

The lives of patients with heart failure are too complicated to expect they will do everything recommended by health care professionals. They will tend to select aspects of advice that best fit their lives (Leventhal *et al.*, 2005). Therefore, the nurse must be prepared to negotiate with the patient – an integral component of concordance. To do this effectively, it is essential that nurses caring for patients with heart failure have a good knowledge of the indications, actions and side effects of drugs prescribed.

Patients themselves feel that learning about their medication is important. Taking medication is viewed as a chore, although a necessary part of living with heart failure, so they welcome information (Cortis and Williams, 2007). Many patients require repeated explanations of the purpose of their medication, and time should be given to answer questions as it has been shown that patients have a persisting need for information (Ekman *et al.*, 2007), and should be guided towards reliable sources of information. Ongoing, regular contact with some patients is necessary to promote concordance (Williams *et al.*, 2008). Community pharmacists can also play a part in this process, but this should be alongside nursing interventions as a recent study has shown pharmacist intervention alone had no impact in preventing hospital readmissions in patients with heart failure (Holland *et al.*, 2007).

Diuretics are the drugs patients find most inconvenient to take, so giving practical advice is valuable. Many elderly patients suffer from stress incontinence or poor mobility which makes it difficult for them to get to the toilet in a hurry. Often they find it embarrassing to discuss this problem, so to alleviate their difficulties they stop their diuretics. It is essential to ask specific questions to assess for urinary problems and to offer continence advice or specialist referral if indicated. Even a simple intervention of providing a commode can help with concordance, and explaining to patients that diuretics work within an hour or two of being taken, can help them plan their day. Also, diuretics do not have to be taken in the morning, but can be taken at any time convenient for the patient, for example when they return from shopping, although taking them after 3 pm may result in disturbed sleep due to waking to pass urine.

Blister packs or dosette boxes are valuable in helping patients organise their medication. However, from my own experience I can report a case in which a blister pack caused poor compliance. A pharmacist reported that a patient's blister pack was being returned with many of the morning doses not having been taken. The patient explained that he liked to go out in the morning, but found this impossible if he took his morning drugs as he needed to pass urine so often. He was unable to identify which of his morning drugs was the diuretic so he omitted them all. The pharmacist was then asked to dispense the diuretics separately from the blister pack, so the patient could take them at a time convenient for him, and the problem was solved. Therefore, an argument could be made for diuretics to be dispensed separately from blister packs other than in patients who are housebound, or those with significant sensory or visual impairment.

Patients should be encouraged to have a commonsense approach to buying over-the-counter medicines and herbal remedies and should always show a list of their medication to the pharmacist for advice. Regarding analgesia, doses of paracetamol, or preparations of paracetamol with codeine are safe to take with heart failure medication, but they should be cautioned against using NSAIDs such as ibuprofen or diclofenac. This is due to the nephrotoxic effects of this group of drugs, and the risk of worsening heart failure (Scott *et al.,* 2008). Generally, herbal remedies should be avoided as their interaction with heart failure medication is unknown, and glucosamine should be avoided in patients taking aldosterone antagonists due to the high potassium content in most preparations. Patients taking digoxin should not take St. John's Wort or ginseng (Kemmerer, 2008).

Device therapy

The use of pacemakers and implanted defibrillators in patients with heart failure is becoming more common. The indications and implications of these devices should be understood by health care professionals caring for these patients, and these issues are addressed in this section.

Patients with heart failure may require a permanent pacemaker for standard reasons such as 2nd or 3rd degree heart block or slow ventricular response AF, but there is evidence that conventional pacing with a transvenous lead in the right ventricle (RV) may worsen symptoms of heart failure. Therefore, a decision needs to be made by the cardiologist as to whether the patient would benefit from cardiac resynchronisation therapy (CRT) pacing (ESC, 2008) where a lead is implanted in both the RV and the coronary sinus, thereby pacing the LV in synchrony with the wire in the RV.

Research studies published over the last few years have shown that patients with symptomatic heart failure with reduced EF ($\leq$35%) and a wide QRS complex $>$120 ms on ECG may benefit from a CRT pacemaker without indication for conventional pacing (NICE, 2007). This device has been shown to improve symptoms in up to 70% of suitable patients

Table 11.9   NICE guidelines (2006) for ICD for primary prevention in patients with heart failure.

• If the patient has a history of previous (more than 4 weeks) myocardial infarction, and
either
• left ventricular dysfunction with an LVEF <35% (no worse than NYHA class III), and non-sustained VT on Holter (24-hour ECG) monitoring, and inducible VT on electrophysiological (EP) testing.
or
• left ventricular dysfunction with an LVEF <30% (no worse than NYHA class III) and QRS duration ≤120 ms

(ESC, 2008). Many patients who could benefit from this treatment are not put forward for consideration, particularly those under community care. Therefore, it is important that patients are checked to assess if they meet the criteria for a CRT pacemaker, and if so, are referred to a cardiac electrophysiologist for expert opinion (Swedberg *et al.*, 2008).

The issue of Implanted Cardioverter Defibrillator (ICD) insertion for primary prevention in heart failure patients has been clarified by guidance (NICE, 2006) (see Table 11.9), as studies have defined the patients who are at highest risk of suffering a life-threatening arrhythmia, showing that ICDs reduce mortality in this group of patients. These devices deliver a small electric shock via a pacing lead in the RV to terminate episodes of sustained ventricular tachycardia, or defibrillate in ventricular fibrillation (VF). Other tachyarrhythmias can be terminated by anti-tachycardia pacing.

There are, however, many ethical issues involved in the decision to proceed with ICD implantation in patients with severe heart failure, and the above guidelines do not take into consideration the patient's quality of life, or prognosis. The recent ESC (2008: 961) guidelines state:

> 'ICD therapy for primary prevention is recommended to reduce mortality in patients with LV dysfunction due to prior MI, who are at least 40 days post-MI, have an LVEF ≤ 35% and NYHA Class II-III, receiving optimal medical therapy, and who have a reasonable expectation of survival with good functional status for more than a year.'

This clearly states the eminently sensible notion that ICD therapy should not be considered for patients who have a very poor quality of life (NYHA, Class IV) and who are likely to die within a year. A patient who has a poor quality of life with severe heart failure in spite of all available medical therapy may prefer to take the risk of sudden death from an arrhythmia, and indeed they may express a view that this is their preferred mode of death. The indication for ICD implantation should be discussed honestly with the patient and their family. Particularly, they need to understand that the ICD alone will not improve symptoms.

Any patient with heart failure who is considered for ICD should have the opportunity to discuss the issues with a specialist in heart failure and a cardiac electrophysiologist in order to make a fully informed decision. Collaborative working is essential if a decision is to be made in the best interests of the individual patient and their family (Swedberg, 2008). A patient's decision not to go ahead should be respected, but if a decision is taken to proceed, discussion should be had regarding the possible future need to deactivate the device as part of end-of-life care. The BHF (2008: 8) has issued excellent guidelines regarding this difficult issue and makes the following recommendations:

- Health professionals working with dying patients should be made aware of the increasing numbers of patients who have an ICD implanted, particularly for the treatment of heart failure.
- Health professionals have responsibility to ensure that the function of the ICD is optimised in the best interests of the patient, particularly for those close to the point of death.
- Open, sensitive communication with patients and their families is essential, to ensure that their expectations are realistic and are compatible with the perceptions of the medical and nursing staff supervising their care.
- There should be close collaboration among medical staff, nursing staff and cardiac physiologists to facilitate timely device management in all care settings. Formal links with electrophysiologists and ICD/arrhythmia nurse specialists may be an advantage.

Nurses should always be aware which of their patients have an ICD (the patient will have a card stating the nature of any device), so when the patient is nearing the end of life plans can be made to deactivate the device to prevent the risk of distressing shocks. This can be undertaken in collaboration with patient's cardiologist or palliative care team.

Patient education

Good medication concordance and the use of modern device therapy can improve the quality of life of patients with heart failure, but most will still have distressing symptoms. Teaching patients to monitor their own condition, thereby assisting them in knowing when to call for medical assistance, can reduce mortality and hospital admissions and improve quality of life (NICE, 2010).

This section discusses the most important issues of patient education in heart failure (see Table 11.10), but some of the education required is not specific to these patients and nurses should remember to include advice regarding stopping smoking, having an annual immunisation against influenza and being immunised against pneumonia.

What is heart failure?

When a patient is diagnosed with heart failure it is essential they receive honest information about their illness. It has been shown that many patients have a poor understanding of their symptoms with some believing, unsurprisingly, that it is due to a lung condition (Rogers *et al.,* 2000). Patients from minority ethnic groups may hold different beliefs

Table 11.10   Essential topics in heart failure patient education.

• What is heart failure?	• Exercise and sexual activity
• Prognosis	• Immunisations
• Monitoring signs and symptoms	• Sleep and breathing disorders
• Drug therapy	• Driving and travel
• Risk factor modification	• Pregnancy and contraception
• Diet	• Psychosocial issues
• Salt and fluid restriction	

Source: Adapted from ESC, 2008.

about the illness and treatment and have difficulties communicating with health and social care professionals (Pattenden *et al.*, 2007). Patients should always have information about their condition given on a one-to-one basis, but this should be supplemented by written information. Good quality Websites should be recommended such as the Heart Failure Association of the European Society of Cardiology (ESC), and younger patients with dilated cardiomyopathy may find the support offered by the Cardiomyopathy Association very helpful.

Prognosis

It is difficult to discuss prognosis with heart failure patients, as in many instances it is very uncertain; however, an explanation that modern drug treatment has improved prognosis may encourage compliance with therapy (ESC, 2008). The majority of patients will suffer a slow deterioration in their symptoms over time, but a number will suffer a sudden death (Mehta *et al.*, 2008). It is essential that questions are answered honestly, and explanations given in a manner the patient and their family can understand. This can help them make realistic future plans. This is particularly important in younger patients with dilated cardiomyopathy as their diagnosis will have a profound impact on all aspects of their lives: employment, getting a mortgage, life insurance and travel. A qualitative study of 10 patients and carers in the United Kingdom showed that few participants reported having been told about their prognosis, but many made realistic statements about their limited life expectancy, and expressed concerns about the future (Aldred *et al.*, 2005). It is vital that patients are given an opportunity to express their worries, and then the options for future care can be discussed openly.

Monitoring signs and symptoms

In order to monitor their condition, patients should be encouraged to weigh themselves every morning on waking. A carer can assist those with poor balance or vision. A record of weight should be kept, and if there is a sudden increase of 1–2 kg over a day or two, the patient should contact the health care professional who is managing their condition (Ekman, 2005). Usually, an increase in diuretics for a few days deals with early signs of congestion, so patients should be encouraged to adhere to daily weighing as this may indicate fluid retention before the obvious physical signs of swollen ankles, breathlessness or abdominal bloating. For patients who are unable to stand on scales, I have found it useful in my practice to teach patients and carers to monitor for ankle swelling before getting out of bed in the morning. If there is no swelling the usual dose of diuretics is taken; however, if there is pitting oedema, an extra diuretic tablet should be taken that day. If the oedema does not resolve within 2 days, the patient should contact their nurse. It is essential that the patient understands the risks of dehydration with excessive diuretic use (ESC, 2008), so should only self-medicate diuretic dosages within preset parameters.

When patients are seeking advice they should be encouraged to contact the health care professional most familiar with them and their condition. The continuity of care offered by chronic disease management programmes, particularly by heart failure nurses and community matrons, enables both patient and health care professionals to get to know each other, to build a trusting relationship, and together formulate a durable plan of care for any deterioration in symptoms. Unfortunately, the health care system itself can militate against patients with chronic heart failure being treated at home. A participant in a qualitative study by Aldred *et al.* (2005: 20) stated: 'you ring the emergency doctor, they ask what the problem is. Next thing an ambulance is here, and you are in hospital', another said, 'I don't go to the doctors because they always send you in'. This concurs with the conclusion reached by Curtis and Williams (2007: 267) whose participants felt they needed to be 'really poorly' before calling the GP.

Diet, salt and fluid restrictions

Patients with heart failure often have a poor appetite, so issuing restrictions on what they should or should not eat can contribute towards malnutrition. To promote a good nutritional intake, patients should be encouraged to avoid excesses of eating and drinking, and small regular meals are preferable to one large meal a day. The most important advice discussed in this section is to limit the intake of dietary salt to help prevent fluid retention, and those with symptomatic heart failure should be advised to limit their fluid intake of no more than 1.5 L per day (Travers *et al.,* 2007).

In obese patients with moderate to severe heart failure, weight loss should not be routinely advised as the development of cardiac cachexia (unintentional weight loss) is common. It has been shown that patients with heart failure who are overweight have a lower mortality than those with a normal or low body mass index (ESC, 2008).

Maintaining fluid restriction can be a problem for some patients, but hints can be given to promote adherence. Using smaller glasses or cups instead of mugs (Falk *et al.,* 2007) is useful, and with practice many patients are able to count their fluid intake in their head. However, it should be emphasised that *all* fluids including soup, should be counted towards their daily intake. I have found numerous instances where patients have been told by other health care professionals to have a high-fluid intake, particularly if they are diabetic or have chronic kidney disease. Written information that the patient can show to others is particularly helpful, which should include a clear explanation as to the reason for the restriction, namely the risk of fluid retention.

Patients with alcohol as a probable cause of their heart failure should completely abstain from alcohol in order to restrict further damage to their heart. Many patients who habitually drink excessively are not dependent, and I have cared for many patients who are so frightened by their condition that they have little problem successfully abstaining from alcohol with little support. However, in those patients who are dependent, early referral to the local substance misuse team should be made to offer expert support and detoxification. Other patients with heart failure due to a different aetiology should be advised to adhere to standard guidelines for alcohol intake per week of no more than 14 units for women and 21 units for men (NHS, 2010). Patients should be reminded that alcohol should be included in their daily fluid allowance.

Adhering to a low salt diet is particularly difficult for many patients. For those who live alone, even if they are able, there is little motivation to cook (Sheahan and Fields, 2008), so they may rely on ready meals which have a high salt content. However, all patients should be advised not to add salt to their food and to try to avoid high salt food by checking food labels. High is more than 1.5 g salt per 100 g (or 0.6 g sodium) and low is 0.3 g salt or less per 100 g (or 0.1 g sodium), with a recommended total daily intake of no more than 6 g (Food Standards Agency, 2008).

To avoid using salt some patients use the potassium-based salt alternative *Lo Salt* (or supermarket own brand equivalent). This must not be used in patients receiving aldosterone antagonists, as the combination could lead to dangerously high serum potassium. Overall, *Lo Salt* should be avoided in patients taking ACE I, and those with diabetes and/or renal dysfunction due to the risk of poor excretion of potassium from the kidneys. Patients who have high serum potassium should be advised to reduce the amount of potassium rich foods in their diet, such as bananas and shellfish (Food Standards Agency, 2008).

Exercise and sexual activity

Physical inactivity in patients with heart failure is common, and can contribute to an exacerbation of symptoms of fatigue and breathlessness. Supervised exercise training is recommended for all stable patients with heart failure, but this should be tailored to the individual's physical capacity (ESC, 2008). Those who are NYHA Class I or II can usually participate in the standard phase 3 cardiac rehabilitation exercise programme, but older patients who are NYHA Class III or with co-morbidities, are likely to gain more benefit from a specific exercise programme, which could be mainly chair based. In my own clinical practice, I have found that the camaraderie of these sessions can also help the psychological, as well as physical well-being of patients.

All patients should be encouraged to engage in some aerobic exercise every day (ESC, 2008), even if this is just walking to nearby shops to buy a newspaper, albeit slowly and with frequent stops. Exercise, such as walking, swimming and cycling is advised for patients with heart failure; however, swimming should only be undertaken in warm water. Cold water causes vasoconstriction and can exacerbate symptoms. Patients should be informed that becoming breathless when exercising is not dangerous; however, they should always be able to carry out activities and talk at the same time. If not, they should rest until they are able, then resume the activity. Heart failure does not preclude going to a gym, and many patients enjoy this; however, they should be encouraged to join a phase 4 cardiac rehabilitation class, or a referral should be made for a local 'Exercise on Prescription' scheme (Department of Health, 2001b), listing all the patient's medical problems, so the exercise physiologist can devise an appropriate exercise regime. Patients should be discouraged from undertaking training with weights.

Sexual activity can be a cause of anxiety to patients and their partners, and the effects of the disease process, medication, fatigue and depression commonly lead to sexual problems. Nurses need to be aware of these issues and feel confident in broaching this topic with patients to allow patients to access available help. Drugs such as Sildenafil (Viagra) should not be prescribed to patients with advanced heart failure without specialist assessment, and should never be used if the patient is taking a nitrate drug. Specialist counselling is recommended, where both the physical and psychological issues can be addressed (ESC, 2008).

Sleep and breathing disorders

Some patients with heart failure experience poor sleep patterns. This can be associated with orthopnoea, and the patient should be encouraged to sleep propped up, and if necessary to obtain a backrest (an occupational therapy department can supply this). During episodes of decompensation, the patient may not be able to sleep in bed and instead will be more comfortable in an armchair, but should always be encouraged to have their legs elevated.

Many patients with heart failure suffer from undiagnosed obstructive sleep apnoea which occurs due to upper airway instability during sleep causing partial or complete obstruction. This is often first noticed by the patient's partner who may report loud snoring with unusual breathing patterns including periods of apnoea followed by the patient waking suddenly. The patient may also complain of constant fatigue and not feeling refreshed from a night's sleep. Lack of ability to concentrate is also a common feature of this condition and this can cause increased risk of accidents, particularly when driving. It is worth being aware that these symptoms are also common symptoms of depression; this highlights the importance of thorough assessments of patient needs to identify the cause of these symptoms. Losing weight, stopping smoking and reducing alcohol intake can help, but referral may be required for a sleep study. If the diagnosis is confirmed, the use of night-time continuous positive airways pressure (CPAP) has been shown to increase energy and reduce daytime sleepiness. It has also been shown in heart failure patients to reduce morbidity and mortality (ESC, 2008).

Some patients suffer from central sleep apnoea, which is an absence of ventilatory effort for more than five times in 1 hour and is associated with increased morbidity and mortality (Rao and Gray, 2005). A recent study has shown that home oxygen therapy at night for patients with central sleep apnoea and heart failure improves symptoms and patient's feeling of well-being, but has no effect on mortality (Sasayama *et al.*, 2009).

Driving and travel

A diagnosis of heart failure does not prevent driving, but patients should be advised against driving long distances due to fatigue. If the patient has a group 2 licence (for lorries or buses), a left ventricular ejection fraction <40% automatically leads to disqualification; however, if the LVEF is equal to or more than 40% the patients must still be able to meet the requirements of an exercise test (Drivers Medical Group, 2010).

Air travel is possible for most people with heart failure, depending on their clinical condition at the time of travel, and is preferable to long journeys by other means of transportation (ESC, 2008). For many people with heart failure, the most difficult part of air travel will be the long walk within the airport, and they may require assistance. It is essential that overseas travel is not undertaken without adequate travel insurance and this can be problematic to obtain, and prohibitively expensive. Travel to destinations which are very hot and humid is best avoided for symptomatic patients.

Pregnancy and contraception

Women of child-bearing age with heart failure who wish to have a child, should be referred to an obstetrician specialising in women with heart disease, where the relative risks can be assessed ideally before they become pregnant. Many drugs used in heart failure are contraindicated in pregnancy due to teratogenic effects, notably warfarin and ACE I. Beta-blockers can cause foetal growth retardation, but can be used with relative safety. Generally, women who have had a previous peripartum cardiomyopathy are counselled against a future pregnancy, even if their LV function has improved, as both maternal and foetal outcomes can be poor (Abboud *et al.*, 2007).

The use of contraception is considered to be of far less risk than that of pregnancy, so the method chosen should be that which is the most reliable for the individual woman. The combined oral contraceptive pill can predispose to thromboembolism, so women with a low cardiac output should avoid this method if possible; also, its efficacy is reliant upon the individual. The most effective and reliable method is the implanted hormonal contraceptive rod, for example Implanon, and this is often recommended to women with heart disease (Thorne *et al.*, 2006).

Supporting patients and carers

This section discusses interventions to empower patients, instil a sense of realistic hope, bolster social support and combat fatigue (Yu *et al.*, 2007). In order to provide comprehensive supportive care to patients with heart failure, it is important to understand the effects this diagnosis can have on the patient and the widespread effects on their family. Assessing the patient at home has many advantages as the physical, psychological and social situation of the patient can be evaluated first-hand, and it is important to use a family-centred approach. In supporting patients and carers, it is essential they receive good education to enable them to make sense of their illness, to prevent feelings of powerlessness and hopelessness.

A diagnosis of heart failure can lead older people in particular to a sense of fear, anxiety and frustration at the loss of independence. They can become physically, psychologically and socially isolated, and suffer a loss of self-esteem and self-worth (Cortis and Williams, 2007). Middle-aged patients report that other people do not understand or believe them when they say they are seriously ill, as signs of the illness can be invisible. They reported that it was no longer possible for them to be the person they used to be as they were unable to maintain their usual role within the family. They often had to take sick leave, work part-time or live on disability benefit (Nordgren *et al.,* 2007).

Patients are often concerned about the 'burden' placed upon their informal carer, who in most instances will be their partner. This is not necessarily how the carer sees the situation, but the social isolation, which can develop due to the condition, is evident to both patients and carers (Aldred *et al.,* 2005). Informal carers of patients with heart failure carry out a range of visible and invisible activities, from bathing and medication management to monitoring for signs of worsening heart failure, and assisting the patient in conserving energy. Their knowledge of the actual disease process may be limited, but they become experts at how the condition affects the patient personally (Clark *et al.,* 2008).

So nurses should take account of the carer's concerns, as they are best placed to notice subtle changes in the patient's condition. The impact of caring for a person with heart failure can affect the physical and psychological health of caregivers (Pattenden *et al.,* 2007), and should also be assessed in the context of family-centred care.

Patients with less socio-economic support find it harder to cope with living with heart failure (Pattenden *et al.,* 2007), so, on a practical level, it is essential to ensure patients are in receipt of benefits to which they are entitled. They often require support in completing applications for Attendance Allowance and Disability Living Allowance, and supporting letters written by health care professionals can be of help. If the patient is expected to live less than 6 months the DS 1500 form should be completed, thus allowing them to claim Disability Living Allowance and Attendance Allowance under what are called 'special rules'.

Occupational therapy assessment of the home situation is vital in patients who have had repeated hospitalisations with heart failure, as often simple adaptations can help an elderly person cope better with their symptoms. Provision of formal carers is often vital to enable an elderly patient to remain in their own home; however, there is sometimes a marked reluctance by patients to accept this help. This may be explained by an interview study of 40 patients with heart failure (Gott *et al.,* 2007), many of whom did not want extra help partly due to the negative experiences of friends. Liaison with all the agencies involved in the care of a vulnerable elderly person who lives alone, is vital to provide safe home care.

Many patients develop social isolation as the unpredictability of their symptoms makes planning activities very difficult (Aldred *et al.,* 2005), and fatigue further exaggerates the problem (Falk *et al.,* 2007). Patients should be encouraged to continue with as many of their favourite activities as possible, for example they may not be able to continue with activities such as crown green bowling due to postural dizziness, but they can still score for their friends. They will need to pace themselves through the day in order to conserve energy, but it has been found that commitment to a preferred activity can reduce the experience of fatigue (Falk *et al.,* 2007). Patients can often do housework or gardening, but must understand they will need to take frequent breaks, and tasks will take longer than usual. Attendance at a day centre can reduce social isolation and raise the mood of those who live alone. Many patients suffer from significant depression and this should be assessed, and discussed with their GP, as the appropriate use of antidepressants can help patients cope better with their symptoms (O'Connor *et al.,* 2008). Referral for clinical psychologist support using cognitive behavioural therapy may also be helpful to enable better coping strategies.

The majority of patients, however, will cope well with their diagnosis and limitations with nursing support. After encouragement and support from a heart failure nurse who paid attention to individual needs and discussed problems, one patient reported, 'After a while I started to ask myself, what can I do? What can't I do? I had thousands of questions so it was great to go to see the nurse.' (Nordgren *et al.*, 2007). In essence, the role of the nurse is to give confidence to the patient and their family to continue to live with heart failure, rather than just exist.

Palliative care

In the recent past, there has been a marked reluctance by primary and secondary care physicians to refer people with heart failure to palliative care services. This led to patients not receiving the care and support patients with cancer have received for many years (Hanratty *et al.*, 2002). Since then, there has been national emphasis on patients without malignant disease accessing palliative care services (Heart Improvement Programme, 2006), and throughout Europe end-of-life care guidelines have been developed (Jaarsma, 2009).

The major problem in the United Kingdom has been that although the prevalence of heart failure was increasing, the service provision for palliative care was not. Therefore, the aim has been to improve access to services provided by the hospice movement, to improve the quality of end-of-life care of patients with heart failure and their family, and to provide a pathway of care for patients by collaborative education of cardiologists, nurses, GPs and palliative care specialists (Lewis and Stephens, 2005, Selman *et al.*, 2007).

The timing of when to refer a patient to palliative care services can be a difficult decision due to the unpredictable prognosis, but some factors (as listed below) can identify that the patient is nearing the end of life, and can assist in decision-making (adapted from Merseyside and Cheshire Cardiac Network guidelines, 2006):

- Recent or multiple admissions with worsening heart failure
- No identifiable reversible precipitant to the worsening heart failure
- Receiving optimal tolerated conventional drugs
- Worsening renal function
- Failure to respond within 2–3 days to appropriate change in diuretic or vasodilator
- Sustained hypotension

It may also become apparent that the patient and/or carer are struggling to cope with the psychological issues of the illness. The support and counselling that can be offered by palliative care services can be invaluable, even if the patient does not yet require physical symptom control.

Addressing the issue of referral to palliative care with a patient and family can be difficult. A study of 31 patients with advanced heart failure found they thought about death infrequently, so when discussing palliative care a path needs to be navigated between inappropriate emphasis on dying, and a collusion of optimism (Willems *et al.*, 2004).

A recent study in the United Kingdom (Selman *et al.*, 2007) has shown that none of the 20 heart failure patients interviewed had discussed their end-of-life preferences with their clinicians. They were not aware of palliative care as a choice, and lived with fear and anxiety about the future.

It has been noted that many palliative care nurses feel they have a lack of knowledge and experience to care for patients with heart failure, and it has been found that joint working between palliative care and heart failure nurses enables them to support each other and work creatively (Pooler *et al.*, 2007). This will also provide continuity of care to the patient.

Symptom control

Many of the symptom control strategies used in cancer care can be readily applied to patients with heart failure. However, due to the paucity of research into symptom control in advanced heart failure some strategies are not evidence based, so should be used on an individual basis according to the patient's needs.

Symptoms of breathlessness, particularly at night, can be helped by using small doses of Oramorph 2.5–5 mg. This has been verified only by a small pilot study of patients with heart failure (Johnson *et al.*, 2002), but extensive clinical experience bears out this conclusion. Similarly, there has been only one experimental study into the use of subcutaneous Furosemide infusions (Verma *et al.*, 2004), but again clinical experience bears out its usefulness in patients who are not able to take oral diuretics and in whom intravenous therapy is not considered appropriate. This can easily be administered at home for palliation, with daily visits from district nursing services.

The use of short burst oxygen in advanced heart failure has no scientific basis, but some patients do find it reassuring to have oxygen available. The guidelines issued by an expert committee suggest individual assessment for the efficacy in individual patients (Booth *et al.*, 2004). Other symptoms such as nausea, constipation, anxiety and depression should be treated appropriately.

Organising services

A review of the studies into models of care for patients with heart failure published between 1999 and 2004 (Hamner, 2005) found that the most effective service models were those with nurses in major roles, having easy access to cardiologist support, with schemes that extended to home visits (Figure 11.3 illustrates an example). This shows patient pathways for those with newly diagnosed or suspected heart failure, movement between primary and secondary care, and medical input as appropriate. Housebound patients can be visited at home, but those who are able, should be encouraged to attend a clinic as it is possible to include more patients in the scheme than if the service is completely home based. The clinic can be sited in either a primary or secondary care setting, and should include on-site access to facilities to take blood tests and record ECGs.

As patients are encouraged to monitor their own condition, it is vital that they have access to their nurse to discuss any changes in their condition. Therefore, a patient

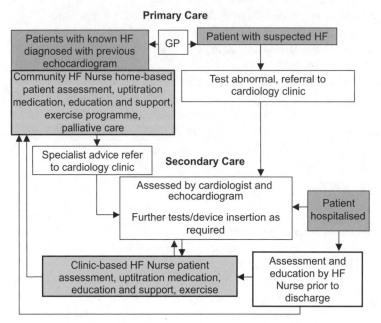

Figure 11.3   Scheme of patient pathways.

'helpline' should be available where patients can leave a message, and the call returned the same day. I have found in my practice that patients do not abuse this facility, and report feeling an increase in confidence as they know they can get advice from someone who knows them.

Specialist nurse interventions

The key components of specialist nurse intervention have been summarised by Stewart and Blue (2001) as follows:

- Assessing patients in their home environment and planning future needs
- Ensuring patients are receiving appropriate therapy in effective doses
- Early adjustment of medication in response to symptoms of clinical deterioration
- Close monitoring of the patient's clinical status and blood chemistry
- Providing tailored education, advice and support about chronic heart failure
- Promoting drug and dietary compliance
- Advising patients on lifestyle changes
- Encouraging patients, families and carers to be actively involved in managing and monitoring their own care
- Being readily available to patients, families and carers in order to detect and treat early clinical deterioration
- Ensuring appropriate and effective communication between patient, GP, hospital and other services

Patient monitoring

Patients who have been hospitalised with heart failure should be seen within 2 weeks of discharge and a comprehensive assessment made of the patient including family support (see Table 11.11), and whether resources available are adequate for caring for the patient at home (Hamner, 2005). Early intervention following hospitalisation contributes to reducing readmission rates, as problems can be identified early and appropriate

Table 11.11   Nursing assessment of heart failure patients – first visit.

Current major problem(s) as reported by the patient, family or carers	
History	**Symptoms**
• Cardiac history • Date of coronary events • Previous investigations • Arrhythmias • Devices • Date of diagnosis of heart failure and aetiology • Past medical history including co-morbidities • Smoking history • Alcohol history • Current medication and any allergies, or prior side effects.	• Degree of breathlessness, for example at rest, on exertion, at night, exercise capacity, etc. • Cough • Chest pain • Palpitations • Dizziness • Pre-syncopal/syncopal episodes • Fatigue • Ankle swelling • Appetite – nausea/abdominal bloating • Itching • Depression
Physical examination	**Vital signs**
• Chest – wheeze, basal crackles • Jugular venous pressure (JVP) • Signs of oedema • Cyanosis • Mobility	• ECG or pulse check • BP • Respiratory rate • Weight
Review latest blood tests	**Home situation**
• Renal function • Liver function • Thyroid function • Serum glucose (if diabetic HbA1c) • Full blood count • BNP (if available)	• Flat/house/stairs to negotiate • Lives alone/support available • Bathroom facilities • Adaptations • Care package
• Patient/carer understanding of condition • Self-monitoring • Medication compliance • Fluid/salt restriction • Immunisation status • Exercise	

interventions instigated. NICE (2010) has made recommendations regarding the minimum monitoring of patients with heart failure, which should include the following:

- A clinical assessment of functional capacity, fluid status, cardiac rhythm, cognitive and nutritional status.
- A review of medication, including need for changes and possible side effects.
- Blood tests for serum urea, creatinine and electrolytes (more detailed monitoring will be required if the patients has co-morbidities), and estimated glomerular filtration rate.

Nurses caring for patients with heart failure will need to use their clinical judgement as to how frequently a patient should be reviewed, and this could be undertaken jointly with other services. In order to provide a comprehensive service, heart failure nurses should be independent prescribers, or work to locally agreed patient group directives (PGDs) (Department of Health, 2007), although in a community setting the latter could be too restrictive. Community nurses need easy access to blood test results, to enable a rapid response to abnormalities, and the ability to perform 12 lead ECGs in the patient's home is useful. The nurse must ensure good communication with the patient's GP, particularly regarding changes in medication.

Conclusion

This chapter has discussed the assessment and management of patients with heart failure, including patient education and support, pharmacological therapies and devices, and end-of-life care.

The care and management of patients with heart failure requires knowledgeable health care professionals, and a coordinated multidisciplinary team if they are to have as good quality of life as possible, in the context of distressing and recurring symptoms. Nurses are best placed to provide that coordination of care, but the labour-intensive nature of nursing intervention for some heart failure patients should not be underestimated nor should the level of hard work which is required to keep these vulnerable patients well cared for in their home environment. However, the success of these interventions is well documented, as is the patients' satisfaction with the care received from their specialist nurses. Therefore, commissioners of health care services should ensure that patients with heart failure have an adequately resourced service, not only to reduce the cost of hospital admissions but also to ensure empathetic individualised care.

References

Abboud, J., Murad, Y., Chen-Scarabelli, C., Saravolatz, L. & Scarabelli, T. M. (2007) Peripartum cardiomyopathy: a comprehensive review, *International Journal of Cardiology*, Jun 12,118(3), pp. 295–303.

Aldred, H., Gott, M., & Garibella, S. (2005) Advanced heart failure: impact on older patients and carers, *Journal of Advanced Nursing*, 49(2), pp. 116–124.

Booth, S., Wade, M., Johnson, M., *et al.* (2004) The use of oxygen in the palliation of breathlessness. A report of the expert working group of the scientific committee of the association of palliative medicine. *Respiratory Medicine*, 98(1), pp. 66–77.

British Heart Foundation (2008) *Coronary Heart Disease Statistics*. British Heart Foundation, London.

British National Formulary (2010) The British National Formulary 59, March. Available at: http://www.bnf.org/bnf/ March 2010 (accessed 18 October 2009).

Burkett, E. L. & Hershberger, R. E. (2006) Clinical and genetic issues in familial dilated cardiomy-opathy, *Journal of the American Journal of Cardiology*, 47(3), pp. 689–690.

Clark, A. M., Reid, M. E., Morrison, C. E., *et al.* (2008) The complex nature of informal home-based heart failure management, *Journal of Advanced Nursing*, February, 61(4), pp. 373–383.

Cortis, J. D. & Williams, A. (2007) Palliative and supportive needs of older adults with heart failure, *International Nursing Review*, 54(3), pp. 263–270.

Department of Health (2001a) *National Service Framework for Coronary Heart Disease*. Department of Health, London.

Department of Health (2001b) *Exercise on Prescription: A Quality Assurance Framework*. Available at: http://www.dh.gov.uk/en/Publicationsandstatistics/Publications/PublicationsPolicyAnd Guidance/DH_4009671 (accessed 18 October 2009).

Department of Health (2002) *Hospital Episode Statistics*. DOH Annual Trust Financial Returns 1998 and 1999. Department of Health, London.

Department of Health (2004) The *National Service Framework for Coronary Heart Disease: Winning the war on heart disease*. Available at: http://www.dh.gov.uk/en/Publicationsandstatistics/Publications/PublicationsPolicyAndGuidance/DH_4077154 (accessed 18 October 2009).

Department of Health (2007) *Non-Medical Prescribing*. Available at: http://www.dh.gov.uk/en/Healthcare/Medicinespharmacyandindustry/Prescriptions/TheNon-MedicalPrescribingProgramme/Nurseprescribing/DH_4123003 (accessed 18 October 2009).

Drivers Medical Group (2010) At a Glance Guide to the Correct Medical Standards of Fitness to Drive. Driver and Vehicle Licensing Agency. Available at: http://www.dft.gov.uk/dvla/medical/ataglance.aspx (accessed 18 October 2009).

Ekman, I., Cleland, J. G., Swedberg, K., Charlesworth, A., Metra, M. & Poole-Wilson, P. (2005) Symptoms in patients with heart failure are prognostic indicators: insights from COMET, *Journal of Cardiac Failure*, 11, pp. 288–292.

Ekman, I., et al. (2007) Standard medication information is not enough: poor concordance of patients and nurse perceptions, *Journal of Advanced Nursing*, 60(2), pp. 181–186.

European Cardiac Society (2001) *Euro Survey on Heart Failure*. Available at: http://www.escardio.org/guidelines-surveys/ehs/heart-failure/Pages/survey-hf1.aspx (accessed 18 October 2009).

European Society of Cardiology (2008) Guidelines in the diagnosis and treatment of chronic heart failure, *European Journal of Heart Failure*, 10, pp. 933–989.

Falk, K., Granger, B. B., Swedberg, K., Ekman, I. (2007) Breaking the vicious circle of chronic fatigue in patients with heart failure, *Qualitative Health Research*, 17(8), pp. 1020–1027.

Food Standards Agency (2008) *Eat Well, be Well Helping you Make Healthier Choices: Salt*. Available at: www.salt.gov.uk (accessed 18 October 2009).

Galasko, G. I. W., Senior, R. & Lahiri, A. (2005) Ethnic differences in the prevalence and aetiology of left ventricular systolic dysfunction in the community: the Harrow heart failure watch, *Heart* 91, pp. 595–600.

Gott, M., Barnes, S., Payne, S., *et al.* (2007) Patient views of social service provision for older people with advanced heart failure, *Health and Social Care in the Community*, 15(4), pp. 333–342.

Hall, C. (2004) Essential biochemistry and physiology of (NT-pro)BNP, *European Journal of Heart Failure*, 6(3), pp. 257–260.

Hamner, J. (2005) State of the science: post hospitalisation nursing intervention in CHF, *Advances in Nursing Science*, 28(2), pp. 175–190.

Hanratty. B., Hibbert, D., Mair. F., *et al.* (2002) Doctors perceptions of palliative care for heart failure: focus group study, *British Medical Journal*, 325, pp. 581–585.

Heart Improvement Programme (2006) *Supportive and Palliative Care in Heart Failure: A Resource Kit.* Available at: http://www.heart.nhs.uk/endoflifecare/resource_kit.htm (accessed 18 October 2009).

Holland, R., Brooksby, I., Lenaghan, E., *et al.* (2007) Effectiveness of visits from community pharmacists for patients with heart failure: heartmed randomised control trial, *British Medical Journal,* 334(7603), p. 1098.

Jaarsma, T., Beattie, J. M., Ryder, M., *et al.* On behalf of the advanced heart failure study group of the hfa of the esc (2009) palliative care in heart failure: a position statement from the palliative care workshop of the heart failure association of the European society of cardiology, *European Journal of Heart Failure*, 11, pp. 433–443.

Jahns, B. G., Stein, W., Hilfiker-Kleiner, D., Pieske, B., Emons, G. (2008) Peripartum cardiomyopathy – a new treatment option of prolactin secretions, *American Journal of Obstetrics and Gynecology.* Oct,199, 4, pp. 5–6

Johnson, M. J., McDonagh, T. A., Harkness, A., McKay, S. E. & Dargie, H. J. (2002) Morphine for the relief of breathlessness in patients with chronic heart failure – a pilot study, *European Journal of Heart Failure*, 4(6), pp. 753–756.

Kemmerer, D. A. (2008) Devious digoxin: a case review, *Journal of Emergency Nursing*, 34(5), pp.487–489.

Leventhal, M. J. E., Riegel, B., Carlson, N. B. & de Geest, S. (2005) Negotiating compliance in heart failure, remaining issues and questions, *European Journal of Cardiovascular Nursing*, pp. 298–307.

Lewis, C. & Stephens, B. (2005) Improving palliative care provision for patients with heart failure, *British Journal of Nursing*, 14(10), pp. 563–568.

Mehta, P. A., Dubrey, S. W., McIntyre, H. F., *et al.* (2008) Mode of death in patients with newly diagnosed heart failure in the general population, *European Journal of Heart Failure*, 10, pp. 1108–1116.

NHS (2010) *NHS Advice on Drinking Limits.* Available at: www.drinking.nhs.uk/questions/recommended-levels (accessed 18 October 2009).

National Institute for Health and Clinical Excellence (NICE) (2006) *Implantable Cardioverter Defibrillators (ICDs) for the Treatment of Arrhythmias.* National Institute for Health and Clinical Excellence, London.

National Institute for Health and Clinical Excellence (NICE) (2007) *Cardiac Resynchronisation Therapy for the Treatment of Heart Failure.* National Institute for Health and Clinical Excellence, London.

National Institute for Health and Clinical Excellence (NICE) (2008) *Chronic Heart Failure (partial update),* National Institute for Health and Clinical Excellence, London.

National Institute for Health and Clinical Excellence (NICE) (2009) *Early and Locally Advanced Breast Cancer: Diagnosis and Treatment.* National Institute for Health and Clinical Excellence, London.

National Institute for Health and Clinical Excellence (NICE) (2010) *Chronic Heart Failure: Full Guideline (CG108).* Available at: www.nice.org.uk (accessed 18 October 2009).

Nordgren, L., Asp, M & Lagerborg G .I (2007) Living with moderate to severe chronic heart failure as a middle aged person, *Qualitative Health Research*, 17(1), pp. 4–13.

O'Connor, C. M., Jiang, W., Kuchibhatla, M., *et al.* (2008) Antidepressant use, depression, and survival in patients with heart failure, *Archives of Internal Medicine,* 168(20), pp. 2232–2237.

Pattenden, J. F., Roberts, H, Lewin, R. J (2007) Living with heart failure: patient and carer perspectives, *European Journal of Cardiovascular Nursing*, 6(4), pp. 273–279.

Pooler, J., Yates, A. & Ellison, S. (2007) Caring for patients dying at home from heart failure: a new way of working, *International Journal of Palliative Nursing*, 13(5), pp. 266–271.

Rao, A. & Gray, D. (2005) Impact of heart failure on quality of sleep, *Postgraduate Medical Journal*, 81, 952, pp. 99–102.

Rogers, A. E. (2000) knowledge and communication difficulties for patients with heart failure: a qualitative study, *British Medical Journal*, 321, pp. 605–607.

Rogers, A. E., *et al.* (2002) A qualitative study of chronic heart failure patients' understanding of their symptoms and drug therapy, *European Journal of Heart Failure*, 4(3), pp. 283–287.

Rutledge, T., Reis, V. A., Linke, S. E., Greenberg, B. H., Mills, P. J. (2006) Depression in heart failure: a meta-analytic review of prevalence, intervention effects and associated clinical outcomes, *Journal of the American College of Cardiology*, 48, pp. 1527–1537.

Sasayama, S., Izumi, T., Matsuzaki, M., *et al.* (2009) Improvement of quality of life with nocturnal oxygen therapy in heart failure patients with central sleep apnoea, *Circulation Journal*, 73(7), pp.1255–1262.

Scott, P. A., Kingsley, G. H, & Scott, D. L. (2008) Non-steroidal anti-inflammatory drugs and cardiac failure: meta-analyses of observational studies and randomised trials, *European Journal of Heart Failure*, 10, pp. 1102–1107.

Selman, L., Harding, R., Beynon, T., *et al.* (2007) Improving end-of-life care for patients with chronic heart failure: "Let's hope it'll get better, when I know in my heart of hearts it won't", *Heart*, 93(8), pp. 901–902.

Sheahan, S. L. & Fields, B. (2008) Sodium dietary restriction, knowledge, beliefs, and decision making behaviour of older females, *Journal of the Academy of Nurse Practitioners*, 20(4), pp. 217–224.

Skotzko, C. E. (2007) Symptom perception in CHF (why mind matters), *Heart Failure Review*, Dec 11 (Epub.), 14(1), pp. 29–34.

Stewart, S. & Blue, L. (eds) (2001) *Improving Outcomes in Chronic Heart Failure. A practical guide to specialist nurse intervention*. BMJ Books, London.

Swedberg, K., Cleland, J., Cowie, M., *et al.* (2008) Successful treatment of heart failure with devices requires collaboration, *European Journal of Heart Failure*, 10, pp. 1229–1235.

Thorne, S., MacGregor, A. & Nelson-Piercy, C. (2006) Risks of contraception and pregnancy in heart disease, *Heart*, 92(10), pp.1520–1525.

Travers, B., O'Loughlan, C., Murphy N. F., *et al.* (2007) Fluid restrictions in the management of decompensated heart failure: no impact on time to clinical stability, *Journal of Cardiac Failure*, 13, pp. 128–132.

University of Nottingham (2007) PRIMIS + Available at: http://www.primis.nhs.uk/pages/prevalence07/comparison-atrialtiaischaemicheartvascular.asp#heart (accessed 18 October 2009).

Verma, A. K., da Silva, J. H. & Kuhl, D. R. (2004) Diuretic effects of subcutaneous furosemide in human volunteers: a randomised pilot study, *Annals of Pharmacotherapy,* 38(4), pp. 544–549.

Vuolteenaho, O., Ala-Kopsala, M. & Ruskoaho, H. (2005) BNP as a biomarker in heart disease, *Advances in Clinical Chemistry*, 40, pp. 1–36.

Willems, D. L., Hak, A., Visser, F. & van de Wal, G. (2004) Thoughts of patients with advanced heart failure on dying, *Palliative Medicine*, 18, pp. 564–572.

Williams, A., Manias, E. & Walker, R. (2008) Interventions to improve medication adherence in people with multiple chronic conditions: a systematic review, *Journal of Advanced Nursing*, pp. 132–143.

Yu, S. F., Lee, D .T. F., Kwong A. N. T., *et al.* (2007) Living with chronic heart failure: a review of qualitative studies of older people, *Journal of Advanced Nursing*, 61, pp. 474–483.

HELPFUL RESOURCES

Attendance Allowance
http://www.direct.gov.uk/en/DisabledPeople/FinancialSupport/DG_10012425
Disability Living Allowance
http://www.direct.gov.uk/en/DisabledPeople/FinancialSupport/DG_10011731
Heart Failure Association of the European Cardiac Society (ESC)
www.heartfailurematters.org
Cardiomyopathy Association www.cardiomyopathy.org.

Chapter 12

Management of respiratory disease

Liz Nicholls
Bexley Care NHS Trust, London, UK

Introduction

Respiratory diseases include diseases of the lung, pleural cavity, bronchial tubes, trachea, upper respiratory tract, and of the nerves and the muscles used for breathing. They are broad in their effect and duration. They can range from mild and self-limiting, such as the common cold, or life-threatening, such as bacterial pneumonia or pulmonary embolism, to those which are long term, such as asthma and chronic obstructive pulmonary disease (COPD), and require extensive adjustments and adaptations to manage and live with the disease.

Respiratory disease can be divided into two main categories: (1) restrictive and (2) obstructive. The two terms refer to the nature of the particular lung disease and the effect it has on the anatomy and physiology of the lung tissue itself. Restrictive lung diseases can come about through differing causal agents, but they all have in common a reduction in the volume of the lung, or the amount of air the lung can hold, and the ability of the lung to diffuse oxygen and carbon dioxide through the alveoli. This category can also be described as diseases that create diffuse interstitial and/or alveolar inflammation leading to progressive fibrosis. Obesity can be classed as a restrictive lung disease as the amount of body fat and stomach size will reduce the amount of lung volume. Restrictive lung diseases are less common, but include, for example, sarcoidosis and idiopathic pulmonary fibrosis. In obstructive lung diseases, there is an alteration in the airways which prevents air from being expelled from the lungs. COPDs include emphysema, bronchiectasis and chronic bronchitis.

Respiratory disease affects approximately 1 in 7 people in the United Kingdom (British Lung Foundation, 2008) – approximately 8 million people – a figure which is expected to increase in the United Kingdom (BTS Report, 2006) and has associated implications for healthcare resources. People living with respiratory disease are intensive users of primary and secondary care services, with an estimated 24 million consultations with GPs, and 1 million hospital admissions in 2004 estimated to be for respiratory disease (BTS Report, 2006). According to the BTS Report (2006), respiratory disease costs the NHS £6.6 billion per year. It is responsible for more deaths than ischaemic heart disease in

Long-Term Conditions: Nursing Care and Management, First Edition. Edited by Liz Meerabeau and Kerri Wright.
© 2011 Blackwell Publishing Ltd. Published 2011 by Blackwell Publishing Ltd.

the United Kingdom. In addition, the symptoms of respiratory disease can be debilitating and terrifying to live with, and can have far-reaching implications for an individual's ability to manage and live with their condition.

Due to the range and scope of management of respiratory diseases, this chapter focuses on the most common long-term respiratory conditions of COPDs and asthma, and discusses the management and care available to support people to live their lives with these conditions.

Epidemiology

There are clear social class gradients in respiratory disease mortality. According to the data, social inequality causes a higher proportion of deaths in respiratory disease than any other disease area. The BTS Report (2006) states that almost a half of all deaths from respiratory disease (44%) are associated with social class inequalities, compared with 28% of deaths from ischaemic heart disease. Furthermore, men, aged 20–64, employed in unskilled manual occupations are around 14 times more likely to die from COPD and nine times more likely to die from tuberculosis than men employed in professional roles. The majority of people living with COPD come from the least affluent sections of the population, and live primarily in urban areas (The Respiratory Alliance, 2003).

Death rates from respiratory disease are higher in the United Kingdom than both the European and EU average. There are only seven other European countries with a worse record than the United Kingdom, five of which are former Soviet Union countries, with relatively underfunded, less sophisticated health services. Data shows that more women than men die from lung disease.

Risk factors

Lung disease can be caused by a wide range of factors. As an adult, exposure to occupational materials such as dust, asbestos fibres and other irritating particles can cause lung disease. For example, exposure to asbestos has been linked to the production of pleural plaques, lung fibrosis, bronchial carcinoma and mesothelioma. Chronic lung disease can also be caused *in utero*, or during the post-natal period. Many mechanisms that protect the lung from injury are poorly developed or not present in a newborn. *In utero*, the baby's lungs are filled with fluid that protects them and allows them to develop. Once born, a baby's lungs are no longer protected and are affected by the environment the baby is developing within. Passive smoking and poor housing conditions can affect lung development, and poor nutrition can increase the risk associated with developing lung disease. Inherited conditions such as cystic fibrosis (CF) are also diagnosed in early childhood.

> *Smoking:* One of the common causes of lung disease is smoking; it has been accepted for many years that the cost of smoking-related illness, both to the economy and to the individual patient, is huge. It is the main cause of COPD, but other environmental

and industrial pollutants can be contributory to the disease process. There is also wide acceptance that passive smoking can and does contribute to respiratory symptoms.

Cannabis: There is relatively little research on the effects of cannabis smoking, but recent studies, such as that published by The British Lung Foundation (2008) *A Smoking Gun?*, suggest that there is a need for further research if lung disease in the younger population is to be avoided. The cannabis smoked today is much more potent than that smoked in the 1960s. Tetrahydrocannabinol (TCH), the ingredient which accounts for the psychoactive properties of cannabis, which was at the level of 10 mg per cigarette in the 60s, is now often in excess of 150 mg. Three to four cannabis cigarettes a day are associated with the same evidence of acute and chronic bronchitis, and the same degree of damage to the bronchial mucosa as 20 or more tobacco cigarettes a day.

Pollution: Outdoor air pollution is believed to contribute to adult and childhood respiratory disease, especially asthma, the causes of which are often multifaceted. The type of disorder encountered depends on the concentration, size and shape of the pollutant as well as the sensitivity of the airways. There are inherited genetic factors that affect susceptibility to various respiratory diseases, such as hay fever or asthma which are triggered by allergens. At risk workers include coal miners, metal workers, grain handlers, cotton workers and paper-mill workers. The introduction of strict occupational health guidelines, such as the wearing of face masks and smoking ban laws recently introduced across the United Kingdom, should impact on reducing the burden of lung disease.

Chronic obstructive lung disease (COPD)

Pathophysiology and diagnosis

The Global Initiative for Chronic Obstructive Lung Disease (GOLD) guidelines (2009: 2) define COPD as 'A preventable and treatable disease with some significant extrapulmonary effects that may contribute to the severity in the individual patient. Its pulmonary component is characterized by airflow limitation that is not fully reversible. The airflow limitation is usually progressive and associated with an abnormal inflammatory response of the lung to noxious particles or gases.' COPD is a disease affecting the airways, which often leads to irreversible airflow obstruction, due to chronic bronchitis, emphysema or chronic asthma.

COPD has two main mechanisms: chronic inflammation of the small airways and gradual destruction of the alveoli. Chronic inflammation results in fibrosis, which in turn leads to narrowing of the airways. Various enzymes released by neutrophils damage the elasticity and support of the alveoli. Terminal bronchioles collapse or are blocked by plugs of mucus, causing the alveoli to die (see Figure 12.1).

The main clinical features of COPD are:

- Chronic cough, which may be daily and productive, but can also be intermittent and unproductive.
- Breathlessness on exertion, initially intermittent and becoming persistent.

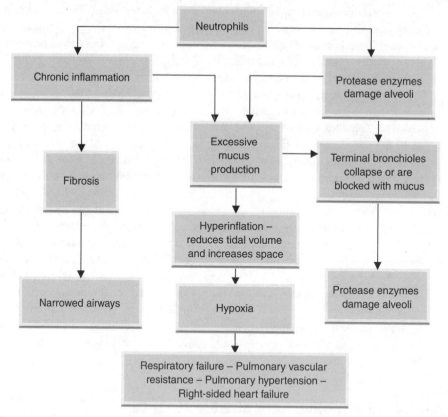

Figure 12.1   Mechanisms and manifestations of COPD (Jones, 2007).

- Sputum production: Any pattern of sputum production may indicate COPD.
- Frequent exacerbations of bronchitis.
- A history of exposure to risk factors, especially tobacco smoke, occupational dusts, and biomass fuels.

COPD is by far the commonest respiratory cause of mortality and morbidity in adults in the United Kingdom. It is managed chiefly in the community; however, in recent years, it has been acknowledged that many patients may have been misdiagnosed and therefore inappropriately treated (Bellamy and Booker, 2008). This is often due to poor education of health care practitioners, who may confuse the symptoms of asthma with those of COPD, especially if there is a significant smoking history. COPD is a chronic progressive debilitating disease which puts a huge burden on individuals, health care systems and the wider economy.

The GOLD international COPD Guidelines (updated 2009), recommend spirometry be used to confirm the clinical diagnosis of COPD with objective measurement. Spirometry is the best way of detecting airway obstruction and making a definitive diagnosis of asthma and/or COPD. Other assessments such as chest X-ray, blood gases and exercise tolerance are also useful in assessing severity, to ensure appropriate and cost-effective management.

Its major uses in COPD as stated in the GOLD Spirometry for healthcare provider's handbook are to:

- confirm the presence of airway obstruction;
- confirm an FEV1/FVC ratio <0.7 after bronchodilator;
- provide an index of disease severity;
- help differentiate asthma from COPD;
- detect COPD in subjects exposed to risk factors, predominantly tobacco smoke, independently of the presence of respiratory symptoms;
- enable monitoring of disease progression;
- help assess response to therapy;
- aid in predicting prognosis and long-term survival; and
- exclude COPD and prevent inappropriate treatment if spirometry is normal.

The standard spirometry manoeuvre is a maximal forced exhalation (greatest effort possible) after a maximum deep inspiration (completely full lungs). Several indices can be derived from this. These values are compared with predicted normal values determined on the basis of age, height, sex and ethnicity, and a measure of the severity of airway obstruction can be determined (see Table 12.1).

- *FVC (forced vital capacity):* The total volume of air that the patient can forcibly exhale in one breath.
- *FEV1 (forced expiratory volume in 1 second):* The volume of air that the patient is able to exhale in the first second of forced expiration.
- *FEV1/FVC:* The ratio of FEV1 to FVC expressed as a fraction.

The spirometric criterion required for a diagnosis of COPD is an FEV1/FVC ratio below 0.7 after bronchodilator. The degree of bronchodilator reversibility can vary; larger changes above 200 mL or 12% do not negate a diagnosis of COPD, although the greater

Table 12.1 GOLD spirometric criteria for COPD severity.

Mild COPD	FEV1/FVC<0.7 FEV1 >80% predicted	At this stage, the patient may not be aware that their lung function is abnormal.
Moderate COPD	FEV1/FVC<0.7 50%<FEV1<80% predicted	Symptoms usually progress at this stage, with shortness of breath typically developing on exertion.
Severe COPD	FEV1/FVC<0.7 30%<FEV1<50% predicted	Shortness of breath typically worsens at this stage and often limits patients' daily activities. Exacerbations are especially seen beginning at this stage.
Very severe COPD	FEV1/FVC< 0.7 FRV1<30% predicted *or* FEV1<50% predicted *plus* Chronic respiratory failure	At this stage, quality of life is very appreciably impaired and exacerbations may be life-threatening.

these changes are the more likely that the patient is asthmatic, either instead of or in addition to COPD.

Physiological changes that characterise the disease include: mucus hypersecretion, ciliary dysfunction, airflow limitation, pulmonary hyperinflation, gas exchange abnormalities, pulmonary hypertension and cor pulmonale, usually developing in that order, resulting in the classic COPD symptoms of chronic productive cough and dyspnoea.

Living with COPD

Whilst there is no cure for COPD, health care professionals can strive to improve patients' symptoms and experience of living with the disease, by listening and responding to how their symptoms affect them. Breathlessness is the major symptom of COPD, and has an insidious onset with compensatory behaviour to reduce symptoms, such as slowing down and having frequent stops when walking or climbing the stairs. Breathlessness or dyspnoea is described as 'a subjective experience of breathing discomfort' (The American Thoracic Society, 1999). Breathlessness is thus experienced uniquely by the individual and does not necessarily correlate with lung function or disease severity. The impact of breathlessness is graphically described here:

'If you want to imagine what it is like to have an exacerbation, pinch your nose and close your mouth and see how long you can do that before you panic. Don't give up when you feel like giving up, keep going until you become desperate and panic. If I was in a situation where I could not get help quickly, that is how I would feel; I would feel this desperate panic. So if a patient is on a ward and they say they need help, this does not mean that they need it in an hour's time; they need it there and then.' (Brownrigg, 2007: 19)

The experience of living with breathlessness and the behaviours and adaptations that people adopt to try to manage this symptom can have a far-reaching impact on their life. Therefore, understanding how the person experiences breathlessness and the effect it has on their life is an important part of the assessment process, before appropriate interventions are considered. There are many different interventions that have been found to be beneficial for people experiencing breathlessness; these are discussed in more detail in the section 'Breathlessness (Dyspnoea)' of Chapter 9.

Despite breathlessness being the main presenting symptom of COPD and the distress that this symptom can cause, people are reluctant to seek help, and often do not present to the health care system until they have lost approximately 50% of their lung function. There are several reasons for this but primarily there is a feeling of guilt and shame that the condition has been self-imposed because of their smoking. Arne *et al.* (2007) interviewed patients with COPD to explore their perspectives at the time of diagnosis. Shame was often the main theme and was related to the belief that their disease was self-inflicted, thus preventing them from seeking advice earlier. Because of this belief patients often perceive themselves to be 'a burden'.

Table 12.2 MRC dyspnoea scale.

Grade	Degree of breathlessness related to activity
1	Not troubled by breathlessness except on strenuous exercise
2	Short of breath when hurrying or walking up a slight hill
3	Walks slower than contemporaries on the level because of breathlessness, or has to stop for breath when walking at own pace
4	Stops for breath after walking about 100 m or after a few minutes on the level
5	Too breathless to leave the house, or breathless when dressing or undressing. Breathless at rest

Source: Blackler *et al.*, 2007.

Many primary care organisations are undertaking projects supporting initiatives that offer smokers with 20 pack years (a pack year is smoking 20 cigarettes a day for 1 year) over the age of 35 the opportunity to attend their local GP practice for COPD screening using spirometry to detect early airflow obstruction before symptoms become apparent. Smoking cessation, if successful at this stage, could mean the patient does not develop the symptomatic disease. If, however, patients are already experiencing some degree of breathlessness, then it is important to assess dyspnoea objectively. The MRC dyspnoea scale can be used to do this and should be recorded yearly as part of an annual review (see Table 12.2).

Addressing social and psychological needs as well as symptom control is vital, as the progression of the disease will result in increasing shortness of breath when washing or getting dressed for example, and even minimal exertion will become more and more difficult. These limitations imposed by the symptoms of COPD can impact on a person's social roles, relationships and self-perception.

Living with COPD can have an effect on the person's psychological well-being, and can result in people experiencing anxiety and depression (Blackler *et al.*, 2007). This can affect their ability to manage their condition optimally as well as their quality of life. Despite the high incidence of psychological effects, it has been reported that 82% of patients with COPD received no treatment for depression (Elkington *et al.*, 2005). The Quality Outcomes Framework (QoF) for GP performance has a process for screening patients with known coronary heart disease (CHD) and/or diabetes for depression, but to date this has not been extended to include routine depression screening for patient with COPD (see section 'Breathlessness (Dyspnoea)' in Chapter 9).

Nurses need to be sensitive to the impact that a COPD diagnosis could have on the individual. While some may adapt well, others find the news devastating. Dudley *et al.* (1980) stated that the expression of emotion is closely linked with dyspnoea and that repressing emotions could limit the experience of breathlessness. This could lead to some people avoiding expressing their emotions as a way of managing their breathlessness which could predispose them to anxiety and depression. It is important then that a clinician making a diagnosis of COPD has the time to explain everything to the patient, in a way that is understandable and supportive, with an opportunity for review within the next few weeks in order to answer any questions and address emerging issues and to offer support.

Anxiety often presents with depression but with effective treatment for the depression the anxiety usually resolves. Giving information is a useful strategy to allay anxiety, as are effective communication and appropriate reassurance. The Patient Health Questionnaire 9 (PHQ 9) score is often used in general practice to assess depression, and the HAD (Hospital Anxiety and Depression Scale) questionnaire can also be used; both are effective tools and can be helpful in identifying patients who may benefit from further assessment of their mental health status (more information about assessment tools is available in Chapter 5).

Aims of management

GOLD (2009) lists the aims of COPD management to be as follows:

- Relieve symptoms.
- Prevent disease progression.
- Improve exercise tolerance.
- Improve health status.
- Prevent and treat complications.
- Prevent and treat exacerbations.
- Reduce mortality.
- Prevent and minimize side effects from treatment.

This can be achieved by structured assessment and monitoring of the disease process, reducing risk factors, such as supporting smoking cessation, the management of stable COPD and early intervention during exacerbations. Self-management plans (SMPs) have also been found to be helpful as the patient has clear instructions as to the indications to initiate oral steroids and antibiotics. The National Institute for Health and Clinical Excellence (NICE) guidance for the management of COPD details a multidisciplinary approach to how this can be implemented in practice.

Long-term oxygen therapy (LTOT)

LTOT improves breathlessness and survival in patients with severe COPD who are in chronic respiratory failure; it needs to be administered for at least 15 hours per day. The most cost-effective way of administering oxygen over long periods is by oxygen concentrator. This allows a certain level of mobility around the home but ambulatory oxygen may be needed as well so the patient can still maintain some kind of social activity outside the home. LTOT aims to increase the concentration of oxygen in inhaled air to around 30%; this provides the best tissue oxygenation without increasing the arterial carbon dioxide and worsening the respiratory failure. LTOT must be provided following locally and nationally agreed guidelines, which entails a full assessment by a nurse specially trained in LTOT assessment and management. Oxygen is a specialist drug that can have adverse effects, so accurate assessment of blood gases needs to be undertaken prior to initiation of LTOT. Oxygen is then provided via a contracting company who are responsible for delivery and maintenance of all equipment and delivery of oxygen. A home oxygen order form (HOOF) has to be completed which is used to provide information to the contractor; patient consent is therefore required so that information can be shared across all parties involved and a supply maintenance agreement established.

Smoking cessation

Cigarette smoking is addictive due to the nicotine content; however, nicotine itself does not cause major health problems, it is the accompanying pollutants that account for most of the harm caused by cigarettes. Cigarettes contain at least 4,000 substances, of which about 400 are toxic. Smoking destroys the tiny hairs (cilia), which line the upper airways and protect against infection. Normally, there is a thin layer of mucus and thousands of these cilia lining the airways. The mucus traps fine particles of dirt and pollution, and the cilia move together like a wave to push the dirt-filled mucus out of the lungs. The more cigarette smoke inhaled the more difficult this becomes, due to damage to the cilia, and increase in mucus production due to the constant irritation of the delicate lining of the airways.

Smoking is the single greatest preventable cause of disease, hospital admissions, GP consultations and death in the United Kingdom (Secretary of State for Health, 1998). One of the major barriers to smoking cessation practice is that many health professionals do not have the skills and knowledge to intervene, or fail to intervene routinely. It should be routine to ascertain smoking status, delivering brief advice and offering further help to smokers interested in stopping. This should now be an established part of the GP consultation as it is strongly supported by the Quality and Outcomes Framework (NHS Employers and British Medical Association, 2008). Cessation of smoking is the only effective long-term intervention in the management of COPD.

Within the United Kingdom, there is considerable variation in smoking prevalence according to gender, age and socio-economic status and ethnicity, with numbers highest among young people (National Centre for Social Research, 2004), but declining (Wardle, 2010). Smoking behaviour is strongly related to socio-economic status; smoking cessation rates also have a strong inverse relation with deprivation. Cessation rates have doubled in the most advantaged groups, but are lower in the most disadvantaged sectors of society (Jarvis 1997; Bauld *et al.*, 2009). Twigg *et al.* (2004) state that in the United Kingdom, cigarette smoking is responsible for more than 2,000 deaths per week. This means, on an individual level, that long-term regular smokers can expect to lose an average of 10 years' life expectancy (Doll *et al.*, 2004). The main causes of death attributable to cigarette smoking are cancers, diseases of the heart and circulation and lung disease.

Nicotine addiction is a recognised disease (WHO, 1992). Nicotine vaporises from smoke particles in the lungs and is rapidly absorbed into the blood and carried to the brain. The nicotine reaches the brain in a 'bolus' with great speed – creating a 'hit' that underpins the addictiveness (Kaul, 2007). About 30% of smokers actively try to stop each year, with an overall quit rate of just 3%; however, many smokers require multiple attempts before they are successful (Ginsberg, 2005). Cessation of smoking at any age has beneficial effects on the lung function of patients with chronic lung disease (Fletcher and Peto, 1997). This can be seen in Figure 12.2 (Kaul, 2007).

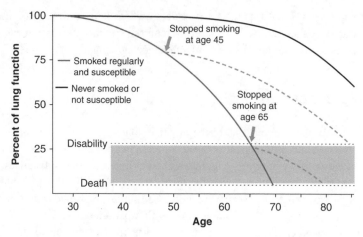

Figure 12.2   Relationship between lung function and smoking status (Kaul, 1997).

All health professionals should encourage smokers to stop at every available opportunity, offering advice in an encouraging, non-judgmental and empathetic manner. Patients with COPD who still smoke need to understand that it may take several attempts to achieve long-term success. If they are not motivated to stop then it is important to explore their reasons for this and encourage them to consider stopping in the future. Often cigarettes are regarded as a 'comforting friend' rather than something harmful, so it is important to explore this thinking and try to explain that it is only pleasurable because it relieves withdrawal symptoms. Counselling is the cornerstone of smoking cessation management, and this can be delivered on the following three different levels depending on the level of both interest and skill of the clinician and the individual needs of the patient:

1. *Brief intervention:* Ask about smoking status and give brief advice. This should be an integral part of most consultations.
2. *Intermediate intervention:* Give in-depth advice, assist in stopping smoking and arrange follow-up appointments.
3. *Specialist services:* Provide expert advice and ongoing support in both quitting and preventing relapse.

The five 'As' of smoking cessation as suggested by The British Thoracic Society are also useful for nurses in providing smoking cessation support:

1. ASK all patients about their smoking history.
2. ADVISE all patients to quit using personalised but non-judgemental language.
3. ASSESS motivation to quit.
4. ASSIST motivated smokers by giving further advice and prescribing nicotine replacement therapy (NRT) or medication.
5. ARRANGE support follow-up with the local smoking cessation service.

NRT is the most common drug treatment to help smoking cessation and increases the chances of quitting by about 1.7-fold. It works by supplying nicotine without the toxic components of cigarette smoke. Since there is no clear evidence that any formulation is more effective than another, the best approach is to follow individual patients' preferences. Heavy smokers may require a combination of products in order to succeed. NRT is available as chewing gum, transdermal patches, an inhalator, a nasal spray, sublingual tablets and lozenges.

Bupropion (Zyban) was initially developed as an antidepressant. It works directly on the addiction pathways in the brain and helps to prevent cravings for nicotine rather than replacing one nicotine delivery system with another. It can be very effective, but it is not a replacement for willpower.

The current NICE guidance (2002) for prescribing NRT and bupropion states that NRT or bupropion should only be prescribed when a patient wants to quit and commits to a target stop date. There is currently insufficient evidence to recommend the use of NRT and bupropion together; choice of replacement therapy depends on the following factors:

- Likely compliance
- Availability of counselling and support
- Previous use of cessation therapies
- Contraindications and adverse effects of the therapies
- Patient preferences

Initial prescriptions should last only 2 weeks past the stop date; this will be 2 weeks of therapy for NRT and 3–4 weeks for bupropion. A second prescription should be issued only if a smoker remains committed to stopping smoking. If the quit attempt fails, smoking cessation therapy should not normally be prescribed for a further 6 months. Varenicline (Champix) has also been approved and works by binding to the same receptor sites as nicotine in order to reduce withdrawal symptoms. It should only be used as part of a programme of behavioural support (NICE, 2002).

Pulmonary rehabilitation

Pulmonary rehabilitation aims to improve the knowledge of their condition of patients with COPD, as well as their ability to live with their LTC, by improving their exercise ability, quality of life (QOL) and functional independence. Pulmonary rehabilitation is a multidisciplinary continuum of services directed to persons with pulmonary disease and their families, usually by an interdisciplinary team of specialists, with the goal of achieving and maintaining the individual's maximum level of independence and functioning in the community (Cole and Fishman, 1994).

Breathlessness on exertion and the fear, anxiety and panic this can invoke often result in patients becoming increasingly inactive. This in turn results in muscle deconditioning and increasing disability and can often lead to social isolation as even short walks can result in leg tiredness. Pulmonary rehabilitation has been shown to reduce breathlessness, improve functional ability and improve health-related quality of life.

Pulmonary rehabilitation may also lead to a reduction in the use of health service consultations, hospital admissions and inpatient stays. Ideally, it should be available to all patients who feel they are functionally disabled by COPD, the cornerstone being an individually prescribed exercise and endurance programme. However, this is very often not the case, either because the patient does not have access to the service or health professionals do not refer into the service appropriately. Exercise for specific muscle groups can improve functional ability and may be particularly useful for patients with severe disease. Education about the disease and its management, nutrition, relaxation and coping strategies, and the management of exacerbations should also be included in the programme. Where possible carers should also be encouraged to participate in the programme, as this is likely to improve long-term benefit by supporting long-term lifestyle changes.

Improved exercise performance and reduced breathlessness associated with exercise can be maintained for up to 12 months, so it may be helpful for some patients to attend on more than one occasion. However, there is very little evidence that this improves disease progression (as judged by decline in FEV1) or long-term survival. Therefore, the overall aim is to improve QOL (Lacasse *et al.*, 2006) and reduce dependence rather than to extend life, and as such it is of huge benefit and should be encouraged and supported by health care professionals.

Diet and nutrition

Patients with respiratory disease and especially those with COPD should be weighed regularly; low body mass index (BMI) is linked to mortality, as there is a loss of lean tissue including respiratory muscle. Unintentional weight loss due to an exacerbation needs to be corrected and a healthy weight restored and maintained. A low BMI and loss of lean muscle is common, especially when emphysema is the predominant pathological problem. Breathlessness can make the process of eating tiring, so underweight patients need to be encouraged to fortify food with extra calories such as butter, cream and sugar, eat small frequent meals and snacks, and sweets and nourishing drinks. This needs to be linked to increased exercise in order to build muscle bulk which is an integral part of pulmonary rehabilitation. Obese patients need support to lose weight as this too will impede good respiratory function.

Management of COPD – NICE guidelines

Following NICE guidelines ensures management is patient centred and multidisciplinary to ensure best outcomes (see Figure 12.3). Most Primary Care Trusts now have specialist COPD teams with open referral criteria; this has greatly improved the QOL as well as end stage care for many patients with severe COPD.

Pharmacological management

Bronchodilators are the most important treatment for symptom relief in COPD; they are discussed in more detail under section 'Asthma'. They are given 'as needed' and work by decreasing bronchomotor tone and decreasing lung hyperinflation. The short-acting beta$_2$

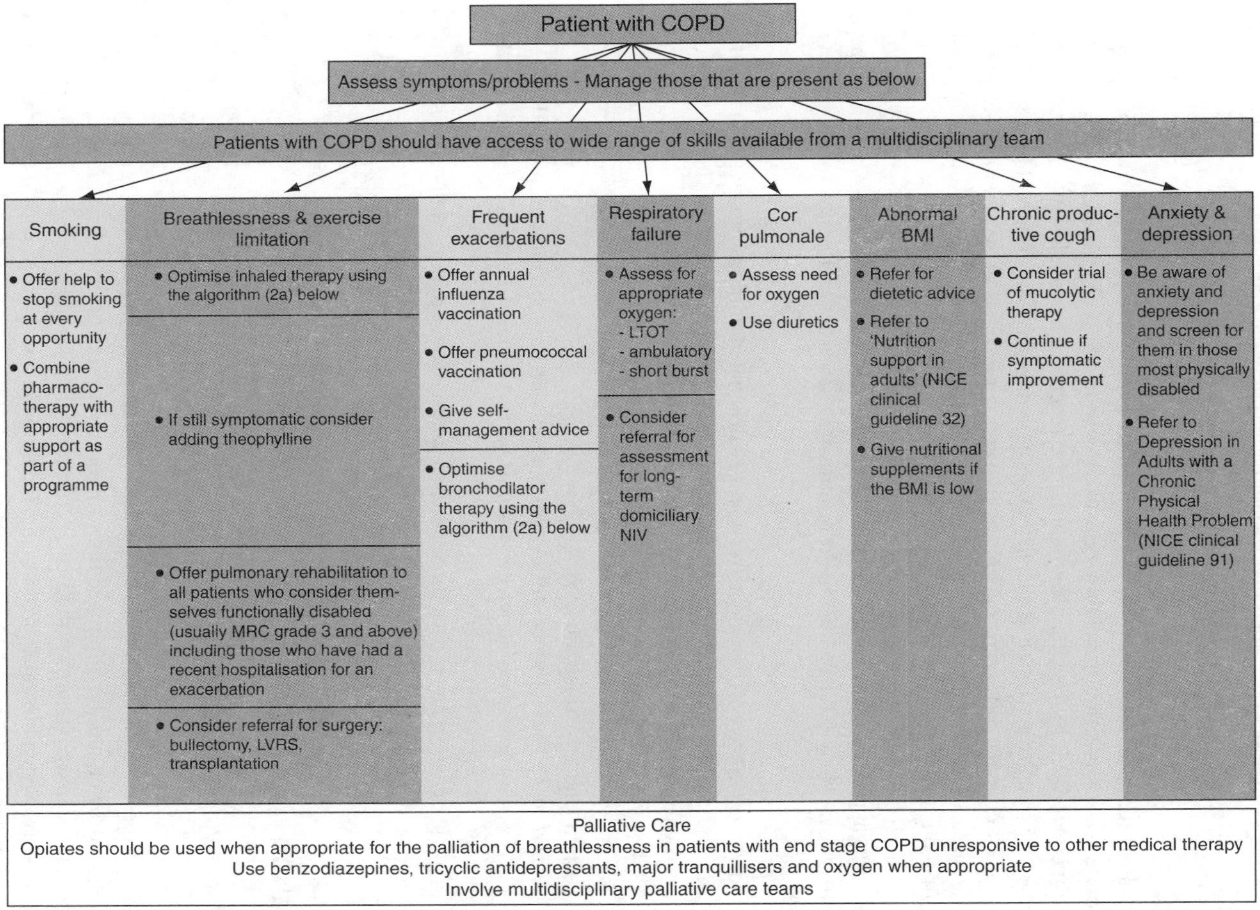

Patient with COPD

Assess symptoms/problems - Manage those that are present as below

Patients with COPD should have access to wide range of skills available from a multidisciplinary team

Smoking	Breathlessness & exercise limitation	Frequent exacerbations	Respiratory failure	Cor pulmonale	Abnormal BMI	Chronic productive cough	Anxiety & depression
• Offer help to stop smoking at every opportunity • Combine pharmaco-therapy with appropriate support as part of a programme	• Optimise inhaled therapy using the algorithm (2a) below • If still symptomatic consider adding theophylline • Offer pulmonary rehabilitation to all patients who consider themselves functionally disabled (usually MRC grade 3 and above) including those who have had a recent hospitalisation for an exacerbation • Consider referral for surgery: bullectomy, LVRS, transplantation	• Offer annual influenza vaccination • Offer pneumococcal vaccination • Give self-management advice • Optimise bronchodilator therapy using the algorithm (2a) below	• Assess for appropriate oxygen: - LTOT - ambulatory - short burst • Consider referral for assessment for long-term domiciliary NIV	• Assess need for oxygen • Use diuretics	• Refer for dietetic advice • Refer to 'Nutrition support in adults' (NICE clinical guideline 32) • Give nutritional supplements if the BMI is low	• Consider trial of mucolytic therapy • Continue if symptomatic improvement	• Be aware of anxiety and depression and screen for them in those most physically disabled • Refer to Depression in Adults with a Chronic Physical Health Problem (NICE clinical guideline 91)

Palliative Care

Opiates should be used when appropriate for the palliation of breathlessness in patients with end stage COPD unresponsive to other medical therapy
Use benzodiazepines, tricyclic antidepressants, major tranquillisers and oxygen when appropriate
Involve multidisciplinary palliative care teams

Figure 12.3 NICE guidance COPD (2010, updated from 2004).

agonists (SABA) – salbutamol and terbutaline – are prescribed to relieve intermittent breathlessness; the short-acting anticholinergic ipratropium can also be used, especially if mucus production is an issue. Both have a rapid onset of action, although ipratropium takes slightly longer; they can be given together and may have an additive effect in some patients. Regular treatment with long-acting beta agonists (LABA), such as salmeterol and formoterol can be effective when symptoms become more persistent. The duration of action is 12 hours so they can be taken twice daily.

Ipratropium bromide (Atrovent) can be used for both asthma and COPD. Tiotropium bromide is a long-acting anticholinergic used only in the management of COPD. Anticholinergics work by blocking the cholinergic receptors in the airways. This leads to reduced cholinergic activation of the airway smooth muscle and subsequent bronchodilation (Blackler *et al.*, 2007). They are also believed to reduce mucus secretion. Tiotropium can be used in combination with a LABA combination in order to maximize relief of breathlessness.

It is also vital that the patient be given a device that can be used effectively. Technique and appropriateness of device should be checked regularly, to ensure maximum effectiveness. Many patients benefit from utilising spacer devices which increases lung deposition.

Inhaled corticosteroids: Regular treatment with inhaled corticosteroids (ICS) is only appropriate for patients with symptomatic improvement and a documented spirometric response to ICS or an FEV1 <50% and repeated exacerbations.

Oral steroids: They are used for acute exacerbations with a locally recommended antibiotic. However, because of the potential side effects the NICE guidelines do not recommend their regular use.

Theophyllines: They produce only small amounts of bronchodilation in COPD; they may increase exercise tolerance but have a narrow therapeutic range, so blood levels need to be monitored regularly.

Mucolytic agents: They are useful in patients with viscous sputum, but overall benefits are small and they should be discontinued if there is no benefit after 1–2 months.

Asthma

Pathophysiology and diagnosis

When a person with asthma comes into contact with something that irritates their airways (asthma trigger), the muscles around the walls of the airways tighten so that the airways become narrower and the lining becomes inflamed and starts to swell. Sometimes sticky mucus builds up which narrows the airways further. All these reactions cause the airways to become narrower and irritated, making it difficult to breathe. Unfortunately, there are still deaths from acute asthma attacks with a reported 1,400 per year. Nine out of ten of these deaths are preventable; however, there are a few cases that are so resistant to treatment that it is a near-insoluble situation. Because of this it is important that the clinician is willing

Table 12.3 Clinical features in adults that influence the probability that episodic respiratory symptoms are due to asthma.

Features in adults that increase the probability of the diagnosis being asthma

More than one of the following symptoms: wheeze, breathlessness, chest tightness and cough, particularly if:

Symptoms worse at night and in early morning

Symptoms in response to exercise, allergen exposure and cold air

Symptoms after taking aspirin or beta-blockers

History of atopic disorder

Family history of asthma and/or atopic disorder

Widespread wheeze heard on auscultation of the chest

Otherwise unexplained low FEV1 or PEF (historical or serial readings)

Otherwise unexplained peripheral blood eosinophilia

Features that lower the probability of the diagnosis being asthma

Prominent dizziness, light-headedness, peripheral tingling

Chronic productive cough in the absence of wheeze or breathlessness

Repeatedly normal physical examination of chest when symptomatic

Voice disturbance

Symptoms when colds only

Significant smoking history (i.e. > 20 pack years)

Cardiac disease

Normal PEF or spirometry when symptomatic

Normal spirometry when not symptomatic does not exclude the diagnosis of asthma. Repeated measurements of lung function are often more informative than a single assessment

---

Source: BTS/SIGN, 2008.

to spend time establishing what triggers each individual person with asthma may have and then discussing how these can be avoided if possible, as well as offering medication. The BTS and Scottish Intercollegiate Guidelines Network (SIGN) guidelines (2008) state that the diagnosis of asthma is a clinical one. There is no standardised definition of the type, severity or frequency of symptoms, nor of the findings on investigation. The absence of a gold standard definition means that it is difficult to make clear clinical evidence-based recommendations on how to diagnose asthma. There are clinical features in a person more likely with asthma and these are listed in Table 12.3.

Inflammation of the airways is central to the pathogenesis of asthma. Airway inflammation can be defined as the presence of activated inflammation cells, and is characterised by bronchial hyper-responsiveness, which is generally defined as an abnormal response of the airways to a provoking stimulus. The most common stimuli are cigarette smoke and allergens, such as pollen, house dust mite and animal dander. In addition cold air, exercise and viral infection can also affect asthma symptoms. In the person without asthma, antibodies are produced which attach themselves to antigens and render them harmless. However, in the asthmatic patient the allergen triggers an abnormally vigorous immune response which causes tissue damage. Under normal circumstances immunoglobulin E (IgE) attaches onto the allergen and prevents any reaction. However, in asthma the IgE binds to mast cells causing a process known as degranulation resulting in the release of histamine, prostaglandins, and leukotrienes from within the cell, causing broncho-constriction and hyper-secretion of mucus (Marieb, 1991).

The inflammation associated with asthma is chronic, and present even when the patient feels well, but responds well to ICS, and short-acting inhaled beta$_2$ agonists, such as salbutamol, to give symptomatic relief. The main difference between asthma and COPD is that asthma symptoms are variable and intermittent, whereas with COPD there is very little symptom variation from day-to-day.

Living with asthma

Asthma is a common disease that affects about 5 million people in the United Kingdom (British Lung Foundation, 2008), often starting in childhood, but it can begin at any age, even in people in their 70s or 80s. Asthma cannot as yet be cured but in the majority of cases it can be controlled. There is a small group of patients, known as brittle asthmatics, for which control is not always the case, often this is described as 'living on a knife edge'. Patients were invited to share their experiences in an Asthma UK survey in 2004, in the report *Living on a Knife Edge* (Asthma UK, 2004): Catherine Tunnicliffe of Derby states that,

> 'On a bad day I feel like I'm drowning and I can't reach the surface of the water and I am going to burst, yet a tiny, tiny bit of air keeps me alive. It's very scary – I feel like I'm living with a time bomb and if I have a bad attack I say to myself: "Is this the one that will kill me?' (Asthma UK, 2004: 8).

Because the range of severity of asthma is so wide, it is difficult to imagine living with that degree of fear day-to-day. This group of patients must have access to, and be managed by, a team of respiratory specialists who have access to the latest evidence and medication. The quote above gives some idea as to what it must be like to live with asthma and how much it can interfere with the activities of daily living (ADL) and/or QOL – even with mild asthma there is some degree of night waking which will affect QOL the next day. It is difficult to hold down a job when sleep is disturbed regularly and the person feels tight chested and wheezy.

Aims of management

The BTS/SIGN (2008) guidelines state that the aim of all asthma management is control of the disease (see Figure 12.4). Control of asthma is defined as:

- No daytime symptoms
- No night-time awakening due to asthma
- No need for rescue medication
- No exacerbations
- No limitation on activity including exercise
- Normal lung function with minimal side effects

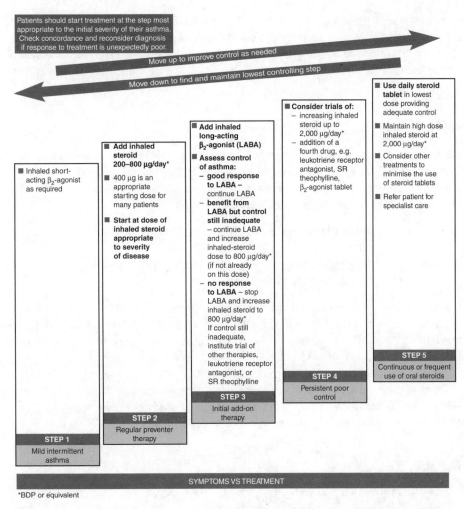

Figure 12.4   The British guidelines on asthma management in adults (BTS/SIGN, 2009).
(Used with permission of the British Thoracic Society.)

Since asthma is a variable condition, the patient may not be symptomatic at the time
of the review, and therefore, it is often helpful as part of the clinic review if the patient is
able to provide peak flow data. The normal diurnal variation of peak flow is around 5%;
if there is a variation of 15% or more then this will indicate that there is the potential to
improve control.

Pharmacological management

The management of asthma is achieved predominantly by the use of medications to reverse the narrowing and inflammation of the airways. These medications can be inhaled,
taken orally or intravenously, depending on the severity of the asthma and control required, and can be divided into two main groups: drugs which relieve symptoms as they

occur, known as 'relievers', and drugs which prevent worsening or progression of the asthma process, known as 'preventers'. The BTS/SIGN guidelines recommend a stepwise approach to asthma management which enables the lowest dose and least medication possible to control the asthma, gradually increasing this as required to ensure appropriate management.

Relievers (bronchodilators)

Relievers in the community setting are administered with inhalers. This can be via a metered dose inhaler (MDI) or a dry-powder device. Relievers have a direct bronchodilator effect and relieve the symptoms of asthma; they are the mainstay drugs for the acute relief of asthma symptoms, and work in the following two ways:

1. On the sympathetic nervous system by stimulating beta$_2$ receptors, causing bronchial smooth muscle to relax
2. On the parasympathetic nervous system by blocking the cholinergic receptors and therefore preventing bronchoconstriction

SABA, such as salbutamol and terbutaline, relax bronchial smooth muscle by stimulating beta$_2$ receptors, primarily in the airways, skeletal muscle and, to a lesser extent, the heart; this is especially important at higher doses as patients may experience the associated side effects, such as palpitation and headache, tachycardia and tremor.

SABA treat the immediate symptoms of asthma, and can help to prevent exercise-induced asthma when used before exercise. They have no anti-inflammatory properties. They should be taken on an as-needed or on-demand basis, rather than regularly. Salbutamol and terbutaline will work within 5–15 minutes of inhalation.

Delivery

- Inhalation is the preferred method of delivery, via a pressurised MDI, breath-activated inhaler or dry-powder inhaler (DPI).
- The onset of action is faster with inhalation and there are fewer adverse effects compared to other delivery methods.
- Delivery via an inhaler plus a spacer is as effective as nebulised therapy, with less time to deliver a dose and reduced equipment maintenance.
- The patient should be given specific instructions about the dosage to be used for minor and acute exacerbations.

As exemplified in Box 12.1, there are several different devices on the market; the important issue is that the patient is happy with the device, how it looks and feels, and the ease with which it can be used. The choice of device for an individual should be based upon patient factors, for example age, strength, vision, cognition, inspiratory flow rate and the patient's personal preference. Manual dexterity should be assessed as some devices require a higher level than others. Spacer devices allow inhaled medication via an MDI to be delivered to most patients, and they can even be given via a third person in this way. Technique is of utmost importance, and this should be checked at each review to ensure correct usage. Inhalers should be prescribed only after patients have received training in the use of the device and have demonstrated satisfactory techniques, since this will improve lung deposition thus reducing the amount of medication required.

Box 12.1   Methods of Delivering Salbutamol.

Metered-dose inhalers (MDI): Ventolin, Airomir, Salamol
Breath actuated inhalers: (BAI) Airomir autohaler, Asmasal clickhaler, Easyhaler salbutamol, Pulvinal salbutamol, Salamol easi-breathe, Salbulin novoliser, Ventolin accuhaler

---

Preventers

Preventer agents have anti-inflammatory properties and are generally taken regularly via an inhaler device; inhaled corticosteroids help reduce symptoms and exacerbations by reducing the inflammation in the airways (see Box 12.2). They remain the most effective agents for gaining and maintaining control of asthma in adults and in children with persistent asthma.

Box 12.2   Preventer medication.

Inhaled corticosteroids

Beclomethasone dipropionate-HFA (Qvar, Asmabec, Beclazone, Becodisks, Clenil) Budesonide (Pulmicort, Novolizert) (brown inhaler); Fluticasone propionate (Flixotide) (orange inhaler); Ciclesonide (Alvesco) (rust-coloured inhaler), Mometasone (*Asmanex*)

Combination medications

Fluticasone and salmeterol (Seretide) (purple inhaler); budesonide and eformoterol (Symbicort) (red and white inhaler) beclomethasone and eformoterol (Fostaire)

The combination of LABA and ICS should be considered when symptoms or suboptimal lung function persist on ICS alone, or it is desirable to reduce the current dose of ICS while maintaining optimal asthma control. The use of combination ICS–LABA inhalers is well tolerated and there is no evidence that the adverse effects of either drug are potentiated by simultaneous delivery (see Box 12.2).

Fluticasone and salmeterol (Seretide) are delivered by MDIs. The Accuhaler is suitable for patients who have good inspiratory flows but coordination difficulties when using MDIs.

Budesonide and eformoterol (Symbicort) is a dry powder delivered via a turbohaler device. This combination inhaler is now licensed for rescue as well as maintenance therapy, and can be used routinely twice daily to maintain control and as required for rescue. This is because eformoterol is both a quick-acting and a long-acting bronchodilator, giving relief from symptoms in 1–2 minutes and lasting for up to 12 hours.

A stepwise approach aims to abolish symptoms as soon as possible (see Figure 12.4). Before initiating a new drug therapy practitioners should check compliance with existing therapies. The successful management in adults involves the practitioner working in partnership with the patient. The individual needs to develop an increasing awareness of the factors in the environment, such as pollen, dust and house dust mite which may trigger attacks, as well as the psychological influences and physiological reasons for their condition.

Self-management plans

The mainstay of a successful SMP is the involvement with the patient in the management of their asthma, based on either symptoms or peak flow readings. The plan will focus on the early recognition of unstable or deteriorating asthma. Written instruction of when to increase therapy must be clearly stated; it is also important that the patient is aware of the need to maintain therapy even when feeling well, in order to reduce acute exacerbation. The SMP should be developed in partnership with the patient and reflect individual cultural needs. Most patients with appropriate education and understanding of their condition will be able to follow an SMP to an individualised level.

Conclusion

This chapter has focussed in particular on the long-term conditions of COPD and asthma. Both are potentially debilitating conditions which require self-management and partnership between the patient and the clinician.

COPD is a progressive disease directly linked to cigarette smoking; the only way prevalence can be reduced is to reduce smoking rates, especially in the 'at risk patient'. The national clinical strategy for services for COPD in England (soon to be published) by the Department of Health (2010) states that everyone diagnosed with COPD should receive equitable, responsive, high-quality health and social care services, seeing the right person in the right place at the right time. This vision is still some way off, but the strategy, which is a 10-year plan, has highlighted the need for a joined up care service that meets the needs of this previously largely poorly managed group of people living with a frightening and debilitating long-term condition.

Asthma is a common chronic condition, the symptoms of which vary from person to person depending on the triggers and severity of acute episodes. Often, people experience asthma symptoms differently, some adapting their lifestyle to accommodate the impact that the disease has on their day-to-day activities. Ideally, with an individualised approach, education, support and understanding of their management patients should be in control of their asthma rather than asthma being in control of them.

References

Arne, M., Emtner, M., Janson, S. & Wilde-Larsson, B. (2007) COPD patients' perspectives at time of diagnosis, *Primary Care Respiratory Journal*, 16(4), pp. 215–221.

Asthma UK (2004) *Living on a Knife Edge. A Powerful and Moving Account of Living with Serious Symptoms of Asthma*. Asthma UK, London.

Bauld, L., Bell, K., McCullough, L., Richardson, L. & Greaves, L. (2009) The effectiveness of NHS smoking cessation services: a systematic review. *Journal of Public Health*. Available at: http://dx.doi.org/10.1093/pubmed/fdp074 (accessed 7 June 2010).

Bellamy, D. & Booker, R. (2008) *Chronic Obstructive Pulmonary Disease in Primary Care All You Need to Know to Manage COPD in Your Practice* (3rd edn). Class Publishing, London.

Blackler, L., Jones, C. & Mooney, C. (eds) (2007) *Managing Chronic Obstructive Pulmonary Disease*. Wiley, Chichester.

British Lung Foundation (2008) *Facts About Respiratory Disease*. Available at: www.lunguk.org (accessed 7 June 2010).

British Thoracic Society (BTS) (2006) *Burden of Lung Disease: A Statistics Report* (2nd edn), The British Thoracic Society, London.

British Thoracic Society (BTS) and Scottish Intercollegiate Guidelines Network (SIGN) (2008) *British Guidelines on the Management of Asthma. A National Clinical Guideline 101* (revised edn 2009). BTS/SIGN, Edinburgh.

British Thoracic Society (BTS) and Scottish Intercollegiate Guidelines Network (SIGN) (2009) BTS/SIGN Guideline on the Management of Asthma, 2009 (http://www.brit-thoracic.org.uk/clinical-information/asthma/asthma-guidelines.aspx).

Brownrigg, E. (2007) The Patients' perspective. In: *The Management of COPD in Primary and Secondary Care* (ed D. Lynes). M&K, Liverpool.

Cole, T. M. & Fishman, A. P. (1994) Workshop on pulmonary rehabilitation research: a commentary, *American Journal of Physical Medicine and Rehabilitation*, 73, pp. 132–133.

Department of Health (2010) *Consultation on a Strategy for Services for Chronic Obstructive Pulmonary Disease (COPD) in England – consultation document*, Department of Health, London. Available at: http://www.dh.gov.uk/en/Publicationsandstatistics/Publications/PublicationsPolicyAndGuidance/DH_116716 (final version not available yet) (accessed 7 June 2010).

Doll, R., Petro, R., Boreham, J. & Sutherland, I. (2004) Mortality in relation to smoking: 50 years' observations on male British doctors, *British Medical Journal*, 328, pp. 1519–1528.

Dudley, D. L., Glaser, E. M., Jorgensen, B. M. & Logan, D. L. (1980) Psychosocial concomitants to rehabilitation in chronic pulmonary disease: part 1: psychosocial and psychological considerations, *Chest*, 77(3), pp. 413–420.

Elkington, H., White, P., Addington-Hall, J., *et al*. (2005) The healthcare needs of chronic obstructive pulmonary disease patients in the last year of life, *Palliative Medicine*, 19(6), pp. 485–491.

Fletcher, C. & Peto, R. (1997) The natural history of chronic airflow obstruction. *British Medical Journal*, 1, pp. 1645–1648.

Ginsberg, D. (2005) *Duloxetine for Smoking Cessation. Psychopharmacology Reviews*. Available at: www.primarypsychiatry.com (accessed 7 June 2010).

Global Initiative for Chronic Obstructive Lung Diseases (GOLD) (2009) *Global Strategy for the Diagnosis Management, and Prevention of Chronic Obstructive Pulmonary Disease*. GOLD. Available at: www.goldcopd.com (accessed 7 June 2010).

Jarvis, M. J. (1997) Patterns and predictors of smoking cessation in the general population. In: *The Tobacco Epidemics* (eds C. T. Bolliger & K. O. Fragerstrom). Karger, Basel.

Jones, R. (2007) *Pocket Science COPD-Evidence and Experience*. CSF Medical Communications, Gloucestershire.

Kaul, S. (2007) Smoking cessation. In: *Managing Chronic Obstructive Pulmonary Disease* (eds L. Blackler, C. Jones & C. Mooney). Wiley, Chichester, pp. 65–83.

Lacasse, Y., Goldstein, R., Lassersin, T. & Martin, S. (2006) Pulmonary rehabilitation for chronic obstructive pulmonary disease. *Cochrane Database of Systematic Reviews*, (4), http://onlinelibrary.wiley.com/o/cochrane/clsysrev/articles/CD003793 (accessed 7 June 2010).

Marieb, E. N. (1991) *Essentials of Human Anatomy and Physiology* (3rd edn). The Benjamin/Cummings Publishing Co Ltd, Wokingham.

National Centre for Social Research (2004) *Health Survey for England 2003: Latest Trends*. National Centre for Social Research, London.

National Institute for Health and Clinical Excellence (NICE) (2002) *Guidance on the Use of Nicotine Replacement Therapy (NRT) and Bupropion for Smoking Cessation*. NICE, London. Available at: www.nice.org.uk (accessed 7 June 2010).

National Institute for Health and Clinical Excellence (NICE) (2010) *Chronic Obstructive Pulmonary Disease (update)*. NICE, London.

NHS Employers & British Medical Association (2008) *Quality and Outcomes Framework Guidance for GMS Contract 2008/09 Delivering Investment in General Practice*. NHS, London. Available at: http://www.wmrlmc.co.uk/gms2/qof/qof_guidance_2008-09.pdf (accessed 7 June 2010).

Secretary of State for Health and Secretaries of State for Scotland, Wales and Northern Ireland (1998) *Smoking Kills: A White Paper on Tobacco*. The Stationery Office, London.

The American Thoracic Society (1999) Dyspnoea. Mechanisms, assessment and management: a consensus statement, *American Journal of Respiratory and Critical Care Medicine*, 159(1), pp. 321–340.

The Respiratory Alliance (2003) *Bridging the Gap. Commissioning and Delivering High Quality Integrated Respiratory Healthcare*. Direct Publishing Solutions Limited Maiden head.

Twigg, L., Moon, G. & Walker, S. (2004) *The Smoking Epidemic in England*. Health Development Agency, London.

Wardle, H. (2010) Smoking, drinking and drug use. In: *Smoking, Drinking and Drug use Among Young People in England in 2009* (eds E. Fuller & M. Sanchez). NHS Information Centre, London. Available at: www.ic.nhs.uk (accessed 7 June 2010).

WHO (1992) *World Health Report 1992, Reducing Risks, Promoting Healthy Life*. WHO, Geneva. Available at: http://www.who.int/whr/2002/en/index.html (accessed 7 June 2010).

Chapter 13

Management of diabetes

Lynne Jerreat
Queen Elizabeth Hospital, London, UK
University of Greenwich, London, UK

Introduction

Diabetes mellitus is a disease defined by hyperglycaemia, caused by a total or partial lack of insulin, with or without insulin resistance. The most common types of the disease in the United Kingdom are type 1 diabetes, type 2 diabetes, secondary diabetes and gestational diabetes; 90% of people with diabetes have type 2 diabetes. This chapter covers type 1 and type 2 diabetes and illustrates the importance of empowering people with diabetes to manage their disease; accurate up-to-date knowledge is essential to enable patients to set goals and make choices. Quotes from patients are used to illustrate how diabetes may affect the individual with the condition; the majority of these are from patients who I have had the privilege of knowing (unless otherwise stated) and are therefore not referenced.

It is predicted that by 2010, 220 million people will have the disease worldwide (McCarty and Zimmet, 1994) and it is amongst the five leading causes of death in most countries (International Diabetes Federation, 2001) despite diabetes being frequently under-reported on death certificates (IDF, 2001). In 2007, the Centers for Disease Control and Prevention in the USA classified the increase in diabetes as an epidemic, unusual for a non-infectious disease (Higgins, 2008). Figures from the Yorkshire and Humber Public Health Observatory (2008) reveal that 11.6% of deaths among 20 to 79 year olds in England can be attributed to diabetes.

Primary Care Trusts (PCTs) with the highest numbers of diabetes related deaths are in areas with a high proportion of the population over age 40 and where a large number of these are of Asian and Black origin, who are more at risk of developing diabetes. They also have high levels of deprivation compared to PCTs with the lowest proportion of deaths (Diabetes UK, 2009).

Definition of diabetes

Type 1 diabetes

Type 1 diabetes is characterised by absolute insulin deficiency, abrupt onset of symptoms, proneness to ketosis and dependency on injected insulin to stay alive. Type 1 diabetes is

Long-Term Conditions: Nursing Care and Management, First Edition. Edited by Liz Meerabeau and Kerri Wright.
© 2011 Blackwell Publishing Ltd. Published 2011 by Blackwell Publishing Ltd.

an autoimmune disease and requires a genetic predisposition and environmental triggers which activate loss of pancreatic β-cells. Possible environmental triggers include a variety of viruses and neonatal exposure to bovine serum albumin in cows' milk. Type 1 disease is relatively rare, affecting 0.4% of the population. There is a 6% risk of type 1 diabetes for siblings, 2–7% risk if one parent has type 1 diabetes, 5–20% risk if both parents have type 1 and a 30–70% risk in monozygotic twins (Pociot and Nerup, 2002). Type 1 diabetes usually occurs in those less than 30 years of age, although it can occur at any age. In older people, it is usually a more slowly progressive form, and is referred to as latent autoimmune disease in adults (LADA).

Type 2 diabetes

Type 2 diabetes is characterised by underlying insulin resistance (the insulin produced doesn't work properly) and a lack of insulin to compensate for this. Over 80% of people with type 2 diabetes are overweight. Obesity, particularly central obesity, increases insulin resistance, as does lack of physical activity (exercise increases the body's sensitivity to insulin). Type 2 diabetes is commonly associated with hypertension, hyperlipidaemia and a tendency to thrombosis, which is often referred to as the metabolic syndrome. β-cell insufficiency (caused by destruction of β-cells by high blood glucose levels and exhaustion due to excessive insulin production in response to insulin resistance) increases over time, requiring an increase in anti-hyperglycaemic medication and often insulin treatment. Fifty per cent of those with type 2 diabetes have no symptoms at diagnosis (United Kingdom Prospective Diabetes Study (UKPDS), 1998). This makes it very difficult for the patient to believe that they have the disease and makes compliance with long-term lifestyle changes, and medication, which may cause more symptoms than the disease itself, very difficult.

Type 2 diabetes is associated with high cardiovascular risk. Complications include: coronary artery disease (heart attacks, angina), peripheral vascular disease (claudication, gangrene) and carotid artery disease (strokes, dementia). The risk of a cardiovascular event for a person with diabetes is equivalent to a person without diabetes who has already experienced a heart attack, while those with diabetes who have experienced a cardiac event have a tenfold increased risk. The management of cardiac risk factors such as hypertension, dyslipidaemia, smoking and obesity is important in the management of type 2 diabetes. Microvascular complications are less common than in type 1 diabetes as the length of time of disease is often shorter, but eye, kidney and nerve damage do occur in type 2 diabetes (Royal College of Physicians, 2008). Table 13.1 summarises the differences between type 1 and type 2 diabetes.

How is diabetes diagnosed?

The WHO (1999) states that in the presence of symptoms, either a random venous plasma glucose of ≥11.1 mmol/L or a fasting venous plasma of ≥7 mmol/L is diagnostic. In the absence of symptoms, diagnosis should not be made on a single glucose determination, but on at least two laboratory samples on different days with a value in the diabetic range.

Table 13.1 Differential diagnosis of type 1 and type 2 diabetes.

Suspicion of type 1 diabetes	Suspicion of type 2 diabetes
• Under 30 years of age • No family history of diabetes or family history of type 1 • Severe symptoms of a short duration • Sudden and marked weight loss • Moderate/large amount of ketones in blood or urine • Presence of autoimmune disease, for example Graves' disease	• 40 years of age and over • Family history of type 2 diabetes • No symptoms or symptoms of long duration • No weight loss or small weight loss • No ketones or ketones associated with starvation • No autoimmune disease

This can be fasting, a random sample or from the 2-hour glucose load in an oral glucose tolerance test.

Common symptoms of diabetes include the following:

- Thirst
- Polyuria/nocturia/incontinence in older people
- Weight loss
- Blurred vision
- Genital irritation/thrush
- Recurrent infections/boils
- Mood changes
- Tingling in hands and feet

Treatment of diabetes

The aim of treatment is to prevent acute and chronic complications of diabetes and minimise side effects from treatment, thereby improving quality of life and the avoidance of premature death. It is important that the nurse effectively communicates to the patient that treatment is not always about relieving symptoms, as many patients will feel better with blood levels significantly higher than the normal range, but about meeting targets which help to reduce the risk of complications.

The daily care of diabetes is in the hands of the person with the disease. For this reason patients must be able to set goals and make frequent daily decisions that are effective and fit their values and lifestyles, while considering multiple physiological and psychosocial factors. Strategies that enable patients to make decisions about goals, therapeutic options, and self-care behaviours and to assume responsibility for daily diabetes care are effective (Funnell and Anderson, 2004).

The Diabetes Control and Complications trial – Type 1 (DCCT, 1993) and the United Kingdom Prospective Diabetes Study – Type 2 (UKPDS, 1998) have both demonstrated the beneficial effects of control of blood glucose (BG) and blood pressure (BP) on the development of diabetic complications. However, even tight control of diabetes cannot guarantee that complications will not occur, or poor control guarantee that they will. There is a cost to controlling diabetes for the patient which may include increased risk of hypoglycaemia (low level of glucose in the blood), frequent injections, blood tests and polypharmacy, with associated side effects of drugs and change in lifestyle, and, in some cases, occupation.

The National Service Framework (NSF) for Diabetes (Department of Health, 2001) Standard 3 concentrates on empowering people with diabetes and recommends that all will receive a service which encourages partnership in decision-making, supports them in managing their diabetes, and helps them to adopt and maintain a healthy lifestyle. This should be reflected in an agreed shared care plan, in which personal goals and targets are agreed and evaluated.

Control of BG, lipids, BP, obesity and smoking and the use of guardian drugs such as aspirin and ACE inhibitors (ACE I) can reduce and prevent complications. It is generally accepted that BG levels as measured by HbA1c (glycated haemoglobin), which give an indication of glucose levels over the last 3 months, should be between 6.5–7.5%. NICE (2008a) recommends that patients should be involved in decisions regarding the target measure of HbA1c and informed that any reduction in HbA1c is advantageous. Once controlled, HbA1c should be measured every 6 months. From 1 June 2009, the reporting of HbA1c results in the United Kingdom changed to the International Federation of Clinical Chemistry and Laboratory Medicine (IFCC) standard which will standardise reporting across the world. How the new and old methods relate and their relationship to capillary BG monitoring are shown in Table 13.2.

Blood pressure should be <130/80 if kidney, eye or cerebrovascular damage is present and <140/80 if it is not. Total cholesterol should be ≤4 mmol/L and ≤LDL 2 mmol/L.

Education

Diabetes is lifelong and impacts on every aspect of life. People with type 2 diabetes often need to make lifestyle adjustments to reduce weight which is difficult if they don't have symptoms. People with type 1 diabetes need to balance the risks of hypoglycaemia against the risks of long-term complications caused by hyperglycaemia; this is difficult when actions have delayed repercussions. The empowerment model acknowledges that

Table 13.2 How HbA1c readings compare to capillary blood glucose results.

HbA1c (%)	HbA1c (IFCC) (mmol/mol)	Average blood glucose (mmol/L)
12	108	19.5
11	97	17.5
10	86	15.5
9	75	13.5
8	64	11.5
7	53	9.5
6	42	7.7

patients have the right to make decisions about their lives. Only the individual can decide whether the benefits of a management plan outweigh its emotional, social, physical, psychological and financial costs (Shillitoe, 1994).

Funnell and Anderson (2004) recommend goal setting as an effective strategy to aid the educational process within the empowerment model. It is a five-step process; the first and second steps allow problem definition and ascertain patient beliefs, thoughts and feelings which may hinder their efforts. The third identifies long-term goals towards which patients will work, including barriers. The fourth involves the patient choosing and committing to a behaviour that helps achieve their goal, and the fifth is evaluation of efforts and identification of what they have learned in the process. Rather than seeing outcomes as success or failure, this framework allows all efforts to be seen as opportunities to learn more about the problem, feelings, barriers and effective strategies. The role of the educator is to provide information, collaborate during the goal-setting process, and offer support for patients' efforts.

The Department of Health and Diabetes UK (2005) recommend that structured patient education, based on formal assessment of needs, is made available to all people with diabetes both at diagnosis and ongoing. This should be provided by a trained specialist team which should include at least a nurse and a dietitian. It recommended that people with diabetes should generally be taught in groups, with one-to-one teaching available. There are several programmes which meet this criterion: The Dose Adjustment for Normal Eating (DAFNE) (type 1) and Diabetes Education and Self-Management for Ongoing and Newly Diagnosed (DESMOND) and XPERT (type 2). These are summarised in Table 13.3.

The Department of Health recommended the DAFNE course for those with type 1 diabetes. DAFNE showed a reduction in HbA1c of 0.7% at 1 year without increasing the risk of severe hypoglycaemia, with 77% of patients who had attended recording an improvement in well-being and 95% recording an improvement in treatment satisfaction. DAFNE is a 5-day course with 8-week, 6-month and yearly updates, which helps participants calculate how much insulin they need for what they eat. Participants learn from experience under the supervision of DAFNE trained nurses and dietitians. Comments from graduates include:

'How have I managed to survive before this week?'

'I've met people who understand what it is like to live with Type 1 diabetes, I've learnt such a lot in a short space of time both from the educators and my fellow delegates, I feel in control and supported.. We all exchanged e-mails..'

Structured education for people with type 2 diabetes includes the XPERT programme and DESMOND. A recent study compared DESMOND, a 6-hour programme delivered by two trained health care professionals, to 'usual care'. The main outcome measure was HbA1c at 12 months, with weight, smoking and a variety of psychosocial measures. There was no statistically significant change in HbA1c at 12 months between the two groups. There was significant weight loss of around 1 kg, there was also a modest

Table 13.3   Content and structure of education courses meeting Department of Health recommendations, 2005.

DAFNE	DESMOND	XPERT
• 5-day course (9 am to 5 pm) with half-day follow-ups at 8 weeks, 6 months and yearly • Yearly audit of patient data – central DAFNE • Training, 1 week observation, 3 days theory, entire first course peer reviewed by an external reviewer • Internal audit of staff within 1 year • External audit every 3 years • Helps patients to count carbohydrate and establish 'ratios' for each meal to allow insulin adjustment • Adult education model used, group work, experiences shared • Covers all aspects of diabetes, including exercise (practical and theory), illness, complications, hypos, social aspects, correct administration of insulin, uses quizzes, case-studies, experiences of participants, feed back of calculating carbohydrate portions, insulin ratios, corrections and BG twice a day throughout the course	• 6 hour programme, may be delivered over 1 day or in two half-day sessions • Delivered by two health care professionals who have attended a 2 day formal training programme with quality assurance at 1 year and every 3 years • Community/primary care venue • Resources such as magnetic board, demonstrating how glucose is used in the body • Content includes the patient story, monitoring diabetes, food choices, what diabetes is, consequences and personal risks, physical activity, food choices, stress and emotions, games, quizzes, questions and formulation of a diabetes self-management plan	• 6 2-hour group sessions (12 hours) • Based on theories of empowerment and discovery learning • Week 1: What is diabetes? • Week 2: Weight management • Week 3: Carbohydrate awareness • Week 4: Supermarket tour • Week 5: Complications and prevention • Week 6: Evaluation and question time • Goal setting – last 20 minutes each week • Patient manual (given at beginning of course)

difference in smoking cessation between the groups, and there were positive improvements in depression and beliefs about illness (Davies *et al.*, 2008).

Patient self-monitoring of blood glucose

The usefulness of self-monitoring of blood glucose (SMBG) is unquestioned for patients taking insulin or oral hypoglycaemic agents who may experience hypoglycaemia (hypos).

There is evidence that when used as an integral part of effective patient education packages, SMBG enables effective lifestyle interventions and the most effective use of therapies (Martin *et al.,* 2006; Karter *et al.,* 2006). However, the SMBG in those not at risk of hypos to provide feedback on the impact of lifestyle measures is controversial and many PCTs have rationed the prescription of strips. The strips are expensive, although the meters are often available free of charge from the pharmaceutical company via the diabetes nurse since profit is made from the strips. Urine testing is an indirect measurement of blood glucose – accuracy depends on renal threshold which increases with age, it is unable to detect hypos and many patients find it unhygienic, inconvenient and less accurate (Lawton *et al.,* 2004).

> 'Doing DAFNE has given me the real reason for doing blood tests, I'm actually doing less tests now – one before each meal and one before bed (I used to do 6–8 a day) and so probably costing the government less but I'm writing them down and acting on them now.'
>
> 'My nurse taught me to test my blood and explained how to increase my tablets if my sugars were high such as during illness, celebrations and the like and how to reduce them for exercise and eating less, it really gave me confidence and stopped the need for me to have to eat to keep up with the gliclazide . . . .The only problem was when I needed more tablets (or even strips) than I was allocated for the month or didn't use enough tablets, the implication was that I was somehow not complying with "medical advice". . . I wish that professionals would communicate . . .'

NICE (2009) suggests that SMBG should only be offered to a person with newly diagnosed type 2 diabetes as an integral part of self-management education; how results should be interpreted and acted upon requires discussion. The latest NICE guideline (2009) re-emphasised that SMBG is not a stand-alone intervention. No guideline on frequency of testing has been given, allowing both excessive use by some and rationing to others or the 'postcode lottery' to continue.

> 'I have no idea why I bother with these tests, no one is really interested in the results and one nurse tells me that they are OK, the next that they are too high. Even when I do everything right they go up and I don't understand why, I feel so frustrated I might as well not bother with the diet or pills either . . .'

As these quotes illustrate, each person with type 2 diabetes should be individually assessed as to whether SMBG is of value. SMBG can be used to diagnose hypoglycaemia, assess the effectiveness of medication and lifestyle changes which can motivate patients to continue. Assessment should be based on the individual goals of the patient, the risk of hypoglycaemia and the ability of the patient to interpret and act on the results. However, it is painful, time consuming to document results and look for patterns, results are not always accurate and poor results can be discouraging. If the goal is weight loss, there is very little risk of hypoglycaemia and HbA1c can be assessed every 3 months, I would suggest that SMBG would offer little value unless the patient specifically wants to perform it and it may be counterproductive if patients are not adequately educated. For example, high fat, low carbohydrate foods are high caloric but would not increase BG, whereas foods relatively high in carbohydrate but low in calories may show an increased BG result and discourage healthy eating.

Type 2 diabetes: treatment of hyperglycaemia

The UKPDS (1998) demonstrated that every 1% reduction in HbA1c reduces microvascular complications by 37% and cardiovascular risk by 10–15%. Type 2 diabetes is a progressive disease; β-cells produce less and less insulin and gradually more drugs are added until insulin treatment becomes inevitable. The progressive nature of type 2 diabetes should be explained at diagnosis and at regular intervals to prevent patients feeling 'failures' and to prepare them if insulin is required. The choice of which order drugs should be added in clinical practice is based on weight, tolerability, whether the patient drives and events such as pregnancy and surgery.

The latest NICE (2009) guidelines recommend an initial trial of lifestyle measures with the addition of metformin if HbA1c remains above 6.5%. This differs from The Joint American and European guidance of 2006 which recommends starting metformin at diagnosis together with lifestyle changes (Nathan *et al.*, 2006).

Diet

Dietary advice has been shown to influence control in both type 1 and type 2 diabetes. In the DCCT, the average HbA1c was significantly lower in those who reported adhering to diet advice than those who did not (Delahanty *et al.*, 1993). In the 3-month diet alone period in the UKPDS (1995), there was evidence of significant improvement in glycaemic control. Intentional weight loss of 11% in overweight people was associated with a 25% reduction in total mortality and a 28% reduction in cardiovascular and diabetes mortality (Williamson *et al.*, 2000). Education should focus on supporting patients to eat a good diet which can positively affect BG and the risk of diabetic complications (see Box 13.1).

Box 13.1   General advice on diet.

- Eat regularly – aim for three meals a day.
- Include some carbohydrate with a low GI at each meal.
- Five portions of fruit and vegetables a day.
- Oily fish such as mackerel, sardines or salmon twice a week.
- Fewer sugary foods and drinks.
- Fewer fatty foods, particularly saturated fats.
- Less salt. Keep to less than 6 g per day.

For the majority of people with type 2 diabetes, the major nutritional consideration is correction or limitation of obesity. All should be advised about the principles of healthy eating as recommended by the Health Education Authority in 1995 (Nutrition Sub-Committee of the Diabetes Care Advisory Committee of Diabetes UK, 2003), thus encouraging high-fibre low glycaemic index (GI) carbohydrates from fruit, vegetables, wholegrains and pulses, reduction in salt intake, the inclusion of low fat milk and oily fish, and control of saturated and trans fatty acid intake. There should be access to a state registered dietitian at diagnosis, usually through structured patient education in groups. The dietitian will tailor advice to the individual based on weight, activity, culture and the ability to buy and cook food. Many education leaflets are available aimed at different cultures and in different languages; Diabetes UK provides many free of charge and they can be downloaded from their website.

Portion size control in addition to knowledge of types of food are important in controlling BG and reducing the risk of macrovascular and microvascular complications (McArdle, 2007). The larger the portion of carbohydrate eaten, the more effect it will have on raising BG levels. Lower GI carbohydrate helps increase satiety and prevents rapid falls in BG levels; this includes wholegrain bread, porridge, pulses, most fruit and low fat yogurt. If several pieces of fruit are eaten at once BG will increase. Therefore, it is important to know how much a portion is, for example, one handful of grapes. It is unnecessary to follow a sugar-free diet; sucrose (refined sugar) can contribute 10% of daily energy (calories) if eaten as part of a healthy diet. Those who are overweight or have hypertriglyceridaemia should consider non-nutritive sweeteners (Nutrition Sub-Committee of the Diabetes Care Advisory Committee of Diabetes UK, 2003). Even low calorie foods eaten in excess will increase body weight.

'My diet was excellent, I obeyed all the rules, I just eat too much! Once the dietician explained how to reduce calories I began to lose weight.'

Fats are high in calories; therefore, reducing fats will help weight loss. Total fat should contribute less than 35% to total energy intake and saturated fat less than 10%. Saturated fats are found in pastry, butter, fatty red meat and cheese and are linked to heart disease. Choosing leaner meat, reducing portion sizes, using lower fat alternatives and using monounsaturated fats, such as olive oil and spreads made from these, can help reduce weight and improve lipid profile and sensitivity to insulin. Monosaturated fats are promoted as the main source of dietary fat due to their lower atherogenic potential (Kratz *et al.,* 2002). Pre-packaged and convenience foods contain a lot of salt. Including more home-cooked foods with no added salt, either in cooking or at the table, will help improve BP and reduce the risk of cardiovascular disease.

Diabetic foods such as diabetic sweets and chocolate are not recommended, since they are often high in fat and calories, are expensive and some cause diarrhoea. Alcohol should be kept to the safe recommended limits for the general population; no more than 14 units a week for women and 21 units for men, observance of 1–2 alcohol free days per week and avoidance during pregnancy. Alcohol is high in calories and can cause or aggravate hypertriglyceridaemia (Bell, 1996); therefore, it should be restricted in those who are trying to lose weight or who have hypertriglyceridaemia.

Low carbohydrate diets were noted to be of unproven safety in the long term and were thus not endorsed by NICE (2008a); similarly high protein diets, although promoting short-term weight loss, were not recommended as safe in the long term.

Table 13.4 Benefits of exercise.

Physical	Psychological
• Increased insulin sensitivity • Less atherogenic lipid profile • Strengthens the heart • Promotes circulation • Lowers BP	• Improved sense of well-being • Greater self-esteem • Aids relaxation and controls stress

This general healthy eating advice is applicable to people with type 1 diabetes. In addition, it is vital that they have some understanding of how to balance carbohydrate intake and insulin doses. If carbohydrate intake is higher or lower than usual, BG levels will either increase leading to hyperglycaemia or decrease leading to hypoglycaemia. Structured education courses such as DAFNE cover carbohydrate estimation and finding the correct ratio of quick-acting insulin needed for every 10 g of carbohydrate eaten.

Exercise

Exercise is beneficial for people with diabetes (see Table 13.4). It does not need to be sport or gym related; gardening, dancing, walking and even chair exercises can improve BG and treatment may require adjustment if exercise is increased. Motivation may be increased if undertaken with a friend or in a group. In many areas, local NHS groups which promote local walks are available free of charge; they also provide advice and education for housebound people in addition to exercise on prescription schemes. The local PCT should be able to advise on availability.

The immediate effect of exercise on diabetes is dependent on the type of diabetes. In type 1 diabetes, exercise may cause BG to fall (most likely outcome), stay the same or increase. If control is good, BG is likely to fall unless the insulin dose is reduced or carbohydrate intake increased. The action of insulin may speed up if it is injected into an exercised limb. Strenuous or prolonged exercise can lower BG for up to 18 hours post exercise. If BG is high before exercise in those with type 1 diabetes, particularly in the presence of ketones, the lack of circulating insulin will cause BG levels to rise due to increased glucose production by the liver. Extra quick-acting insulin may therefore be needed prior to exercise. In those with type 2 diabetes, unless sulphonlyureas or insulin is used, hypos are unlikely and there is enough circulating insulin to prevent increase in BG.

'They told me to increase exercise, I even got a prescription for cheap gym membership but initially it was a nightmare. I had to eat so much to stop hypos that my weight went up, I was on insulin twice a day and if I cut the dose in the morning before aquarobics my blood glucose was high in the afternoon! We sorted it out though by using a different insulin regime.'

Antihyperglycaemic medication

It is likely that those with type 2 diabetes will require a number of drugs to control BG. NICE recommends an order in which these should be used. This may require adjustment according to individual needs such as co-morbidity, side effects experienced or type of employment and patient preference. Non-concordance with medication is common. In one study among newly treated patients with diabetes, only 53.8% adhered to their treatment regime (Hertz *et al.*, 2005), and concordance decreases as the regime becomes more complex (Odegard and Capoccia, 2007). Nurses need to help educate patients regarding the benefits of treatments, the potential side effects and how best to minimise them (Jerreat, 2009). The benefits of the medication are often long term and do not always result in any positive change in how the patient feels, making long-term concordance difficult.

Metformin

The main effects are to inhibit gluconeogenesis and decrease hepatic glucose output. It also increases peripheral uptake of glucose and delays gastrointestinal absorption of glucose. It does not cause weight gain and cannot cause hypoglycaemia. The most serious side effect is the risk of lactic acidosis which is extremely rare and can be largely avoided by not using it if the glomerular filtration rate is <40, creatinine >150 mmol/L, or the patient is in hepatic or cardiac failure. The most common side effects are gastrointestinal (nausea, abdominal pain and diarrhoea); these can be minimised by starting on a small dose and taking it after food. If side effects occur, a slow release version is available which is associated with fewer side effects.

Sulphonylurea

Sulphonylureas (SUs) are recommended as second-line treatment by NICE; like metformin they are inexpensive and reduce HbA1c by about 1% (UKPDS, 1998; NICE, 2008a). They work by stimulating β-cells to produce insulin. Their main side effects are weight gain and hypoglycaemia and therefore they are less desirable if the person is overweight. They are often used as first line in those who are slim, or if glucose levels are particularly high (NICE, 2009). Examples include gliclazide, glimepiride and glipzide. Glibenclamide is no longer recommended except in pregnancy due to the increased risk of hypos. An SU should be added to metformin if BG remains or becomes uncontrolled. If drug compliance/concordance is a problem, a once daily SU such as gliclazide MR should be offered. It is important to educate about the risks, prevention and recognition of hypoglycaemia.

Rapid-acting insulin secretagogues

Examples of these drugs include repaglinide and nateglinide. They too stimulate insulin production, but have a rapid onset of action and a short duration of activity. They are particularly useful when post-prandial peaks (high BG levels 1/2–2 hours after food) occur or in non-routine lifestyle patterns. They need to be taken before meals and require multiple dosing which may limit compliance, and they are more expensive than SUs.

Acarbose

Acarbose is the only α-glucosidase inhibitor available; it delays and reduces carbohydrate absorption in the small intestine and reduces post-prandial peaks. The main side effect is flatulence with abdominal distension and pain. It does not cause weight gain. NICE (2008a) recommends that acarbose be considered for a person unable to use other glucose lowering medications. It concluded that acarbose has lower glucose-lowering efficacy, a higher rate of intolerance and dropout from therapy and relative expense compared to generic metformin and SUs.

Thiazolidinedione (glitazones)

There are two glitazones licensed in the United Kingdom: rosiglitazone and pioglitazone. Rosiglitazone is licensed for use as monotherapy, combination therapy with metformin or an SU, or as part of triple therapy with metformin and an SU in the United Kingdom. Pioglitazone is additionally licensed with the use of insulin. Their main function is to reduce insulin resistance and thus improve glucose uptake; they have also been shown to improve pancreatic β-cell function. They are contraindicated in liver disease, cardiac failure, severe renal impairment and pregnancy. Side effects include weight gain (0.7–2.3 kg), oedema, and anaemia. Rosiglitazone is associated with increased risk of distal fractures in women and cardiac failure. NICE recommends that glitazones be added to metformin and an SU where insulin would otherwise be considered, but is considered unacceptable due to the following reasons:

- Employment, for example driving restrictions.
- Patient barriers to insulin, for example needle phobia.
- Negative associations.
- If SU or metformin is not tolerated.
- If the risk of hypoglycaemia is unacceptable.

Dipeptidyl-peptidase-4 (DPP4) inhibitors

NICE (2009) recommends metformin as second-line therapy instead of an SU if control of BG remains inadequate or if the patient is at significant risk of hypoglycaemia or an SU is not tolerated. DPP4 inhibitors can also be used with an SU if metformin is not tolerated, or third line (with metformin and SU) if insulin or glitazones are undesirable (e.g. due to risk of weight gain). DPP4 inhibitors are incretins or peptide hormones that are released from the gut in response to the ingestion of food and enhance glucose-stimulated insulin secretion from the pancreas; examples include sitagliptin and vitagliptin. They are weight neutral, orally administered and have been demonstrated to lower HbA1c by 0.6–0.8% (Elrishi *et al.*, 2007). They are not associated with nausea and have a low risk of hypoglycaemia. However, long duration trial data is unavailable.

Glucagon-like peptide-1 agonists (GLP-1)

Exenatide is a glucagon-like peptide-1 (GLP-1). It is administered by twice daily sub-cutaneous injection and has been shown to lower HbA1c by 0.9–1.1% with significant progressive weight loss and an increase in β-cell mass. GLP-1 slows gastric emptying, inhibits glucagon secretion, and stimulates insulin secretion in a glucose-dependent manner. Gastrointestinal side effects are common, particularly nausea which tends to lessen over time. A rare side effect is acute pancreatitis. It is licensed in the United Kingdom for use with metformin or an SU. NICE (2009) does not recommend routine use, and it should be used only if the following all apply:

- A BMI of >35 kg/m^2.
- Problems of a specific psychological, biochemical or physical nature arising from a high BMI.
- Inadequate control with metformin and SU.
- If other high cost medications such as glitazones would otherwise be used.

It should only be continued if HbA1c reduction at 6 months is at least 1% and weight loss is 5% per year. Liraglutide has recently been introduced and is a once daily GLP-1.

Use of glucose-lowering medication

'I was told by the nurse that I am overweight. I tried to explain that all my family are big, we are big boned. I hardly eat. Anyway apparently my blood tests are still high so they gave me metformin. No one told me that it could make me ill. I think that they were trying to punish me cause I couldn't manage the diet, they are huge to swallow too. . . . I know now that I should take them after food and that they can help control my diabetes and protect my heart.'

'I weighed 120 kg and my blood sugar was too high, I was taking metformin and 120 units of insulin a day. I felt trapped, if I didn't eat I had hypos, if I did eat I couldn't stop and just got fatter. I had tried Xenical (a fat busting drug) but it gave me diarrhoea and I was told that the other drugs which could help me lose weight would be dangerous due to my blood pressure and depression. My only hope was bariatric surgery or exenatide. I chose the exenatide. Well I feel great! I was nauseous for the first month, and a little when the dose was increased, but I'm now feeling great, I've lost 8 Kg and my HbA1c has decreased by 2%, I am taking all my metformin and other drugs now as I can see the effects.'

Treatment with insulin

It is important firstly to understand how insulin is secreted in people without diabetes to understand how each insulin regime compares to this. It allows us to see and explain to the patient the advantages and disadvantages of each insulin regime more clearly. Insulin is secreted at two rates in response to rising blood glucose levels: a slow basal rate over 24 hours, and as a bolus in response to rising blood glucose such as after meals (see Figure 13.1). Figures 13.2 to 13.8 show the duration of action of various forms of insulin.

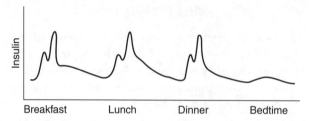

Figure 13.1 Normal insulin response to food.

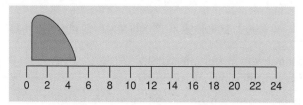

- Onset 5–15 minutes (e.g. Apidra, Humalog, Novorapid).
- Duration of clinically effective action 4–5 hours.
- Can be injected immediately before meals or up to 15 minutes after.
- May cause less hypoglycaemia due to shorter duration of action than soluble insulin.
- Effective in reducing post-prandial hyperglycaemia.
- Used pre meals with intermediate or long-acting background insulin (basal bolus therapy) or as part of a mixture, e.g. Humalog mix 25, Novomix 30.

Figure 13.2 Rapid-acting analogues.

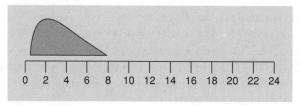

- e.g. Actrapid, Humulin S.
- Onset 30–45 minutes.
- Peaks 2–4 hours.
- Duration 5–8 hours.
- Often used pre meals, combined with intermediate or long-acting background insulin (basal bolus) or in a 'free-mix" or part of a mixture, e.g. Mixtard 30, M3.

Figure 13.3 Soluble insulin.

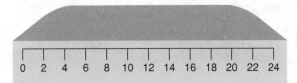

- e.g. glargine, detemir.
- Duration of action up to 24 hours used once/twice daily (care in pregnancy).
- Less variation in absorption than isophane.
- Used as basal insulin in Type 1 diabetes with quick acting analogue or soluble to cover carbohydrate-containing meals. In Type 2 may be used once a day with sulphonylureas and metformin.
- Detemir has a peak 5–7 hours, often used as twice daily basal insulin in those with Type 1 diabetes, it is flexible and can be adjusted for exercise (DAFNE, 2007).
- Glargine has a peakless profile and is used once a day.

Figure 13.4 Long-acting analogue.

Technique for insulin administration

In order for insulin to act predictably, correct injection technique is vital and nurses have a responsibility to ensure that the advice that they give and the technique used is consistent with current recommendations.

Insulin must be given subcutaneously not intramuscularly (IM), so it is important that the correct size of needle and site is chosen. Recommended sites are upper thighs, abdomen or buttocks. The sites have different rates of absorption with the abdomen being the quickest and the buttocks the slowest. It is generally recommended that quick sites

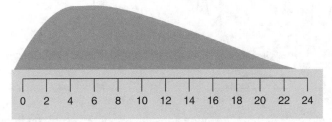

- Looks cloudy and must be mixed well before use.
- Onset of action 2 hours, peaks 4–8 hours.
- Duration 22 hours.
- Can be used once (usually twice) daily as part of a basal bolus regime or once a day as a basal insulin with tablets or as part of a twice-a-day regime with soluble or quick acting analogue insulin.

Figure 13.5 Medium-acting isophane insulin.

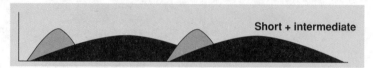

- Pre-mixed short-acting and intermediate insulin, e.g. Mixtard 30/70 or Humulin M3.
- Or analogue insulin combined with intermediate acting insulin, e.g. Humalog Mix 25, Humalog mix 50 or NovoMix 30.
- Available as 25/75, 30/70, 50/50 mixtures.
- Generally used twice daily, occasionally three times.
- Suits people with regular lifestyle pattern.
- Not re-suspending alters mix.

Figure 13.6   Mixed insulin.

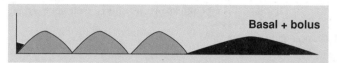

- Intermediate or long-acting analogue insulin, usually before bed (twice a day background insulin, may be necessary in Type 1 diabetes).
- Can be tailored to individual needs, for example dose adjusted for changes in carbohydrate eaten or exercise.

Figure 13.7   Basal bolus.

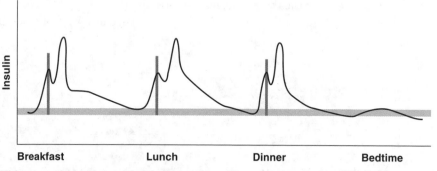

This most closely resembles the normal insulin response; a constant infusion of rapid-acting insulin is delivered by a pump attached by tubing to a cannula under the skin, and the cannula is changed every 2–3 days. The basal rates can be varied for different times of the day, reducing the risk of hypoglycaemia. Bolus doses can be given when carbohydrate is eaten, or in response to hyperglycaemia. The treatment is expensive (around £2,500 for the pump and £2,000 for consumables per year) and proficient carbohydrate counting and SMBG is required. The pump is also a visible reminder of diabetes 24 hours a day.

Figure 13.8   Continuous subcutaneous infusion of insulin (CSSI).

be used for quick-acting insulin and thighs and buttocks for basal insulin or for twice daily regimes, abdomen in the morning and thighs in the evening. Arms are no longer recommended as there is less fat, no pinch up can be used and IM injection is more likely. However, if other sites are 'lumpy' it may be necessary using the smallest needle available (5 mm or 6 mm). Needles are available in lengths of 5 mm, 6 mm, 8 mm and 12.7 mm. It is suggested that children, adolescents and thin adults use 5 or 6 mm needles without a skin fold (although a skin fold can be used), and normal weight adults use an 8 mm needle with a lifted skin fold or 5 mm or 6 mm with no lifted skin fold.

Insulin should be injected at a 90° angle, and skin should be pinched up using the thumb and index finger/middle finger to ensure insulin is not injected into the muscle. Swabbing skin is unnecessary; it may toughen the skin, and stings if the spirit is not left to dry. If using a pen rather than a syringe the needle should be left in for at least 6 seconds after the plunger is depressed to allow the entire dose to leave the needle.

Lipohypertrophy (lumpy injection sites) causes erratic insulin absorption; therefore, injection sites should be rotated to prevent lumps and sites regularly observed to identify lumps. If sites are moved insulin doses may need reduction to prevent hypos.

The timing of insulin in relation to food is important. For example, if soluble insulin (Actrapid, Humulin S, Mixtard 30) is used, it must be given 30 minutes before food. If given with or after food, BG is likely to be very high 2 hours after food and too low before the next meal as the peak of insulin will have missed the peak glucose level. If quick-acting analogue is given more than 15 minutes before food, a hypo is likely before the meal. Basal insulin should be given at a similar time each day to prevent overlap with the insulin given the day before (or after) or gaps in cover if more than 24 hours are left between basal injections.

> 'Starting on insulin has been amazing. The injections don't hurt, the pen is so easy to use and I feel great. I had been losing weight and I was very underweight I looked like I was anorexic, the tablets weren't working, my HbA1c was 15.8% but I didn't have ketones . . . The nurse at the diabetes centre took one look at me and just said insulin. . . . The dietitian actually suggested an increase in calories. I'm now normal weight, have lots of energy and other than two injections a day, eating fairly frequently to avoid hypos, informing the DVLA and a few blood tests I'm completely back to my old self.'

Chronic complications of diabetes

Diabetes can lead to long-term complications damaging both large and small blood vessels; these are grouped into macrovascular and microvascular complications. Macrovascular complications include coronary heart disease, stroke and peripheral vascular disease. Microvascular disease includes nephropathy (kidneys), retinopathy (eyes) and neuropathy (nerves). In type 2 diabetes vascular complications and hypertension commonly exist at diagnosis. In type 1, complications usually emerge 10–20 years after diagnosis. Regular monitoring and assessment of people with diabetes can help in the detection and prevention of complications. Education should focus on the positive interventions that can be made to prevent or slow down complications. Regular clinic attendance, at least yearly, enables not only assessment of BG, BP, lipid and weight, but also early signs of complications. For example, detection of microalbuminuria if treated can prevent renal failure, eye photography can identify changes which can be treated with improved BG or BP control or laser to prevent blindness and identification of neuropathic or ischaemic feet can promote better self-care of feet or podiatry attendance. It is often easier for patients to take medication and/or change lifestyle if screening shows that diabetes is affecting them. Involving patients by sharing results, explaining what is happening and revising goals and clinical management plans to reflect findings is therefore vital. Nurses need to have a good understanding of what the results of screening tests mean and how these affect the progression of disease. To set goals the complication status of the patient needs to be known by both the patient and the health professionals involved.

Microvascular disease

People with type 1 and type 2 diabetes are prone to microvascular disease but there are differences in how these are expressed. There is evidence implicating hyperglycaemia in the development of microvascular complications in both types of diabetes and the benefits of good glycaemic control in preventing microvascular complications and their progression have been clearly demonstrated in the DCCT (1993) and the UKPDS (1998).

Diabetic retinopathy (DR)

Diabetes is the commonest cause of blindness in working age in the Western world. Risk factors for the development of retinopathy include: duration of diabetes, type of diabetes, level of glycaemic control, hypertension, nephropathy, hyperlipidaemia, pregnancy, smoking and ethnic origin (higher in people of African and Afro-Caribbean origin).

DR is very responsive to treatment if found early and yearly attendance for retinal photography is vital. Visual loss from diabetic retinopathy is caused by either maculopathy leading to impairment of central vision or retinal ischaemia resulting in proliferative diabetic retinopathy. The prevalence of diabetic retinopathy increases with the duration of diabetes; therefore, it is more prevalent in those with type 1 diabetes, whereas maculopathy is ten times more common in those with type 2 (Shotliff and Duncan, 2006). In addition to the retina, other eye problems are common such as cataracts and glaucoma.

DR is classified as background, pre-proliferative, proliferative, advanced eye disease (retinal detachment, rubeosis (in which new blood vessels grow on the iris), neovascular glaucoma) and maculopathy. An alternative broad classification is non-sight threatening or sight threatening. Sight-threatening DR occurs in 10% of diagnosed patients and includes exudative maculopathy, proliferative retinopathy or retinal ischaemia (Mackinnon and Forrester, 2002). In background retinopathy, the small vessels of the retina become blocked and other vessels dilate to compensate. It is not a threat to vision and does not require treatment, nor are symptoms apparent to the patient. Proliferative retinopathy is sight threatening and is characterised by the development of new blood vessels in response to ischaemia. Maculopathy is also sight threatening and endangers central vision.

Screening for DR

The NSF (Department of Health 2001, 2003) recommends annual retinal screening for all those with diabetes using digital photography. This allows prompt laser treatment of advanced retinopathy. Pregnant women with diabetes should be screened in each trimester.

Treatment of DR

Treatment is focused on minimising the risk factors such as glycaemic control, hypertension or hyperlipidaemia and actively reducing further sight deterioration using laser treatment.

Glycaemic control is important. The DCCT (1993) demonstrated that an HbA1c of 7% or less reduced the risk of developing retinopathy by 76% and slowed the risk of progression in those with retinopathy by 54%. The UKPDS (1998) showed a 21% reduction in progression and a 29% reduction in the need for laser therapy. A BP of 144/82 or less showed a 35% reduction in the need for laser treatment (UKPDS, 1998). The use of ACE I may alter local growth factor levels and lessen the production of new vessels, and therefore has other benefits in addition to reducing BP.

Hyperlipidaemia is associated with increased risk of proliferative retinopathy and worse outcome from laser therapy; therefore, aggressive lipid lowering is advocated. Lifestyle changes such stopping smoking are also advised (Shotliff and Duncan, 2006).

Laser treatment aims to prevent further visual loss rather than restore vision and it may reduce night vision or affect visual fields. Topical local anaesthetic drops are used and treatment is usually performed over a number of sessions. Kohner *et al.* (1996) claim that early laser treatment can prevent blindness in 90% of patients with proliferative retinopathy if applied adequately. Vitreous surgery may be needed for end-stage disease.

Nephropathy

Between 25 and 50% of people with diabetes develop kidney disease and diabetic nephropathy is now the single most common cause of renal failure in the Western world. Nephropathy is closely linked to retinopathy, and 75% of people with proliferative retinopathy will also have nephropathy. Diabetic renal disease is characterised by changes in both albuminuria and the glomerular filtration rate. In diabetic nephropathy the small vessels in the kidney become abnormal and protein leaks into the urine. Initially, this is below the level which is detectable by routine 'dipstick' testing for albumin but it can be detected in a laboratory and is expressed as an albumin:creatinine ratio. If positive this stage is called microalbuminuria; protein loss increases to proteinuria which then becomes persistent and indicates overt nephropathy. This is followed by uraemia and end-stage renal failure. Microalbuminuria is an early component in progressive increases in albumin excretion rates and should be tested at least yearly as treatment at this stage could prevent progression. The DCCT (1993) showed that the development of microalbuminuria was reduced by 34% with an HbA1c of 7% or less. The UKPDS (1998) showed that reducing HbA1c to 7% was associated with an absolute risk reduction of developing nephropathy of 11% over 12 years.

Treatment of Nephropathy

Control of hypertension has been shown to slow the rate of decline in glomerular filtration rate (GFR) (Bakris *et al.,* 2000). If persistent proteinuria is present, BP targets should be reduced to 120/75 (MacIsaac and Watts, 2006). There is evidence that using an ACE I or an angiotensin receptor blocker (ARB) results in renal and cardiovascular effects over and above controlling BP alone (MacIsaac and Watts, 2006). A meta-analysis (ACE I in Diabetic Nephropathy Trialist Group, 2001) concluded that in normotensive type 1 patients with microalbuminuria, treatment significantly reduced progression to macroproteinuria and increased the chances of remission to normoalbuminuria. ACE I or ARBs should therefore be used as first-line antihypertensive treatment and in those without hypertension with microalbuminuria.

It is controversial whether restriction in dietary protein in those without advanced renal failure is necessary as trial data is contradictory. Smoking should be discouraged as there is an association between smoking and the development of nephropathy.

Once the GFR has reduced to <30 mL/min/1.73^2, referral to a nephrologist is required to prepare for renal replacement therapy. Renal transplantation should be the aim for all patients with diabetes in end-stage renal failure (ESRF). Patient survival and rehabilitation is superior when compared to dialysis (Trevisan and Viberti, 2002). Haemodialysis remains the most common form of treatment for those with diabetes and ESRF. Unfortunately, the formation of fistulas and shunts may be more difficult due to atheromatous peripheral vessels, and dialysis may be complicated by postural hypotension and fluid retention. Continuous ambulatory peritoneal dialysis avoids rapid volume fluctuations and is therefore more suitable for people with ischaemic heart disease and elderly people.

Neuropathy

Neuropathy refers to nerve damage; however, the mechanisms for this are poorly understood. The UKPDS suggests that both microvascular and macrovascular disease contribute; impaired blood supply to the nerves may contribute to peripheral neuropathy. Hyperglycaemia is known to contribute to the risk and tight glycaemic control reduced the risk of neuropathy by 69% and slowed progression by 57% in the DCCT. The prevalence of neuropathy is related to age, duration of diabetes and glycaemic control (Tesfaye *et al.,* 1996) and to other microvascular complications. Other risk factors include smoking, hypertension and hyperlipidaemia. Prevalence rates (30%) are similar in both types of diabetes (Tesfaye, 2002).

Watkins and Edmonds (1997) classify neuropathies into the following three main groups:

1. Progress steadily with increasing duration of diabetes and are associated with other complications of diabetes, for example distal symmetrical neuropathy (usually affecting feet in stocking distribution) and small fibre neuropathies such as Charcot joint, autonomic neuropathy.
2. Abrupt in onset, often occurring at diagnosis of diabetes, unrelated to disease duration or other complications of diabetes. They are expected to resolve completely, for example acute diffuse painful neuropathy and mononeuropathies such as amyotrophy.
3. Pressure palsies not specific to diabetes but more common in diabetes, for example carpal tunnel syndrome.

Distal symmetrical neuropathy is the most common. It is often symptomless, causing reduced pain sensation and putting the feet at risk of tissue injury and damage. Some people complain of pins and needles or numbness, others of contact sensitivity, particularly at night. Pain can be extremely severe and last for years, although the most severely affected usually recover within 12 to 18 months. Drug and non-drug treatments are not fully effective. NICE (2008a) recommends that patients be asked directly about neuropathic symptoms annually and that clinicians be alert to the psychological consequences of chronic neuropathic pain, providing psychological support as necessary. Therapeutic options should be discussed and agreed with the person with diabetes.

First-line drug treatment should be with a tricyclic drug, for example amitriptyline; if ineffective, a trial of duloxetine, gabapentin or pregabalin should be given. If side effects limit effective dose titration, another drug from this group should be tried. Opiates and referral to the local chronic pain management service should be considered.

'It started about a week after I started insulin, the pain was unbearable, particularly at night. I couldn't even have a sheet on my feet. The amitriptyline helped me sleep but I felt "thick headed" all day. The next drugs didn't really help as much with the pain but at least I could get to work. . . . After a year or so it did get better, they said that it would!'

Autonomic neuropathy can manifest in a number of ways, including gustatory sweating, postural hypotension, diarrhoea, erectile dysfunction, gastroparesis, neuropathic bladder, respiratory arrests and subclinical abnormalities such as blunted counter-regulatory responses to hypoglycaemia and increased blood flow to the feet. Treatment concentrates on relieving the symptoms.

'I felt embarrassed discussing it [erectile dysfunction], it's not really an illness – but my wife was always thinking that I didn't find her attractive anymore and even that I was having an affair. . . . Thankfully I did mention it, Tadalafil 20 mg has been prescribed three times a week and now our sex life is as good as ever.'

Macrovascular disease

Macrovascular complications refer to disease affecting the arteries supplying the heart, brain and legs, which may result in heart disease, stroke and peripheral vascular disease.

Cardiovascular complications are the commonest cause of death in both types of diabetes (Goh and Tooke, 2002). Diabetes affects the coronary, cerebral and peripheral circulation, the predominant disturbance being atherosclerosis or atheroma. The cause is multifactorial and is strongly related to conventional cardiovascular risk factors which are cumulative. Fisher and Shaw (2006) argue that the presence of diabetes at least doubles the risk for each combination of factors – be it single or multiple and that modifying these leads to improved outcome.

The DCCT (type 1) (1993) failed to demonstrate reduced macrovascular disease with improved control, although the participants were <39 years old. However, even in the UKPDS (type 2) (1998) the reduction in myocardial infarction of 16% in the intensively treated group was not statistically significant, although it is now, on longer follow-up. Metformin improved cardiovascular outcomes compared to all other treatments (including insulin) in type 2 diabetes at similar levels of HbA1c, suggesting that factors other than glycaemic control are important in preventing macrovascular complications.

Hypertension

If BP is above 140/80 or above 130/80 with kidney or cerebrovascular damage, NICE (2008a) recommends treatment. Their recommendations are based on a large body of clinical evidence including the Hypertension in Diabetes Study (part of UKPDS, 1998), Hypertension Optimal Treatment Study (Kjeldsen *et al.*, 1998) and Heart Outcomes Prevention Evaluation (HOPE, 2000). NICE recommends lifestyle measures initially such as reduced sodium intake, calorie and alcohol reduction (if overweight), smoking cessation and increased exercise. BP should be monitored 1–2 monthly, and, if still high, pharmaceutical intervention commenced. First line should be an ACE I (unless the person is African -Caribbean in which case an ACE I plus either a diuretic or calcium-channel blocker should be used). If planning pregnancy, a calcium-channel blocker should be the first line. If the ACE I is not tolerated, it should be replaced by an ARB. Second-line therapy if BP continues to be elevated is a calcium channel blocker or a diuretic. Third line should be the drug not added as second line. Fourth line are alpha-blockers, beta-blockers or a potassium sparing diuretic.

Cardiovascular risk

Most people with type 2 diabetes have a high enough cardiovascular risk to justify statin therapy without further assessment (Haffner *et al.*, 1998). NICE recommends treatment with simvastatin unless cardiovascular risk from non-hyperglycaemic factors is low. Cardiovascular risk should be assessed using the UKPDS risk engine (Stevens *et al.*, 2001); if the cardiovascular risk exceeds 20% over 10 years, simvastatin should be initiated. Treatment of patients <40 years old should be considered where there are multiple features of the metabolic syndrome, a strong family history of premature cardiovascular disease, smoking, an at-risk ethnic group or microalbuminuria is present. The dose of simvastatin should be increased to 80 mg until total cholesterol is below 4.0 mmol/L or LDL below 2.0 mmol/L. A more effective statin such as atorvastatin or rosuvastatin or ezetimibe should be used if simvastatin ineffective. They should not be used if the patient is planning pregnancy.

Fibrates should be used if triglycerides remain above 4.5 mmol/L despite alcohol reduction, improved glycaemic control, control of thyroid or other underlying factors. Fenofibrate is recommended as first- line. Fibrates and statins should not be commenced at the same time, although they can be used together. Nicotinic acid derivatives are reserved for those who are intolerant of other therapies and have extreme disorders of lipid metabolism, likewise omega-3 fish oils should not be used first line (NICE 2008a).

Antiplatelet therapy

Diabetes UK continues to recommend the use of aspirin in patients with high cardiovascular risk despite recent controversy (Belch *et al.*, 2008). Recent NICE guidance (2008a) suggests that low dose aspirin (75 mg daily) should be offered to people of 50 years plus if BP is 145/90 mm Hg. If significant other cardiovascular risk factors exist in those under 40 years of age, it should be given. Clopidogrel should be used instead where there are aspirin intolerance and post-coronary events.

Smoking cessation

Coronary heart events occur more frequently and more severely in those with diabetes who smoke, ironically people with diabetes are more likely to smoke (Fisher and Shaw, 2006). Nicotine replacement therapy and smoking cessation clinics should be offered routinely.

Treatment of obesity

Android distribution of fat or 'apple shape' is an independent indicator of cardiovascular risk. Treatment strategies should include referral to a dietitian and exercise programmes. Pharmacological intervention may be necessary. This involves careful consideration; side effects may be unpleasant (oily leakage from the rectum in the case of orlistat) or dangerous (hypertension with sibutramine). Bariatric surgery is approved for those with diabetes and BMI >35 kg/m^2, if all other measures have failed and strict criteria are met (NICE, 2002).

Damage to feet

25% of people with diabetes will develop at least one foot ulcer in their lifetime; 15–20% of these will require a lower limb amputation (McIntosh *et al.*, 2003). The estimated cost of diabetes-related amputation is between £20,000 and £45,000 (Lefebvre, 2005), while the psychological distress is immeasurable (McAleese, 2006). There is loss of mobility and freedom and restriction of social activities. Being housebound can cause social isolation as can periods of unemployment (Kinmond *et al.*, 2003).

There are two main syndromes: the neuropathic foot, in which neuropathy predominates, but the major arterial supply to the foot is intact, or the neuro-ischaemic foot, where both neuropathy and ischaemia resulting from a reduced arterial supply contribute. Neuropathic feet have palpable pulses, sweating is diminished and the skin may be dry. Motor neuropathy may contribute to structural deformities such as high arch and claw toes, leading to prominence of the metatarsal heads. There are two main complications: the neuropathic ulcer and the Charcot joint (painful, swollen hot foot, often after a small injury followed by a destructive phase leading to bone resorption and softening and deformity). The neuro-ischaemic foot is cool and pulseless with poor blood supply. Ulcers in the neuro-ischaemic foot develop on the margins of the foot at sites made vulnerable to pressure often from poorly fitting shoes. Peripheral vascular disease, hypertension, dyslipidaemia and hyperglycaemia all contribute to the development of the at-risk foot (Edmonds and Foster, 2000, 2002). Leucocytes, essential in fighting and preventing infection, are dysfunctional in the presence of hyperglycaemia (Anderson *et al.*, 2004). Delayed healing encourages infection which can lead to gangrene or amputation (see Table 13.5).

Diabetic foot care depends on effective patient education, thorough foot examination at least yearly, referral of the person with at-risk feet to podiatry, well-fitting footwear and

Table 13.5 Six stages of the diabetic foot based on Edmonds and Foster (2000).

Stage	Description	Action needed
1. Normal foot	No risk factors (after testing with 10 g monofilament or vibration, palpation of pulses and inspection of feet and footwear)	Control BG, lipids Stop smoking Well-fitting shoes
2. The high-risk foot	Oedema, neuropathy, plantar callus, ischaemia, deformity not accommodated in footwear	Extra depth shoe in case of deformity Felt padding to relieve plantar pressures Education to patient to recognise danger signs, for example redness, heat, swelling, discharge Educate need to check inside shoes for foreign objects Podiatry needed for thickened or ingrown nails, corns or calluses Moisturiser for dry skin, daily washing of feet in lukewarm water and thorough drying
3. The ulcerated foot	Pivotal state on the route to amputation	Wound control with regular debridement of neuropathic ulcers Microbiological control with inspection of the foot, swabs and antibiotics Mechanical control: casts, insoles in shoes, special shoes, palpation of pulses, measurement of brachial pressure index and perhaps angiography/revascularisation for an ischaemic foot Pain control in the ischaemic foot Metabolic control of BG, BP, lipids and smoking Patient education – danger signs, how to inspect the ulcer and how to clean, dress, rest or use special shoes or casts
4. The cellulitic foot	Infection has taken hold	Swabs for laboratory analysis and appropriate prescription of systemic antibiotics
5. The necrotic foot	Gangrene	Necrotic toes on the neuropathic foot could be amputated and most feet heal quickly Ischaemic patients may need a distal bypass and require wound care for the large leg wounds left after the graft is harvested
6. The foot that cannot be rescued	Major amputation	Rehabilitation of patient and the return of the other foot to an earlier stage of risk

antibiotics as soon as infection is identified; referral to a multidisciplinary foot clinic is vital (NICE, 2004). Diabetic foot ulceration is largely avoidable if good metabolic control and foot care can be maintained (Valk *et al.*, 2005). Protocols should be developed with input from the microbiologist, pharmacists, diabetes team and accident and emergency staff.

'I know that I shouldn't have done it, but I just couldn't wear my special shoes to my daughter's wedding. I had a hat and everything, I brought pink shoes to match. . . . .it was only for a few hours, the ulcer was healed but I'm now back to that awful boot again and weekly visits to podiatry.'

Acute complications of diabetes

Diabetic ketoacidosis (DKA)

Alberti (1974) defines DKA as 'severe uncontrolled diabetes requiring emergency treatment with insulin and emergency fluids with a blood ketone concentration of greater than 5 mmol/l.' The Association of British Clinical Diabetologists (ABCD) (2006) states diagnostic criteria as: BG >11.1 mmol/L, significant ketonuria, or blood ketones (measured with an Optium Xceed meter) and significant acidosis, either a serum venous bicarbonate level of <15 mmol/L or an arterial pH <7.3. Huriel *et al.* (1997) claim that DKA is the largest single cause of death in patients with diabetes under the age of 40 years. They estimate mortality rates to range between 2% and 22 %. The precipitating factors and clinical features of DKA are given in Boxes 13.2 and 13.3.

Box 13.2   Precipitating factors in DKA.

1. Infection.
2. New presentation of type 1.
3. Mismanagement of diabetes by either patient or professional Huriel *et al.* (1997) found that of 23 patients in whom infection precipitated DKA, 10 had omitted insulin.
4. No obvious cause.

Box 13.3   Clinical features of DKA.

Thirst, polyuria, nocturia, blurred vision, weight loss, deep rapid breathing (Kussmaul respiration), nausea, vomiting, abdominal pain, drowsiness and, if untreated, coma.

Treatment of DKA (as advised by ABCD, 2006)

- IV insulin and fluids should be given immediately.
- Essential investigations include laboratory BG, urea and electrolytes, venous bicarbonate, ECG, chest X-ray, urine and blood cultures.

- Arterial gases should be measured if there is reduced consciousness, respiratory distress or hypotension.
- Strict fluid balance needs to be maintained; a urinary catheter should be inserted if the patient is incontinent, or there is no urinary output after 2 hours.
- A nasogastric tube should be inserted if consciousness is impaired.
- A central venous pressure line should be considered if the patient is elderly, and thromboprophylaxis if there is severe dehydration or the patient is elderly.
- Broad-spectrum antibiotics should be given if there is evidence of infection.
- Saline should be replaced with 5–10% glucose once BG falls to 15 mmol/L, or given concomitantly if the blood volume is still depleted. Potassium will fall as acidosis is corrected, and should be monitored 2–4 hourly until stable.
- Capillary glucose should be measured hourly and the dose of insulin adjusted accordingly (never less than 0.5 units/hour).
- When the patient is clinically well, subcutaneous insulin should be started with a meal and IV insulin discontinued 30 minutes after subcutaneous insulin has been given.

Hyperosmolar non-ketotic coma (HONK)

HONK is characterised by marked hyperglycaemia which may exceed 60 mmol/L without significant ketones and acidosis. Onset is slow over weeks rather than days. It usually affects middle-aged or elderly patients who are previously undiagnosed, and mortality is high. Precipitating factors in HONK are: infection, treatment with thiazide diuretic, and large intake of glucose drinks.

Treatment for HONK is the same as for DKA with the exception of the following:

- If serum sodium is >155 mmol/L, 0.45% sodium chloride is given rather than 0.9%.
- High risk of thromboembolic disease, so anticoagulation is required, for example tinzaparin.
- Once the patient is eating and drinking, subcutaneous insulin is initiated and used for a few weeks, after which diet and tablet treatment is usually adequate.

Hypoglycaemia

Hypoglycaemia occurs when the BG concentration falls below 3.6–3.8 mmol/L. Autonomic symptoms (sweating, pounding heart, shaking and hunger) develop at approximately 3.2 mmol/L and neuroglycopenic symptoms (confusion, drowsiness, speech difficulty, incoordination, visual disturbances, atypical behaviour and coma) start to occur at approximately 3 mmol/L (Williams and Pickup, 2004). These levels vary according to the level of control and how many hypos have occurred. Diabetes UK recommend 'make 4 the floor' and that any BG <4 mmol/L on insulin or SUs be treated. People with poor control may feel hypo when their BG levels are within normal limits, and those who have had frequent hypos and/or have had diabetes for many years may fail to recognise hypos. Hypoglycaemic unawareness is defined as 'the onset of neuroglycopaenia before the appearance of autonomic warning symptoms' (de Galan *et al.*, 2006).

Causes of hypos

- Dose of insulin or sulphonylureas too high
- Inadequate amounts of carbohydrate
- Delayed/missed meal (without dose adjustment)
- Unplanned or sustained exercise
- Alcohol (inhibits gluconeogenesis)
- Change of injection site

Prevention of hypos

- Regular meals (if on twice daily insulin or sulphonylureas)
- Insulin should be given at correct time in relation to food, for example rapid-acting analogue no more than 15 minutes before food
- Balance insulin dose and carbohydrate portions
- Accurate regular monitoring of BG
- Reduce insulin/sulphonylureas or increase carbohydrate if exercising

Treatment of hypos

This depends on severity. If the patient is unconscious, nothing should be given by mouth:

- Give 15–20 g of high GI (rapid acting) carbohydrate, for example 5–6 dextrose tablets, 150–200 mL Coca Cola, 100 mL lucozade, 1.5–2 25 g tubes of glucogel.
- If a meal is delayed by more than 1 hour, a snack of 10 g of medium or low GI carbohydrate should be given, for example digestive biscuit or if longer than 2 hours, 20 g should be given.

If unconscious, glucagon should be given subcutaneously or IM; consciousness should be regained after 10 minutes, if not an ambulance will be required. Since glucagon does not provide additional glucose but stimulates glucose release from the liver, 20 g of rapid-acting carbohydrate followed by 40 g of longer acting carbohydrate should be taken orally when conscious. If the patient is in hospital, IV glucose 50% can be given instead.

Driving

If the person is treated with diet or tablets and there are no complications of diabetes, the Driver and Vehicle Licensing Agency (DVLA) does not need to be informed (except for a group 2 licence). However, many insurance companies insist that the DVLA is informed. If a group 2 licence (large goods vehicles and passenger carrying vehicles) is held and the holder is treated with medication which may cause hypoglycaemia, the DVLA must be informed. C1 licences (vehicles weighing 3.5–7.5 tonnes) can be issued to those on insulin following medical assessment by a hospital consultant. Most insurance companies no longer increase premiums for diabetes. Those treated with insulin must inform the

DVLA, who contact the diabetic consultant or GP for medical information and issue a licence for 1, 2 or 3 years. If hypoglycaemic unawareness occurs, driving must stop until warning symptoms have returned (Diabetes UK, 2009).

'I hold a group 2 licence a LGV licence and I drive a lorry for a living. I have been told that my blood glucose is too high and that I need insulin. I have told them I can't have insulin because I would lose my job. I'm 50 and I can't see myself finding another job I have four kids, a wife and a mortgage.'

The law does not bar insulin users from driving taxis (providing there are fewer than nine seats); however, some taxi licensing authorities do.

'I have been driving for 20 years and had Type 1 diabetes for 10 years. I usually test my blood before driving, but it was only a short journey and I was late. Work had been awful and I had grabbed a sandwich on the run. I usually get warnings of hypos but I was in such a rush I didn't notice that my sugar had dropped. I got confused and couldn't decide which turnoff to take at the roundabout. I just kept driving round and round the roundabout. Luckily a police car arrived stopped me, they realised that I wasn't OK and I managed to tell them that I had diabetes. I had glucose in the glove compartment and the police patiently fed me glucose tablets and contacted the school to hold onto the kids. I was so lucky, I didn't hurt anyone and I wasn't prosecuted.'

Advice regarding driving if the patient is on medication which can cause hypoglycaemia

- Measure BG level before getting into the car.
- Do not drive if BG is <4 mmol/L.
- Keep rapid-acting carbohydrates at hand.
- Prior to driving if BG is less than 5 mmol/L have a snack containing carbohydrates.
- Stop every 2 hours to recheck BG levels and take slow-acting carbohydrates as required to keep blood glucose above 5 mmol/L.

If a hypo occurs:

- Pull over to the side of the road.
- Take keys out of the ignition.
- Move into the passenger seat.
- Treat the hypo.
- Recheck BG level.
- Do not drive for 45 minutes once blood glucose is above 5 mmol/L.

Failure to do this is legally seen as being under the influence of drugs (DAFNE, 2007).

Situations which make diabetes more difficult to control – hospital admission or illness

Many people with diabetes fear hospital admission. The Working Party for Improving Emergency and Inpatient Care for People with Diabetes (2007) collated patient experiences under the headings of disempowerment, limited access to food and medication, staff's lack of knowledge and experience, medicine mismanagement and lack of communication. I have included at least one quote from each category:

'I was put on "sliding scale" and after the operation I asked to return to my usual regime. The request was refused . . . I was told that as it was a bank holiday, if my levels were still high on Tuesday they would call somebody in. So I made the decision to discharge myself on the Saturday. Within 24 hours of being at home my levels were back to where they were before the operation.'

'On several occasions I found food delivered to eat when blood sugar was high and no insulin had been given and the insulin dose was not given for another hour . . . had to let the food get cold and wait for the insulin . . . On other occasions insulin had been given when blood sugar was at a moderate or low level an there was no food in sight.'

'Metformin was handed out sometime mid morning and evening, of course nowhere near injection/meal times.'

'I had frequent hypos and staff were always too busy to get me bread until they finished what they were doing. Hypos were always deemed to be my fault. I wasn't allowed to reduce my insulin.'

'I became very nervous of treatment I was receiving as within the ward it was obvious that the left hand did not know what the right hand was doing . . . . I felt like a hospital tick box, confused and feeling very ill and scared.'

There were some positive experiences and these were usually when patients were allowed some control of their condition and or when the diabetes team were involved. Recommendations from the patients included:

'If the NHS wishes to save money, it perhaps should first look at diabetics who do not want to stay in hospital for yet another night, but who are unable to get out because their insulin is impounded, with nobody with sufficient authority to return diabetic control to the patient.'

'Incentives to keep experienced and committed nurses in clinical care rather than management needs consideration as well as more trained specialist diabetic nurses with time to train and respond to ward and community situations.'

Illness can have dramatic effects on diabetes control. During infection, levels of counter-regulatory hormones, for example adrenaline, noradrenaline, glucagon, cortisol and growth hormone rise. These hormones act directly on the liver, stimulating glycogen and fat breakdown and causing BG to rise. In those without diabetes, increased insulin is produced and BG levels remain within the normal range. In those with diabetes, insulin levels cannot be increased resulting in hyperglycaemia; with type 1 diabetes, unless insulin doses are increased ketones may be produced due to a breakdown of fat and muscle. The accumulation of ketones is potentially dangerous and can lead to DKA.

'I felt so ill, I had diarrhoea and was sick a few times during the night. I thought that I'd had a dodgy curry after the pub last night. I rang in sick at work and just went back to bed, as I wasn't eating I didn't take any quick acting insulin, I'm not sure whether I had my long-acting insulin as I was a bit tipsy and I didn't test my blood as I was too rough. My girlfriend came back from work in the evening, my breathing was heavy and fast and I smelt of pear drops. She knew immediately what was wrong and called an ambulance. Hindsight is a great thing – obviously I should have tested injected extra insulin if my blood glucose was high.'

How should illness be managed?

People with type 1 diabetes are totally dependent on injected insulin. The accumulation of ketones is potentially dangerous and can lead to DKA. People with type 2 diabetes can produce some insulin of their own, although an increase in treatment is usually required during illness.

General advice (sick day rule advice)

- Discuss illness before it happens. Ideally, written information should be given.
- Seek prompt medical treatment, for example antibiotics for infections and paracetamol or aspirin to relieve pyrexia.
- Cough mixtures and cold remedies should be sugar free.
- If unable to eat normally, carbohydrates should be replaced with cereals, soups or liquid carbohydrate. Withholding carbohydrate because of high BG levels may make ketosis worse.
- Take plenty of sugar-free liquids.
- If vomiting and unable to tolerate liquid carbohydrate, medical attention should be sought.
- Tablets and insulin should be continued with the exception of metformin if diarrhoea occurs.
- It is likely that the dose of insulin and/or tablets will need increasing during illness, with care not to exceed the maximum recommended dose for tablets. Some people treated with tablets may require treatment with insulin for the duration of the illness.
- BG (particularly if treated with insulin) should be tested more frequently, at least four times a day.

The aim is to prevent DKA. Historically, patients have been told to test blood glucose levels before each meal and before bed and to inject usual doses of insulin with additional doses of rapid-acting insulin at these times if BG is greater than 13 mmol/L. Urine or blood ketones are tested if BG is 17 mmol/L or above. Ideally, the doses of extra rapid-acting insulin were based on total daily insulin requirements but usually ranged from 6–10 units, with 10 units given if BG was 20 or above or if moderate or large levels of ketones were present in the urine or blood (Jerreat, 2003).

If the patient is DAFNE trained, the amount of additional quick-acting insulin is dependent on the level of ketones. If ketones are ≤trace or <1.5 mmol/L on an optium meter, glucose and ketones are tested every 4–6 hours and corrective doses of insulin are used (1 unit of insulin to reduce BG by 2–3 mmol/L, although it is acknowledged that slightly higher doses may be required). If ketones are moderate in the urine or >1.5 mmol/L in the blood and BG is greater than 13 mmol/L, 10% of the total daily dose of insulin is given every 2 hours in addition to the usual background quick-acting insulin needed to cover carbohydrate eaten in meals. If ketones are ≥3 mmol/L or large, 20% of the total daily dose should be given every 2 hours (in addition to usual doses).

'My asthma was bad again and so my GP gave me 40 mg prednisolone. I've had them so many times before that when she asked me if I knew how to take them and their effects I said I knew . . . but that was before. I've got diabetes now. My blood went up to 30!'

Large doses of steroids increase BG dramatically. 'Sick day rule advice' should be followed, as above, and if steroids are used frequently, it is vital that the patient be advised on how to increase his/her tablet or insulin regimes.

Pregnancy

There is insufficient space to discuss gestational diabetes and its management; more information can be found in *NICE Clinical Guideline 63 Diabetes in Pregnancy* (2008b). The care of women who have pre-existing diabetes is discussed here. The control and management of diabetes has been found to impact significantly on both the mother and the baby (see Box 13.4). Providing appropriate care and advice is therefore imperative in improving the outcomes for women who are diabetic and their babies.

Box 13.4   Key findings of Confidential Enquiry into Maternal and Child Health (CEMACH), 2005.

1. Babies of women with diabetes have four times greater risk of perinatal mortality and three times greater risk of congenital malformation.
2. Women with Type 2 diabetes are more likely to live in a deprived area, come from an ethnic minority, less likely to have received pre-conception counselling, less likely to have taken folic acid.
3. Women with diabetes are poorly prepared for pregnancy; only 39% took folic acid pre-conception, only 35% had pre-pregnancy counselling.
4. Only 38% had an HbA1c <7% by 13 weeks' gestation.
5. There is a 36% pre-term delivery rate and 67% caesarean-section rate for women with diabetes.
6. Over 50% singleton babies' birth weights were over the 90th centile for birth weight. A twofold increase in the incidence of shoulder dystocia, and Erb's palsy was increased tenfold.
7. One-third of babies were admitted to neonatal units.

Risks to the baby

- Congenital abnormality – usually heart, central nervous system, face, genito-urinary or gastrointestinal tract
- Spontaneous abortion/miscarriage
- Macrosomia (increasing risk of emergency caesarean section, birth trauma, birth asphyxia, still birth and hypoglycaemia)
- Still birth (four times increased risk)
- Hypoglycaemia (hyperinsulinaemia, β-cell hyperplasia)
- Small for dates (poor placental blood supply)
- Maternal ketoacidosis (foetal mortality rate 50%)
- Respiratory distress syndrome
- Inheritance of diabetes – type 1: 6% father, 1% mother, 30% both; type 2: 15% one parent, 75% both parents

Risks to the mother

- Nausea/vomiting – ketoacidosis risk (type 1)
- Hypoglycaemia – care with driving
- Pre-eclampsia (10% compared to 4% in general population)
- Ketoacidosis if dexamethasone is used in pre-term labour
- Increased mortality (0.1% compared to 0.001% in the general population)
- Increased caesarean-section rate (earlier induction may contribute)

Pre-pregnancy advice/counselling

- Aim for HbA1c within normal range (may need insulin in type 2).
- 5 mg folic acid pre-conception until 13 weeks pregnant (prescription only drug). The risk of neural tube defects is higher in women with diabetes.
- Check retina; progression of retinopathy common due to improved control and pregnancy hormones.
- Reduce alcohol/stop smoking.
- Check urea and electrolytes (if creatinine >250, only 50% pregnancies result in successful outcome).
- Stop ACE I, sartans, beta-blockers and substitute methylodopa, nifedipine or labetalol and stop statins.
- Contact diabetes team as soon as pregnancy is confirmed.

Antenatal care (based on NICE (2008b) and local protocol)

- SMBG at least four times per day. Aim for pre-meal BG of between 3.9–5.9 and less than 7.8 mmol/L 1 hour after food.
- Folic acid.
- Change antihypertensives as necessary.
- Change from long-acting analogue to isophane.

- Stop sulphonylureas other than glibenclamide (metformin can be continued). Likely to need basal bolus regime. CSSI pump may be necessary for some women with type 1 diabetes.
- Glucagon kit and glucogel provided and ketone strips if type 1 diabetes.
- See at least every 2 weeks for insulin/medication adjustment, weight and urine estimation. Aim for weight gain of less than 15 kg.
- HbA1c or fructosamine estimation monthly.
- Eye photography each trimester.
- Scans (viability/dating, nuchal translucency for Downs at 11–14 weeks, anomaly at 23 weeks, detailed cardiac scan at 24 weeks, foetal growth scans every 4 weeks from 28–36 weeks).

Labour

- Intravenous insulin (10% dextrose 100 mL/h) at hourly rate of insulin based on daily insulin requirements (total daily dose divided by 24).
- Pre-pregnancy insulin dose to be commenced post delivery, although further reduction may be needed during breastfeeding.

'I used gliclazide and metformin before I was pregnant but stopped gliclazide and used insulin during pregnancy. I intended to breastfeed but was told that if I did I might need to have insulin if my blood tests are high as gliclazide is unsafe.'

Conclusion

This chapter has examined the treatment and management strategies currently recommended for type 1 and type 2 diabetes. Empowering the patient to self-manage their condition relies on patients having access to and understanding of the best screening and treatments and help to set relevant and achievable goals. The nurse is in an excellent position to help patients to set goals, provide practical help and advice and assist patients to access structured education, exercise programmes and specialised care when necessary.

Unfortunately, word 'restriction' has not allowed me to include all subjects relating to diabetes or to provide detail on insulin injection devices and adjustment. I recommend the Diabetes UK website: www.diabetes.org.uk.

References

Association of British Clinical Diabetologists (ABCD) (2006) *920060 Guidelines for the Management of Hyperglycaemic Emergencies (Diabetic Ketoacidosis and Hyperosmolar Non-Ketotic State) in Adults.* Available at: http//www.diabetologists.org.uk (accessed 30 September 2008).

ACE Inhibitors in Diabetic Nephropathy Trialist Group (2001) Should all patients with type 1 diabetes and microalbuminuria receive ACE inhibitors. A meta-analysis of individual patient data, *Annals of International Medicine*, 134, pp. 370–379.

Anderson, S. K., Gjedsted, J., Christiansen, C. & Tonnesen, E. (2004) The roles of insulin and hyperglycaemia in sepsis pathogenesis, *Journal of Leukocyte Biology*, pp. 413–421.

Alberti, K. G. M. M. (1974) Diabetic ketoacidosis – aspects of management. In: *Tenth Advanced Medicine Symposium* (ed J. G. Ledingham). Pitman Medical, Tunbridge Wells, pp. 68–82.

Bakris, G. L., Williams, M., Dworkin, L. *et al.* (2000) Preserving renal function in adults with hypertension and diabetes: a consensus approach. National Kidney Foundation Hypertension and Diabetes Executive Committees Working Group, *American Journal of Kidney Disease*, 200(36), pp. 646–661.

Bell, D. S. H. (1996) Alcohol and the NIDDM patient, *Diabetes Care*, 19, pp. 509–513.

Belch, J., MacCuish, A., Campbell, I. *et al.* (2008) The prevention of arterial disease and diabetes (POPADAD) trial: factorial randomised placebo controlled trial of aspirin and antioxidants in patients with diabetes and asymptomatic peripheral arterial disease, *British Medical Journal*, 337, a1840.

Confidential Enquiry into Maternal and Child Health (CEMACH) (2005) *Pregnancy in Women with Type 1 and Type 2 Diabetes*. CEMACH, London.

DAFNE (2007) *DAFNE curriculum for people with type 1 diabetes*, T02.002, 9 May.

Delahanty, L., Simkins, S. W. & Camelon, K. (1993) Expanded role of the dietitian in the Diabetes Control and Complications Trial: implications for clinical practice, *Journal of the American Dietetic Association*, 93, pp. 758–764.

Davies, M. J., Heller, S., Skinner, T. C. *et al.* (2008) Effectiveness of the diabetes education and self-management for ongoing and newly diagnosed (DESMOND) programme for people with newly diagnosed type 2 diabetes: cluster randomised control trial, *British Medical Journal*, 336, pp. 491–495.

Department of Health (2001) *National Service Framework for Diabetes – Standards*. HMSO, London. Available at: http//www.doh.gov.uk/nsf/diabetes (accessed 16 April 2010).

Department of Health (2003) National Service Framework for Diabetes – Delivery Strategy. HMSO, London. Available at: http//www.doh.gov.uk/nsf/diabetes (accessed 16 April 2010).

Department of Health and Diabetes UK (2005) *Structured Patient Education in Diabetes. Report from the Patient Education Working Group*. Department of Health, London.

Diabetes Control and Complications Trial Research Group (1993) The effect of intensive treatment of diabetes on the development and progression of long-term complications in insulin-dependent diabetes mellitus, *New England Journal of Medicine*, 329, pp. 977–986.

Diabetes UK (2009) *Driving and Diabetes*. Diabetes UK Information. Available at: https://www.diabetes.org.uk/OnlineShop/Legal-Issues/ (accessed 26 June 2010).

Edmonds, M. E. & Foster, A. V. M. (2000) *Managing the Diabetic Foot*. Blackwell Science, Oxford.

Edmonds, M. E. & Foster, A. V. M. (2002) The diabetic foot. In: *Oxford Textbook of Endocrinology and Diabetes* (eds A.H. Wass, S.M. Shalet, E. Gale & S.A. Amiel). Oxford University Press, Oxford.

Elrishi, M. A., Khunti, K., Jarvis, J. & Davies, M. J. (2007) The dipeptidyl-peptidase-4 (DPP-4) inhibitors: a new class of oral therapy for patients with type 2 diabetes mellitus, *Practical Diabetes International*, 24(9), pp. 474–482.

Fisher, M. & Shaw, K. M. (2006) *Diabetes and the Heart in Diabetes Chronic Complications* (2nd edn) (eds K.M. Shaw & M.H. Cummings). Wiley & Sons Ltd., West Sussex.

Funnell, M. & Anderson, R. (2004) Empowerment and self-management of diabetes, *Clinical Diabetes*, 22(3), pp. 123–127.

de Galan, B. E., Schouwenberg, B. J. J. W., Tack, C. J. & Smits, P. (2006) Pathophysiology and management of recurrent hypoglycaemia and hypoglycaemia unawareness in diabetes, *The Netherlands Journal of Medicine*, 64(8), pp. 269–279.

Goh, K. L. & Tooke, J. (2002) Abnormalities of the microvasculature. In: *Oxford Textbook of Endocrinology and Diabetes* (eds A.H. Wass, S.M. Shalet, E. Gale & S.A. Amiel). Oxford University Press, Oxford.

Haffner, S. M., Lehto, S., Ronnemaa, T. *et al.* (1998) Mortality from coronary heart disease insubjects with type 2 diabetes and in nondiabetic subjects with and without prior myocardial infarction, *New England Journal of Medicine*, 339(4), pp. 229–234.

Heart Outcomes Prevention Evaluation (HOPE) Study Investigators (2000) Effects of ramipril on cardiovascular and microvascular outcomes in people with diabetes mellitus: results of the HOPE study and MICRO-HOPE substudy, *Lancet*, 355(9200), pp. 253–259.

Hertz, R. P., Unger, A. N. & Lustik, M. B. (2005) Adherence with pharmacotherapy for Type 2 diabetes: a retrospective cohort study of adults with employer-sponsored health insurance, *Clinical Therapeutics*, 27(7), pp. 1064–1073.

Higgins, B. (2008) Type 2 *Diabetes, National Clinical Guideline for the Management in Primary and Secondary Care (update NICE Guidelines, 2002)*. Available at: http://www. nice.org.uk/nicemedia/pdf/CG66NICEGuideline.pdf (accessed 16 April 2010).

Huriel, S., Orr, A., Arthur, M. *et al.* (1997) Diabetic ketoacidotic diabetes education and health beliefs, *Practical Diabetes International*, 14(1), pp. 9–11.

International Diabetes Federation (2001) Diabetes Atlas 2000. Available at: http://www. diabetesatlas.org/sites/default/files/IDF%20Diabetes%20Atlas-2000%20(1st%20edition).pdf (accessed 16 April 2010).

Jerreat, L. (2003) *Diabetes for Nurses*. Whurr Publishers, London.

Jerreat, L. (2009) Treatment of hyperglycaemia in patients with type 2 diabetes, *Nursing Standard*, 9 September, 24(1), pp. 50–57.

Karter, A. J., Chan, J., Parker, M. M. *et al.* (2006) Longitudinal study of new and prevalent use of self-monitoring of blood glucose, *Diabetes Care*, 29(8), pp. 1757–1763.

Kjeldsen, S. E., Hedner, T., Jamerson, K. *et al.* (1998) Home blood pressure in treated hypertensive subjects, *Hypertension*, 31, pp. 1014–1020.

Kinmond, K., McGee, P., Gough, S., Ashford, R. (2003) 'Loss of self': a psychosocial study of the quality of life of adults with diabetes ulceration, *Journal of Tissue Viability*, 13(1), pp. 6–16.

Kohner, E., Allwinkle, J., Andrews, R. *et al.* (1996) Report of the Visual Handicap Group, *Diabetic Medicine*, 13(Suppl 4) pp. S13–S26.

Kratz, M., Cullen, P., Kannenberg, F. *et al.* (2002) Effects of dietary fatty acids on the composition and oxidizability of low density lipoprotein, *European Journal Clinical Nutrition*, 56, pp. 72–81.

Lawton, J., Peel, E., Douglas, M. *et al.* (2004) 'Urine testing is a waste of time': newly diagnosed type 2 diabetes patients' perceptions of self-monitoring, *Diabetic Medicine*, 21(9), pp. 1045–1048.

Lefebvre, P. (2005) *Amputations Linked to Diabetes. Available at:* http://www.hospitalmanagement. net/features/features627 (accessed 9 November 2008).

McIntosh, A., Peters, J., Young, R. *et al.* (2003) *Prevention and Management of Foot Problems in Type 2 Diabetes: Clinical Guidelines and Evidence*. University of Sheffield, Sheffield. Available at: http://www.nice.org.uk/nicemedia/pdf/CG10fullguideline.pdf (accessed 9 November 2008).

MacIsaac, R. J. & Watts, G. F. (2006) Diabetes and the kidney. In: *Diabetes Chronic Complications* (2nd edn) (eds K. M. Shaw & M. H. Cummings). Wiley & Sons Ltd, West Sussex.

MacKinnon, J. R. & Forrester, J. V. (2002) Diabetic retinopathy. In: *Oxford Textbook of Endocrinology and Diabetes* (eds A. H. Wass, S. M. Shalet, E. Gale & S. A. Amiel). Oxford University Press, Oxford.

McAleese, J. (2006) Diabetic foot care in the secondary care setting, *Journal of Diabetes Nursing*, 10(9), pp. 346–349.

Martin, S., Schneider, B., Heinemann, L. *et al.* (2006) Self-monitoring of blood glucose in type 2 diabetes and long-term outcome: an epidemiological cohort study, *Diabetologia*, 49(2), pp. 271–278.

McArdle, P. (2007) *Your Food Choices and Diabetes. Food Fact Sheet*. The British Dietetic Association. Available at: http://www.bda.uk.com/foodfacts/Diabetes.pdf (accessed 16 April 2010).

McCarty, D. & Zimmet, P. (1994) *Diabetes 1994 to 2010: Global Estimates and Projections*. International Diabetes Institute, Melbourne.

Nathan, D. M., Buse, J. B., Davidson, M. B *et al.* (2006) Management of hyperglycemia in type 2 diabetes: a consensus algorithm for the initiation and adjustment of therapy, *Diabetes Care*, 29, pp. 1963–1972.

National Institute for Health and Clinical Excellence (NICE) (2002) *Guidance on Surgery for Morbid Obesity 2002/041*. 19 July. Available at: www.nice.org.uk (accessed 16 April 2010).

National Institute for Health and Clinical Excellence (NICE) (2004) *Type 2 Diabetes Prevention and Management of Foot Problems. Clinical Guideline*. Available at: www.nice.org.uk. (accessed 10 January 2004).

National Institute for Health and Clinical Excellence (NICE) (2008a) Clinical Guidelines 66: Management of Type 2 Diabetes. May. Available at: www.nice.org.uk (accessed 16 April 2010).

National Institute for Health and Clinical Excellence (NICE) (2008b) *Diabetes in Pregnancy Management of Diabetes and its Complications from Pre-Conception to the Post-Natal Period*. NICE Guideline 63. Available at: www.nice.org.uk (accessed 16 April 2010).

National Institute for Health and Clinical Excellence (NICE) (2009) *Type 2 Diabetes: Newer Agents for Blood Glucose Control in Type 2 Diabetes. National Institute for Health and Clinical Excellence Short Clinical Guideline 87*. Available at: www.nice.org.uk (accessed 16 April 2010).

Nutrition Sub-Committee of the Diabetes Care Advisory Committee of Diabetes UK (2003) The dietitian's challenge: the implementation of nutritional advice for people with diabetes. The British Dietetic Association Ltd., *Journal of Human Dietetics*, 16, pp. 421–452.

Odegard, P. S. & Capoccia, K. (2007) *Medication Taking and Diabetes: a Systematic Review of the Literature*. University of Washington School of Pharmacy, Washington. Available at: http://www.ncbi.nlm.nih.gov/pubmed/18057270 (accessed 16 April 2010).

Pociot, F. & Nerup, J. (2002) Genetics of type 1 (insulin dependent diabetes mellitus). In: *Oxford Textbook of Endocrinology and Diabetes* (eds A. H. Wass, S. M. Shalet, E. Gale & S. A. Amiel). Oxford University Press, Oxford.

Royal College of Physicians (2008) *Type 2 Diabetes. National Clinical Guideline for Management in Primary and Secondary Care*. The National Collaborating Centre for Chronic Conditions, London.

Shillitoe, R. (1994) *Counselling People with Diabetes*. The British Psychological Society, Exeter.

Shotliff, K. & Duncan, G. (2006) Diabetes and the eye. In: *Diabetes Chronic Complications* (2nd edn) (eds K.M. Shaw & M.H. Cummings). Wiley & Sons Ltd, West Sussex.

Stevens, R. J., Kothari, V., Adler, A. l. *et al.* (2001) The UKPDS risk engine: a model for risk of coronary heart disease in type II diabetes (UPDS 56), *Clinical Science*, 101(6), pp. 671–679.

Tesfaye, S., Stevens, L. K., Stephenson, J. M. *et al.* (1996) The prevalence of diabetic neuropathy and its relation to glycaemic control and potential risk factors; the EURODIAB IDDM Complications Study, *Diabetologia*, 39, pp. 1377–1384.

Tesfaye, S. (2002) Diabetic neuropathy. In: *Oxford Textbook of Endocrinology and Diabetes* (eds A. H. Wass, S. M. Shalet, E. Gale & S. A. Amiel). Oxford University Press, Oxford.

Trevisan, R. & Viberti, G. (2002) Diabetic nephropathy. In: *Oxford Textbook of Endocrinology and Diabetes* (eds A. H. Wass, S. M. Shalet, E. Gale & S. A. Amiel). Oxford University Press, Oxford.

United Kingdom Prospective Diabetes Study Group (UKPDS) (1995) 13: Relative efficacy of randomly allocated diet, sulphonlyurea, insulin or metformin in patients with newly diagnosed non-insulin dependent diabetes followed for 3 years, *British Medical Journal*, 310, pp. 83–88.

United Kingdom Prospective Diabetes Study (UKPDS) group (1998) Intensive blood glucose control with sulphonlyureas or insulin compared with conventional treatment and risk of complications in patients with type 2 diabetes (UKPDS 33), *Lancet*, 352, pp. 837–853.

Valk, G. D., Kriegsman, D. M. & Assendelft, W. J. (2005) Patient education for preventing diabetic foot ulceration, *Cochrane Database of Systematic Reviews*, (4), CD001488.

Watkins, P. J. & Edmonds, M. E. (1997) Clinical features of diabetic neuropathy. In: *Textbook of Diabetes* (2nd edn) (eds J. C. Pickup & G. Williams). Blackwell Science, Oxford.

Williams, G. & Pickup, J. C. (2004) *Handbook of Diabetes* (3rd edn). Blackwell Publishing, Oxford.

Williamson, D. F., Thompson, D. J., Thun, M. *et al.* (2000) Intentional weight loss and mortality among overweight individuals with diabetes, *Diabetes Care*, 23, pp. 1499–1504.

World Health Organisation Department of Noncommunicable Disease Surveillance (1999) *Report of a WHO Consultation. Definition, Diagnosis and Classification of Diabetes Mellitus and its complications. Part 1 Diagnosis and Classification of Diabetes Mellitus*. World Health Organisation, Geneva.

Working Party for Improving Emergency and Inpatient Care for People with Diabetes. Diabetes UK (2007) *Collation of Inpatient Experiences*. Available at: http://www.diabetes.org.uk/ Professionals/Publications-reports-and-resources/Reports-statistics-and-case-studies/Reports/ Improving-Emergency-and-Inpatient-care-for-People-with-Diabetes/ (accessed 16 April 2010).

Yorkshire and Humber Public Health Observatory (2008) Diabetes Attributable Deaths: Estimating the Excess Deaths among People with Diabetes. Available at: http://www.yhpho.org.uk/ resource/item.aspx?RID=9909 (accessed 26 June 2010).

Index

Note: Locators followed by *b*, *f* and *t* refer to boxes, figures and tables respectively.

acarbose, 258
accept reality of loss, 92–3
acceptance, 90, 138
  and adaptation, 64–5
accuhaler, 243
ACE inhibitors (ACE I), 200, 250, 266
  and angiotensin receptor blockers, 201–2
  doses in heart failure, 202*t*
acupuncture, 39–40, 157
adaptation modes, 53
adaptive decision making, 125–6
ADHD. *See* attention deficit hyperactivity disorder
  (ADHD)
affective disorders, 69
An Ageing World: 2008, 4
airway inflammation, 239–40
alcoholic cardiomyopathy, 196
aldosterone antagonists, 203–4
ambulance services, 15
amlodipine, 206
amyotrophic lateral sclerosis, 88
anger, 89
angiotensin receptor blocker (ARB), 200, 201–2,
  266
  doses in heart failure, 202*t*
anticoagulants, 205
anti-depressants, 142–3
antihyperglycaemic medication, 248, 257
  acarbose, 258
  dipeptidyl-peptidase-4 (DPP4) inhibitors, 258
  glucagon-like peptide-1 agonists (GLP-1), 259
  glucose-lowering medication, 259
  metformin, 257
  rapid-acting insulin secretagogue, 257–8
  sulphonylureas (SU), 257
  thiazolidinedione (glitazones), 258
antiplatelet therapy, 268–9
anxiety, 232
  and depression, 197
anxiolytics, 165–6
aspirin, 250
assistive technology, 14
asthma, 228, 236, 239*t*, 244
  control of, 240
  living with, 240–44
  pathophysiology and diagnosis, 238–40
atenolol, 203

attention deficit hyperactivity disorder (ADHD),
  38
autonomic neuropathy, 267

BACP. *See* British Association for Counselling and
  Psychotherapy (BACP)
basal bolus, 262*f*
behaviour, emotions and thinking (BET), 68
bereavement
  journey, 94
  model, 89
  theory, 103
BET. *See* Behaviour, emotions and thinking (BET)
beta-blockers, 202–3
  dosage in heart failure, 203*t*
BHF. *See* British Heart Foundation (BHF)
Bismarck system, 9
bisoprolol, 203
blister packs, 207
blocks in practitioner, 97–8
blood glucose (BG), 249
blood pressure (BP), 249
BMA. *See* British Medical Association (BMA)
BNF. *See* British National Formulary (BNF)
BNP. *See* B-type natriuretic peptide (BNP)
Bowlby's attachment theory, 93
breathing exercises, 159–60
breathlessness, 158, 230–31, 231*t*, 232, 235
  on exertion, 227–8
  non-pharmacological interventions for
    breathing exercises, 159–60
    chest physiotherapy, 164
    environment, 161
    NEMS, 165
    oxygen, 161–2
    pacing and planning, 162–4
    physical exercise, 162
    positioning, 161
    psychological management, 164
    pursed-lip breathing, 160
    removing secretions, 160–61
    saline nebulisers, 162
  pharmacological interventions for
    anxiolytics, 165–6
    bronchodilators, 165
    opioids, 165
    steroids, 165

British Association for Counselling and Psychotherapy (BACP), 97, 143
British Guidelines on Asthma Management in Adults (BTS/SIGN, 2008b, 241*f*
British Heart Foundation (BHF), 166, 195, 209
British Household Panel Survey, 5
British Lung Foundation, 225
British Medical Association (BMA), 141
British National Formulary (BNF), 191, 205
British Thoracic Society, 234
brittle asthmatics, 240
bronchitis, exacerbations of, 228
bronchodilators, 165, 236
BTS and Scottish Intercollegiate Guidelines Network (SIGN) guidelines (2008a), 239, 240
BTS report, 225, 226
B-type natriuretic peptide (BNP), 198
budesonide, 244
bumetanide, 204
bupropion (zyban), 235

calcium channel blockers, 206
cannabis, 227
cardiac cachexia, 197
cardiac electrophysiologist, 208
cardiac function, 197
cardiovascular complications, 267
cardiovascular risk, 268–9
Care Quality Commission, 14
care services improvement partnership (CSIP), 140
carer
    act, 12
    financial benefits for, 12
Cartesian dualism, 36–7
carvedilol, 203
case management
    aim of, 23–4
    approaches, 27–9
        core models, 27, 28*t*
        CPA and LTC agenda, 29
    case finding
        case managers and PCTs, 31
        Combined Predictive Model, 32
        goal of, 31
        PARR case finding algorithm, 32*t*
        PARR tool, 31–2
    case managers, 26, 29–30
    community matrons, 26
    evaluations of
        evercare pilot sites, 26–7
        systematic Cochrane review, 27
    health and social care infrastructure
        financial incentives, 31
        links with secondary care, 30–31
    LTC case management models, 24*t*, 26
    mental health teams, 26
    risk, 32–3
        EBP, 33
    structure
        caseload size, 30
        telemedicine, 24, 25*b*
        virtual community wards, 25*b*
case managers, 26, 29–30
    psychosocial interventions, 30
caseload size, 30

catastrophising/awfulising, 106
CBT. *See* cognitive behavioural therapy (CBT)
β-cell insufficiency, 248
CFS. *See* chronic fatigue syndrome (CFS)
Change4Life, 6
Changes To Primary Care Trusts, 16
changing faces, 52
chest physiotherapy, 164
chronic cough, 227
chronic fatigue syndrome (CFS), 37
chronic illness, 53
chronic inflammation, 227
chronic obstructive pulmonary disease (COPD), 5–6, 111, 124, 135
    living with, 230–32
        anxiety, 232
        MRC dyspnoea scale, 231*t*
        nurses, 231
        smoking cessation, 231
    mechanisms, 227
    NICE guidelines, 236
    pathophysiology and diagnosis, 227–30
        clinical features of, 227–8
        GOLD spirometric criteria, 229*t*
        mechanisms and manifestations of, 228*f*
        standard spirometry manoeuvre, 229
    pharmacological management, 236–8
chronic stress, biopsychosocial effects, 150–51
    physiological effects of, 151*t*
    signs and symptoms, 150*t*
cigarette smoking, 233
co-creating health, 14
cognitive appraisals, 74
cognitive behavioural perspectives, 104
    catastrophising/awfulising, 106
    mind-reading/jumping to conclusions, 106
    personalisation and labelling, 106–7
    selective abstractions, 106
cognitive behavioural therapy (CBT), 71, 139
Colin Murray Parkes work, 90–92
combined predictive model, 32
Commission for Healthcare Audit and Inspection, 13
Commissioning a Patient-Led NHS, 16
common sense model, 122
communication skills, 98–100
    body language and postures, 99
    non-verbal communication, 98–100
    prolonged steadfast eye contact, 99
    voice tone, 100
community matrons, 16, 26
    policy for, 30
community pharmacists, 206
complementary therapies, 39–40
compulsory altruism, 12
confidence and belief, loss of, 70–71
conflict theorists, 46–7
    affective neutrality, 47
    epidemiological evidence, 47
    US system of care, 47
congruence, 95, 96–7
consumerism, 58–9
continuous subcutaneous infusion of insulin (CSSI), 262*f*
COPD. *See* chronic obstructive pulmonary disease (COPD)

coping, 55–6, 122–3
coronary heart disease (CHD), 13, 231
counselling skills, 108
  cognitive behavioural perspectives, 104
    catastrophising/awfulising, 106
    mind-reading/jumping to conclusions, 106
    personalisation and labelling, 106–7
    selective abstractions, 106
  Colin Murray Parkes work, 90–92
    disorganisation and despair, 91
    emotional pining and longing, 91
    grief phases, 91*f*
    numbness, 91
    reorganisation and recovery, 91–2
  Elizabeth Kübler-Ross theory, 89–90
    acceptance, 90
    anger, 89
    bargaining, 90
    denial and isolation, 89
    depression, 90
    grief stages, 89*f*
  Grief theory and adapting to change, 87–9
    adjustment and accommodation, 89
    health care professional, 87
    model of bereavement, 89
  J. William Worden contribution, 92–4
    accept reality of loss, 92–3
    adjust to environment, 93
    bereavement journey, 94
    emotionally relocating, 93–4
    expressing emotional affect, 93
  person-centred perspectives, 94
    blocks in practitioner, 97–8
    challenging skills, 102
    communication skills, 98–100
    congruence, 96–7
    empathy, 95
    probing skills, 102
    reflecting skills, 101–2
    unconditional positive regard, 95–6
  psychodynamic perspectives, 102
    denial, 103
    displacement, 104
    projection, 104
    regression, 103
CSIP. *See* care services improvement partnership (CSIP)
cystic fibrosis (CF), 226

DAFNE, 251, 252*t*, 253
Darzi report, 3
day-to-day care, 120
DCCT (type 1), 267
deaf culture, 51*b*
death, 5–6
  rates, 226
decision-making, 129, 130*t*
deep breathing, 152
deep muscle relaxation, 152
degranulation, 239–40
denial, 103
  and isolation, 89
Department of Health and Physical Activity, 166
depression, 39, 66–70, 90, 116–17, 140–44
  debilitating and isolating illness, 141–2
  national quality indicator, 141

NICE guidelines, 141
  psychological distress, 141*t*
  strategies for
    exercise, 143
    social interaction, 143–4
    talking therapies, 142–3
    validation and education, 142
  symptoms of, 140*t*
DESMOND, 251, 252*t*
deviance, 50–51
  behaviour, 50
  chronic illness, 53
  deaf culture, 51*b*
  disability, 51
  oppression paradigm, 50–51
  paradigm, 50–51
  primary and secondary, 50
  radical disability movement, 51
  rejecting label of, 50*b*
diabetes, 247
  acute complications
    hyperosmolar non-ketotic coma (HONK), 272
    hypoglycaemia, 272–3
  antihyperglycaemic medication, 257
    acarbose, 258
    dipeptidyl-peptidase-4 (DPP4) inhibitors, 258
    glucagon-like peptide-1 agonists (GLP-1), 259
    glucose-lowering medication, 259
    metformin, 257
    rapid-acting insulin secretagogue, 257–8
    sulphonylureas (SU), 257
    thiazolidinedione (glitazones), 258
  chronic complications of, 263–4
    cardiovascular risk, 268–9
    damage to feet, 269–71
    diabetic retinopathy (DR), 264–5
    hypertension, 268
    macrovascular disease, 267–8
    microvascular disease, 264
    nephropathy, 265–6
    neuropathy, 266–7
  diagnosis, 248–9
  diet, 254–6
  driving, 273–4
  education, 250–52
  exercise, 256
  hospital admission, 275–6
  insulin, treatment with, 259–63
  mellitus, 247
  NSF, 13
  pregnancy, 277–9
  self-monitoring of blood glucose (SMBG), 252–4
  symptoms, 249
  treatment of, 249–50
  type 1 diabetes, 247–8
  type 2 diabetes, 248, 254
Diabetes Control and Complications trial – Type 1 (DCCT), 249
diabetic foods, 255
diabetic foot, 270*t*
diabetic ketoacidosis (DKA), 271–2
diabetic retinopathy (DR), 264–5
diastolic dysfunction, 200
diet and nutrition, 236, 254
digoxin, 205

dilated cardiomyopathy, 194, 196
dipeptidyl-peptidase-4 (DPP4) inhibitors, 258
disability, 51
Disability Living Allowance and Attendance
    Allowance, 215
Disease Management Clinics, 178
disease trajectories, 125–6
disorganisation and despair, 91
displacement, 104
distal symmetrical neuropathy, 267
district nursing service, 9
diuretics, 204–5, 206–7
DKA. *See* diabetic ketoacidosis (DKA)
doctor–patient relationship
    conflict theorists, 46–7
        affective neutrality, 47
        epidemiological evidence, 47
        US system of care, 47
    negotiation model
        compensation, 48
        formal contractual relationship, 48
        social characteristics, 47–8
    sick role, 45–6
        rights and obligations, 46
doctors and nurses, 59–60
domiciliary services, 10–11
doses, 187
drug effect, 187
drug interactions, 187
dumping diabetes, 111
dyslipidaemia, 248
dyspnoea. *See* breathlessness

EBP. *See* evidence based practice
    (EBP)
eformoterol (Symbicort), 244
e-health information, 49
ejection fraction, 200
Elizabeth Kübler-Ross theory, 89–90
emotional management, 127
emotional pining and longing, 91
emotional strategies
    acceptance, 138
    cognitive behavioural therapy, 139
    self-efficacy, 139
emotionally relocating, 93–4
empathetic understanding, 124
empathy, 95
emphysema, 111
end-stage renal failure (ESRF), 266
environment, 161
epirubicin, 196
eplerenone, 204
EPP. *See* expert patients programme (EPP)
ESC. *See* European Society of Cardiology (ESC)
ethnic communities, 7
ethnic groups and LTC, 7
etiologic trait approach, 72
European Society of Cardiology (ESC), 210
evercare pilot sites, 26–7
evidence-based medicine or care, 37, 39
evidence based practice (EBP), 33
exercise, 138, 143, 162
    benefits of, 256*t*
    and endurance programme, 236

expert patient
    community nurse visit, 42*b*–43*b*
    concept, 14
expert patients programme (EPP), 110, 127, 192
expressing emotional affect, 93

facial disfigurement, 52
fatigue, 135–9
    COPD, 135
    emotional strategies
        acceptance, 138
        cognitive behavioural therapy, 139
        self-efficacy, 139
    frustration, 135–6
    invisibility of, 136
    problem-based strategies
        exercise, 138
        pacing, 137–8
        rest, 138
    RhA, 135
financial incentives, 31
fluticasone, 243
formoterol, 238
frustration, 135–6
funding model, 12–13
furosemide, 204

GDP per capita, 9
general health questionnaire (GHQ-12), 77
    scoring, 77–8
GHQ-12. *See* general health questionnaire (GHQ-12)
glomerular filtration rate (GFR), 266
glucagon-like peptide-1 agonists (GLP-1), 259
glucose-lowering medication, 259
GOLD international COPD Guidelines, 228–30
GOLD spirometric criteria for COPD severity, 229*t*
GP drug prescription, 206
Grief Counselling and Grief Therapy, 92
Grief theory
    adapting to change, 87–9
    dual process model of bereavement, 89
    phases, 91*f*
    stages, 89*f*
guided visual imagery, 152

HADS. *See* hospital anxiety and depression scale
    (HADS)
HbA1c, 253
health care professionals, 87, 124–5
    partnership with, 131
health practitioner, 75–6
heart failure, management, 194
    aetiology, 195–6
        alcoholic cardiomyopathy, 196
        dilated cardiomyopathy, 196
        heart muscle function, 196
        muscular dystrophy, 196
        peripartum cardiomyopathy, 195–6
        thyrotoxicosis, 196
        viral myocarditis, 195
    causes of, 195*t*
    concordance to patient, 205–7
        blister packs, 207
        calcium channel blockers, 206
        community pharmacists, 206

diuretics, 206–7
  GP drug prescription, 206
device therapy, 207–9
  ICD for primary prevention, 208*t*
  pacemaker, 207
diagnosis, 198–200
  blood samples, 198
  diastolic dysfunction, 200
  ejection fraction, 200
  24 hour Holter monitoring, 200
  recommendations for, 199*f*
epidemiology, 195
organising services, 217
  nursing assessment, 219*t*
  patient monitoring, 219–20
  patient pathways scheme, 218*f*
  specialist nurse interventions, 218
palliative care, 216
  symptoms control strategies, 217
patient education, 209, 210*t*
  diet, salt and fluid restrictions, 211–12
  driving and travel, 213–14
  exercise and sexual activity, 212–13
  monitoring signs and symptoms, 210–11
  pregnancy and contraception, 214
  prognosis, 210
  sleep and breathing disorders, 213
pharmacological treatment, 200
  ACE inhibitors and angiotensin receptor blockers, 201–2
  aldosterone antagonists, 203–4
  algorithm, 201*f*
  anticoagulants, 205
  beta-blockers, 202–3
  digoxin, 205
  diuretics, 204–5
supportive care to patients and carers, 214–16
symptoms and classification, 196–8
  anxiety and depression, 197
  cardiac cachexia, 197
  NYHA classification, 198*t*
  PND, 197
  SOB, 196
heart failure with preserved systolic function (HFPSF), 200
heart muscle function, 196
HFPSF. *See* heart failure with preserved systolic function (HFPSF)
High Quality Care for All, 6
high-risk population, 32–3
home oxygen order form (HOOF), 232–3
hospital anxiety and depression scale (HADS), 140
hospital-based care, 9
24 hour Holter monitoring, 200
House of Commons Health Committee, 7
huffing, 160
hyperglycaemia, 247
  unawareness, 272
hyperkalaemia, 204
hyperlipidaemia, 248
hyperosmolar non-ketotic coma (HONK), 272
hypertension, 248, 266, 268
hypertriglyceridaemia, 255
hypoglycaemia, 253, 272–3

ICD for primary prevention, 208*t*
ICD therapy. *See* implanted cardioverter defibrillator (ICD) therapy
illness
  behaviour approach, 72
  narratives, 121–2
  representation, 122
immunoglobulin E (IgE), 239
implanted cardioverter defibrillator (ICD) therapy, 208
income inequalities, 8
informal care, 11
inhaled corticosteroids, 238, 243*b*
injections and dietary management, 41
INR. *See* international normalised ratio (INR)
insulin, 260*f*
intensive and assertive community treatment (ACT), 28*t*
International Association for the Study of Pain, 154
International Federation of Clinical Chemistry and Laboratory Medicine (IFCC) standard, 250
international normalised ratio (INR), 205
Ipratropium bromide (Atrovent), 238

J. William Worden contribution, 92–4

Kaiser Permanente model, 15

labour, 279
LADA. *See* latent autoimmune disease in adults (LADA)
latent autoimmune disease in adults (LADA), 248
long-acting analogue, 261*f*
long-acting beta agonists (LABA), 238
long-term conditions (LTCs)
  global challenge, 4–5
  health care demand, 5–6
    cardiovascular diseases, 5–6
    Change4Life, 6
    chronic obstructive pulmonary disease, 5–6
    death, 5–6
    medical interventions, 5
  health care systems, 8–9
    bills, 9
    Bismarck system, 9
    district nursing service, 9
    GDP per capita, 9
    hospital-based care, 9
    political power, location of, 8*f*
  health inequalities, 6–8
    categories of explanation, 6–7
    ethnic groups and, 7
    housing conditions, 6–7
    income inequalities, 8
    racism, impact of, 8
    relative poverty, 8
    social exclusion, 8
    variations in health, 7
  home care, 9–11
    domiciliary services, 10–11
    formal help, 10
    international statistics, 10
    key factors, 10
    patient safety and quality assurance, 11
    personal budgets, 11
    policies, 9–10

long-term conditions (LTCs) (*Continued*)
    primary care trusts (PCT), 11
    public funding, 10
  informal care and social care, 11–13
    carers, 12–13
    compulsory altruism, 12
    funding model, 12–13
    unpaid care, 12
  nursing provision, 16–17
    clinical indicators, 16
    community matrons, 16
    skills, 16–17
  policy and practice developments, 13–16
    ambulance services, 15
    Care Quality Commission, 14
    case management of people, 14–15
    Co-creating Health, 14
    community services, 15–16
    expert patient concept, 14
    NSFs, 13–14
    patient and public engagement, 13–14
    pharmacy services, 15
    polyclinics concept, 15
    PSA target, 14
    self-care support, elements of, 14
    self-management programme, 14
  third sector role, 17–18
    mixed economy of care, 17–18
    organisations, 17
long-term oxygen therapy (LTOT), 232–3
low self-esteem, 67
LTC case management models, 24*t*, 26
LTOT. *See* long-term oxygen therapy (LTOT)
lung disease, 226. *See also* respiratory diseases
lung function
  association, 160
  and smoking status, 234*f*

macrovascular disease, 267–8
managing people, approach to
  biopsychosocial model, 41–3
    expert patient, community nurse visit, 42*b*–43*b*
    health care professional role, 42
    initial difficulties, 42
    LTC management, 41
    passive recipients, 42
  medical model, 36–41
    ADHD, 38
    biological management, 41
    Cartesian dualism, 36–7
    CFS, 37
    clinical iatrogenesis, 39
    complementary therapies, 39–40
    depression, 39
    dominance of medicine, 38
    evidence-based medicine or care, 37, 39
    injections and dietary management, 41
    limitations, 40
    medical approach to LTCs, 40–41
    medicalisation of life, 40
    mental processes and emotions, 37
    Rose Perkins experience, 37*b*–38*b*
    scientific revolution, 37
    self-management, 40
    sick role, 37

MBSR programmes, 153–4
medication review, 184–9
  clinics, 178
  doses, 187
  drug effect, 187
  drug interactions, 187
  patient's medication, 187
  schemes and checklists, 185–6
  side effects, 187
  specific indications, 186–7
  targeting, 185*t*–186*t*
  types of, 184–5
medicines management, 173–5
  drug-related falls, 189
  information resources, 190–92
    BNF, 191
    expert patient programme, 192
    medicines information services, 191
    medicines partnership programme, 191
    NHS Direct, 191
    NICE, 191
  medication, 184–9
    doses, 187
    drug effect, 187
    drug interactions, 187
    patient, 187
    schemes and checklists, 185–6
    side effects, 187
    specific indications, 186–7
    targeting, 185*t*–186*t*
    types of, 184–5
  medicines non-adherence, categories of, 181
  multi-compartment compliance devices, 183
  NICE medicines adherence clinical guideline, 182*b*
  patients and, 175–8
    adverse effects, 178
    with chronic heart failure, 174*t*
    with chronic obstructive pulmonary disease, 175*t*
    definition of, 175*b*
    expert patients programme, 176
    information sources, 177
    medicines partnership programme, 176–7
    questions, 175*b*
    recommended treatment, 176
    regular medication, 178
    supply of medication, 177
    with type 2 diabetes, 174*t*
  problems, 178–80
  services, 190
  stages in, 180–84
    ensuring and enabling medicines partnerships, 181–3
    outcome monitoring, 184
    right drug to right patient at right time, 183
    selection of correct and appropriate drug, 181
  swollen ankles, 189
medicines partnership programme, 191
medium-acting isophane insulin, 261*f*
men's participation, 49
mental health teams, 26
mental illness, 50, 69
mental processes and emotions, 37
metabolic syndrome, 248
metered-dose inhalers (MDI), 243*b*
metformin, 257

metoprolol, 203
microalbuminuria, 265
microvascular complications, 248
microvascular disease, 264
mind-reading/jumping to conclusions, 106
mixed economy of care, 17–18
mixed insulin, 262*f*
mucolytic agents, 238
muscular dystrophy, 196
myocardial infarction (MI). *See* heart failure, management

National and Primary and Care Trust Development Centre (NatPaCT), 24*t*
National Health Service (NHS), 54
National Health Service and Community Care Act, 12, 26
National Institute for Health and Clinical Excellence (NICE), 5, 13, 140, 191, 195
    adherence to medicines, 181
    guidelines, 141, 200
    selection of correct and appropriate drug, 181
National Prescribing Centre (NPC), 184, 185
National Primary Care Research and Development Centre, 27
national quality indicator, 141
National Services Frameworks (NSF), 4, 13–14
    for Coronary Heart Disease, 12
    for older people, 173
    standardising care and promoting innovation, 13
National Strategy for Carers, 12
NatPaCT. *See* National and Primary and Care Trust Development Centre (NatPaCT)
nebivolol, 203
nephropathy, 265–6
neuro–electrical muscle stimulation (NEMS), 165
neuropathy, 266–7
New York Heart Association (NYHA), 197
    classification, 198*t*
NHS. *See* National Health Service (NHS)
NHS Direct, 191
NICE guidance, 235
    COPD, 232, 237*f*
nicotine addiction, 233
nicotine replacement therapy (NRT), 234–5
NPC. *See* National Prescribing Centre (NPC)
numbness, 91
nurses, 137–8, 144
    counsellors and, 144
    supporting people with fatigue, 139*b*
nursing assessment, 219*t*
NYHA. *See* New York Heart Association (NYHA)

obesity, 248, 269
obstructive lung diseases, 225
OECD. *See* Organisation for Economic Co-operation and Development (OECD)
older dependency ratio, 4
ontological deficit, 53
opioids, 165
oral steroids, 238
Organisation for Economic Co-operation and Development (OECD), 4
outcome monitoring, 184
oxygen, 161–2

pacemaker, 207
pacing, 137–8
    and planning, 162–4
        suggestions, 163*t*–164*t*
pain
    classification, 154
    definition, 154
    interventional treatments, 157–8
    misconceptions about treatment, 156*t*
    non-pharmacological treatments for
        acupuncture, 157
        physical therapy, 157
        psychological therapy, 157
        stepwise ladder, 155, 156*f*
        TENS, 156–7
    persistent pain, 154–5
    pharmacological treatment of, 155–6
pain management programmes (PMP), 158
panic attack, 166
PARR case finding algorithm, 32*t*
PARR score, 31
PARR tool. *See* patient at risk of re-hospitalisation (PARR) tool
passive recipients, 42
passive smoking, 226. *See also* smoking
patient
    chronic heart failure, 174*t*
    chronic obstructive pulmonary disease, 175*t*
    concordance to, 205–7
        blister packs, 207
        calcium channel blockers, 206
        community pharmacists, 206
        diuretics, 206–7
        GP drug prescription, 206
    education, 119, 120*b*, 209, 210*t*
        diet, salt and fluid restrictions, 211–12
        driving and travel, 213–14
        exercise and sexual activity, 212–13
        monitoring signs and symptoms, 210–11
        pregnancy and contraception, 214
        prognosis, 210
        programmes, 127
        sleep and breathing disorders, 213
    as experts, 58–9
        careful experimentation, 58
        consumerism, 58–9
        relief and apprehension, 58
    medication, 187
    medicines management
        adverse effects, 178
        definition of, 175*b*
        expert patients programme, 176
        information sources, 177
        medicines partnership programme, 176–7
        recommended treatment, 176
        regular medication, 178
        supply of medication, 177
    monitoring, 219–20
    pathways scheme, 218*f*
    public engagement and, 13–14
    safety and quality assurance, 11
    type 2 diabetes, 174*t*
patient at risk of re-hospitalisation (PARR) tool, 31–2
Patient Health Questionnaire 9 (PHQ 9), 232
Payment by Results (PbR), 30–31

PbR. *See* Payment by Results (PbR)
PCT. *See* primary care trusts (PCT)
peripartum cardiomyopathy, 195–6
persistent pain, 154–5
personalisation and labelling, 106–7
personality, 72
person-centred care
  doctors and nurses, 59–60
person's personality traits, 71
PGWBI. *See* psychological general well-being index
    (PGWBI)
pharmacy services, 15
physical activity
  classification, 166
  definition, 166
  exercise, 162
  strategies to increase, 167
    motivation, 168
physical therapy, 157
PMP. *See* pain management programmes
    (PMP)
pollution, 227
polyclinics concept, 15
positioning, 161
potential tissue damage, 154
practitioner, 96
pregnancy and diabetes, 277–9
preventers, 242
primary care trusts (PCT), 11, 247
  financial incentives, 30
probing skills, 102
projection, 104
psychological effects
  availability of support, 76
  behavioural aspects
    tearfulness and depression, 68–9
  being ill long-term, 64–6
    acceptance and adaptation, 64–5
    self identity, 66
    stress response, 65
    three-stage model of LTC and response, 65*f*
  cognitive aspects
    CBT, 71
    loss of confidence and belief, 70–71
    self-perceptions and self-concept, 70–71
  consequences of LTC, 66–7
    depression, 66–7
    low self-esteem, 67
    relationship, 66*t*
  consequences to person, 75
  emotional aspects, 69–70
    affective disorders, 69
    depression, 69–70
    mental ill-health, 69
    SPD, 69
    in younger populations, 70
  experience, individual's BET, 68
  interventions in LTCs, 73–5
    cognitive appraisals, 74
    self-efficacy behaviour, 74–5
  mental health assessment
    general health questionnaire, 77, 77*t*,
      78*t*
    GHQ-12 scoring, 77–8
    PGWBI, 78, 79*t*–81*t*

nature of relationship, 67
  psychological make-up, long-tem condition and
      mental impairment, 67*f*
personality and its role
  generality approach, 72
  LTCs and influence on, 72–3
  specificity approach, 71
  transactional theory, 72
planning and providing care
  health practitioner, 75–6
  therapeutic relationships, 76
  type A personality, 76
psychological general well-being index (PGWBI), 78
psychological management, breathlessness, 164
psychological therapy, 157
psychosocial transition theory, 72, 91
public funding, 10
public service agreement (PSA) target, 14, 26
pulmonary rehabilitation, 235–6
pursed-lip breathing, 160

QALY. *See* quality-adjusted life years (QALY)
QoF. *See* quality outcomes framework (QoF)
quality outcomes framework (QoF), 231
quality-adjusted life years (QALY), 5

racism, 8
radical disability movement, 51
rapid-acting analogues, 260*f*
rapid-acting insulin secretagogue, 257–8
readers, 181, 190
reflecting skills, 101–2
reflexology, 39–40
regression, 103
reiki, 39–40
Rejuvenating Ageing Research, 4
relative poverty, 8
relief and apprehension, 58
relievers, 242
removing secretions, breathlessness, 160–61
reorganisation and recovery, 91–2
resources utilisation, 130
respiratory diseases, 225–6
  asthma
    living with, 240–44
    pathophysiology and diagnosis, 238–40
  categories, 225
  chronic obstructive lung disease (COPD)
    living with, 230–32
    NICE guidelines, 236
    pathophysiology and diagn, 227–30
    pharmacological management, 236–8
  diet and nutrition, 236
  epidemiology
    death rates, 226
  long-term oxygen therapy (LTOT), 232–3
  management, 232
  pulmonary rehabilitation, 235–6
  risk factors, 226–7
    cannabis, 227
    pollution, 227
    smoking, 226–7
  smoking cessation, 233–5
rest, 138
restrictive lung diseases, 225

rheumatoid arthritis (RhA), 32, 54, 55, 69, 70, 76, 135
role management for self-management, 127
role theory, 48–9
  bureaucratic format, 48–9
  ceremonial order, 48
  concept of role format, 48
  multiplex relationships, 48
Rose Perkins experience, 37b–38b
Royal Commission on Long-term Care, 13

salbutamol, 238
saline nebulisers, 162
salmeterol, 238, 243
seeking help
  e-health information, 49
  internet access, 49
  men's participation, 49
  particular problem, 49
  triggers, 49
selective abstractions, 106
self identity, 66
self-care, 120b
self-efficacy, 131–2, 139
  behaviour, 74–5
  factors, 131
  modelling, 132
  performance mastery, 131–2
  social persuasion, 132
  symptom interpretation, 132
self-management and current health care policies
  ability to manage symptoms, 120
  approaches
    decision-making, 129, 130t
    emotional management, 127
    EPP, 127
    medical management of condition, 126
    partnership with health care professionals,
      131
    patient education programmes, 127
    problem solving, 127–9
    resources utilisation, 130
    role management, 127
    self-efficacy, 131–2
  day-to-day care, 120
  definitions of, 120b
  patient education, 119, 120b
  professional practice, implications for, 123–6
    adaptive decision making, 125–6
    disease trajectories, 125–6
    empathetic understanding, 124
    health care professional, 124–5
  self-care, 120b
  shattered life and self-identity, 120–23
    coping behaviours, 122–3
    illness narratives, 121–2
    illness representation, 122
    self-regulation model, 123f
self-monitoring of blood glucose (SMBG), 252–3,
    252–4
self-perceptions and self-concept, 70–71
self-regulation model, 122, 123f
serious psychological distress (SPD), 69
shattered life and self-identity, 120–23
short-acting beta2 agonists (SABA), 238
shortness of breath (SOB), 196

sick role, 37, 45–6
  patterns of illness, 46
  rights and obligations, 46
Sickle Cell Society, 40
side effects, 187
smoking, 117–18, 226–7, 248
smoking cessation, 231, 233–5, 269
  counselling, 234
  five 'As' of, 234
  lung function and smoking status, 234f
SOB. *See* shortness of breath (SOB)
social exclusion, 8
social interaction, 143–4
social persuasion, 132
sociological insights
  deviance, 50–51
    behaviour, 50
    deaf culture, 51b
    disability, 51
    oppression paradigm, 50–51
    paradigm, 50–51
    primary and secondary, 50
    radical disability movement, 51
    rejecting label of, 50b
  doctor–patient relationship
    conflict theorists, 46–7
    negotiation model
    sick role, 45–6
  illness as biographical disruption, 54–6
    coping, 55–6
    experience, 55b
    experimentation and sense of humour, 56
    meaning, 55
    visitors, 56
  long-term illness
    economic effects of, 54
    experience of, 56–8
  patients as experts, 58–9
    careful experimentation, 58
    consumerism, 58–9
    relief and apprehension, 58
  person-centred care
    doctors and nurses, 59–60
  role theory, 48–9
    bureaucratic format, 48–9
    ceremonial order, 48
    concept of role format, 48
    multiplex relationships, 48
  seeking help, 49–50
    e-health information, 49
    internet access, 49
    men's participation, 49
    particular problem, 49
    triggers, 49
  stigma, 51–4
    changing faces, 52
    in chronic illness, 53–4
    disattention, 52
    effects of, 52
    facial disfigurement, 52
    ontological deficit, 53
    types of, 51
soluble insulin, 260f
SPD. *See* serious psychological distress (SPD)
specialist nurse interventions, 218

special rules. *See* Disability Living Allowance and
    Attendance Allowance
specific skills, 95
spirometry, 228–9
spironolactone, 204
sputum production, 228
stepwise ladder, 155, 156*f*
steroids, 165
stigma, 51–4
stress
    adaptive syndrome, 144–9
        stages, 149
    challenging depressive symptoms, 145*t*–148*t*
    chronic stress, biopsychosocial effects, 150–51
        physiological effects of, 151*t*
        signs and symptoms, 150*t*
    hormones and their functions, 149*f*
    response, 65
    strategies for reducing, 151
        deep breathing, 152
        deep muscle relaxation, 152
        guided visual imagery, 152
        MBSR programmes, 153–4
        yoga, 153
stress-moderator approach, 72
sulphonylureas (SU), 257
swollen ankles, 189
systematic Cochrane review, 27

talking therapies, 39, 142–3
tearfulness and depression, 68–9
telemedicine/telecare, 24, 25*b*
TENS. *See* transcutaneous electrical nerve stimulation
    (TENS)
terbutaline, 238
theophyllines, 238
thiazolidinedione (glitazones), 258
third sector role, 17–18
    businesses with primarily social objectives, 17

mixed economy of care, 17–18
    organisations, 17
thrombosis, 248
thyrotoxicosis, 196
tiotropium bromide, 238
tobacco smoke, 228
transactional theory, 72
transcutaneous electrical nerve stimulation (TENS),
    156–7
Transforming Community Services, 16
triggers, 49
type 1 diabetes, 247–8, 249*t*
type 2 diabetes, 248, 249*t*
type A personality, 73, 76
type C personality, 73

unconditional positive regard, 95
United Kingdom Prospective Diabetes Study – Type 2,
    249
unpaid care, 12

validation and education, 142
varenicline (champix), 235
victim blaming, 6–7
viral cardiomyopathy, 195
viral myocarditis, 195
virtual community wards, 25*b*
visitors, 56

welfare bill, 53
Winning the War on Heart Disease, 194
working age, 4
Working for a Healthier Tomorrow, 54

XPERT, 252*t*

yoga, 153